THE Juicing BIBLE

PAT CROCKER
& SUSAN EAGLES

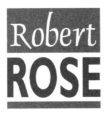

Robert
ROSE

The Juicing Bible

For complete cataloguing data, see page 4.

Design, editorial and production:	Matthews Communications Design Inc.
Illustrations:	Kveta
Photography:	Mark T. Shapiro
Art direction, food photography:	Sharon Matthews
Food stylist:	Kate Bush
Prop stylist:	Charlene Erricson
Managing editor:	Peter Matthews
Index:	Barbara Schon

We acknowledge the financial support of the Government of Canada through the Book Publishing Industry Development Program (BPIDP) for our publishing activities.

Published by: Robert Rose Inc. • 120 Eglinton Ave. E., Suite 800

Toronto, Ontario, Canada M4P 1E2 Tel: (416) 322-6552

Printed and bound in Canada by Canadian Printco Limited

6 7 8 9 CPL 09 08 07 06 05

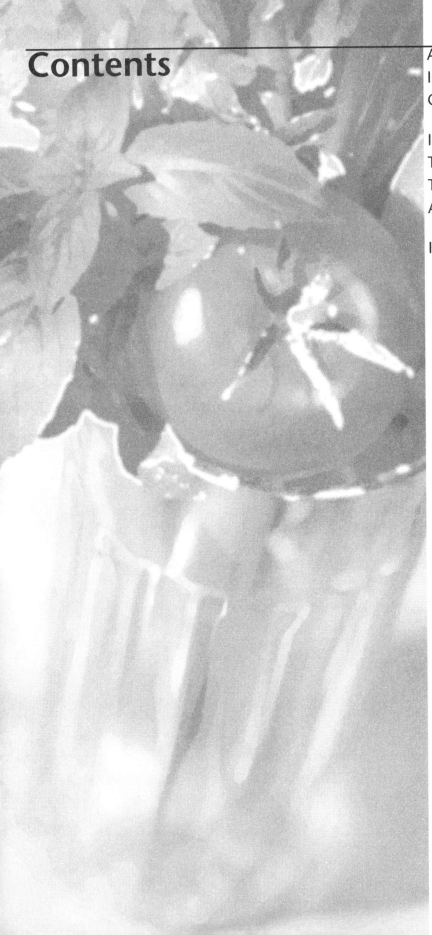

Contents

Canadian Cataloguing in Publication Data

Crocker, Pat L.
   The juicing bible

Includes index.
ISBN 0-7788-0019-9

1. Fruit juices. 2. Vegetable juices.   I. Eagles, Susan. II. Title.

TX840.J84C76 2000   641.8'75   C00-931304-4

To my very dear friend, Joanna.
– P.C.

For Patrick and Colleen.
– S.E.

In Taoist philosophy, shen, *one of the Three Treasures means "spirit" or "mood." It refers to the radiance that comes from someone who is truly healthy. This book is dedicated to good health. May you always show bright* shen *and vibrate with the salubrious energy that comes from healthy living.*

ACKNOWLEDGEMENTS

Every book has its own distinct personality, and this book is no exception. As a book is written, it seems to take on a life of its own, nourished by the common goals of the author(s), the publisher and all the people who support them — family, friends, colleagues and business associates.

While Bob Dees at Robert Rose Inc. always had a broader vision for this book, our original intention was not to write the Juicing "Bible." We simply wanted to provide some healthful drinks for a broad range of individuals — whether or not they had health concerns — and to make sure those recipes would be appealing, delicious and easy to use.

But as we progressed, it soon became apparent that recipes alone were not enough. We began to explore all the helpful drinks that can be used to help alleviate or prevent specific health conditions, as well as the many other ways to use juices and their pulp by-products.

The result was what you see now — an all-inclusive, multi-layered approach to vegetable, fruit and herb drinks. Thanks to Bob and his group for seeing what this book could really be.

SPECIAL THANKS

Generous help was provided by the marketing team at Vitamix® who, early on, sent their wonderful machine and made available background research information. Not a morning has gone by since receiving the Vitamix® that we haven't enjoyed a wake-up fruit drink to start our day. This machine has taken center stage on our counters and in our hearts. (For more information, visit www.vitamix.com)

Our thanks to Chris Wilson of Fay Clack Communications Ltd., who was most helpful in linking us with the Apple Commission, which was most generous in supplying the apples used in testing the recipes.

For organic herbs and tinctures to use in the tea recipes, we turned to Monteagle Herb Farm, located just north of Bancroft, Ontario. Particular thanks to Peter Benner and herbalist Tina Sentoukas, who offered both their herbs and their help. (For more information visit www.go.to/MonteagleHerbfarm)

Hemp seeds, oil and frozen products were supplied by Christina's Hemp Products (see Sources section, page 270).

We have made and tasted a lot of juices — literally hundreds of different combinations — most of them using the powerful L'Equip® juice machine. Easy to use and able to handle a continuous flow of fruit or vegetables, we can say without reservation that the L'Equip® juicer is one of the best on the market today. (For more information visit www.lequip.com)

INTRODUCTION

With juice bars and "elixir cafés" springing up in cities throughout North America, it's tempting to think that juicing is a new trend. But it's really just the latest manifestation of a centuries-old health practice. And in this new age of genetically modified, over-refined, chemical-laden non-food, this "rediscovery" of juicing has never been more welcome.

Research consistently shows that people who eat the greatest quantity of fruits and vegetables are about half as likely to develop cancer as those who eat little or no fresh fruits and vegetables. So it's not surprising that the United States Cancer Institute recommends eating 5 servings of fresh vegetables and 3 servings of fresh fruit each day. In fact, the phytochemicals in fruit and vegetables hold the keys to preventing many other modern diseases, such as heart disease, as well as debilitating conditions such as asthma, arthritis and allergies.

Still, even the most disciplined person can find it difficult to eat all those fruits and vegetables every day. So why not drink them? Raw fresh juices, blended drinks and homemade frozen treats are an easy and a tasty way to ensure that adults and children get their "daily eight."

BENEFITS OF JUICING

Easy assimilation. In whole fruits and vegetables (or even in drinks that contain pulp), some enzymes, phytochemicals, vitamins A, C and E — along with minerals like iron, copper, potassium, sodium, iodine and magnesium — are trapped in the indigestible fiber and cannot be assimilated by the body. But once "liberated" from the cellulose in the pulp, those nutrients can be taken into the cells of the body within 15 minutes (as compared to the hour or more it takes for nutrients to be assimilated from drinks with the pulp intact). This saves the energy required for digestion and allows the body to rest while detoxifying or cleansing, before or after physical activity, or while recovering from an illness.

Water supply. Our cells consist mostly of water, which is essential to their proper function. That's why we should consume at least 8 glasses of water a day. Raw juice — unlike coffee, soft drinks and alcohol (which take water from the body in order to metabolize) — supplies the water you need to replenish lost fluid, while providing all the necessary vitamins, minerals, enzymes and phytochemicals. In addition, juices promote the alkalinity of body fluids, which is vital for proper immune and metabolic function.

Cleansing action. Because the fiber is removed by extraction, raw juice has a laxative effect (more evident in fruit juices) which helps to rid the body of toxins. Detoxifying the system, and cleansing the digestive tract and colon, helps clear the mind and balance your moods. Cleansing also causes your metabolism to become more efficient and, if a whole-food diet is followed, the body will revert to its natural weight.

The spark of life. The living "greenpower" that is present in all living plants is available to the body when raw fresh juices are consumed. This "life force" is a natural, vital quality that is lost in processing and when fruit and vegetables are stored.

Antioxidants. Herbs, fruits and vegetables are high in antioxidants, which counteract the free radicals that can cause cellular damage, aging and susceptibility to cancers.

Natural sugars. The sugars in fruits and vegetables come bundled with the goodness of vitamins, minerals, enzymes and other phytochemicals that aren't found in refined sugar. They deliver the same energy as pastries, candy and soft drinks, but without the chemicals and fat.

Chlorophyll. Found only in plants, chlorophyll has a unique structure that allows it to enhance the body's ability to produce hemoglobin which, in turn, enhances the delivery of oxygen to cells.

BENEFITS OF PULPING

Full of fiber. Fruit and vegetables contain fiber in the form of cellulose, pectin, lignin and hemicellulose — all of which are essential to health. Combined, these types of fiber slow absorption of food (increasing absorption of nutrients), help lower cholesterol, reduce the risk of heart disease, help eliminate toxins and carcinogens, prevent hemorrhoids, varicose veins, constipation, colitis (and possibly colon cancer), and help to prevent gallstones. When fruit and vegetables are blended or pulped, their fiber is retained, along with all the vitamins, minerals, enzymes and phytochemicals.

Keeping you satisfied. By pulping different fruit and vegetable combinations and combining with herbs, nuts, seeds and whole grains, the body is nourished and the bulk in the fiber gives a sense of satisfaction that lasts longer than what you get from fast food snacks, soft drinks or coffee.

Water. See page 7.

More cleansing action. Fiber in pulped juices cleanses the body in a manner different from that of extracted juices. Insoluble fiber adds bulk to fecal matter, facilitating its rapid elimination through the colon. As a result, there is no undue multiplication of bacteria with production of toxins.

The spark of life. See page 8.

Antioxidants. See page 8.

Natural sugars. See page 8.

Chlorophyll. See page 8.

JUICING AS PART OF A HEALTHY DIET

Juicing plays a major role in ensuring a healthy diet by making it easier to consume the recommended 8 daily servings of fruits and vegetables. One large glass of pure, raw, fresh juice per day will help improve the immune system, increase energy, strengthen bones, clear skin and lower the risk of disease. For maximum benefit, it is wise to consume a wide variety of juices from different types of organic herbs, fruits and vegetables.

Be sure to incorporate juices into a well-balanced, high-fiber, whole food diet. Extracted juices should not completely replace whole fruits and vegetables since their fiber is important for eliminating toxins and preventing cancer.

A healthy diet includes protein, carbohydrates, fat, vitamins, minerals, enzymes and phytochemicals, fiber and water in proportions that promote growth and maintain vibrant, salubrious cells. Eat food in its natural and whole state where possible, avoiding packaged, refined, preserved, colored, pickled, salted, sweetened and artificially flavored foods.

Use the chart on pages 10 and 11 as a guide to structuring your diet to provide the maximum nutrients.

GUIDELINES TO GOOD HEALTH

What	Why	How
1. Make **complex carbohydrates** the main part of your meals; 60% of calories should come from complex carbohydrates.	Complex carbohydrates (found in fruits, vegetables and whole grains) also supply vitamins, minerals, enzymes, phytochemicals and fiber. Simple, refined carbohydrates, (found in white sugar and flour) are stripped of nutrients and deliver only "empty" calories. White sugar can also decrease immune functioning.	Eat five different vegetables per day, one of which should be red or orange. Eat two fruits per day, one of which should be citrus. Drink at least one glass of raw, fresh fruit or vegetable juice or pulped drink per day. Eat five servings of whole grains or cereals every day: whole grain muesli or oatmeal for breakfast; whole wheat bread with meals; add rice, barley, amaranth or spelt to soups and stews; cook with whole wheat pastas and make whole grain salads.
2. Protein should comprise 20% of total daily calories. Half (or more) of the protein should come from plant sources – preferably raw.[1]	The body needs protein to maintain growth and health of cells. For more information on protein, see Glossary, page 264. Meats contain saturated fat, which clogs blood vessels and, if not organic, can add toxins to the diet.	Eat more plant food proteins and reduce animal protein. Eat foods in combinations to provide complete protein: whole grains with legumes; dairy products with nuts and seeds; legumes with nuts and seeds; dairy products and legumes. Substitute tofu, soy milk or soy-based foods for meat products; use powdered soy protein in smoothies. Use lean chicken and fish as "accents" to meals of grains, legumes and vegetables.
3. Fat should comprise 20% (or less) of total daily calories. Eat polyunsaturated fat, restricting the saturated fat in the diet. Ensure that essential fatty acids (such as Omega 3) are part of the diet.	Protein, carbohydrates and fat all supply food energy (calories) but fat contains twice as many calories as equal quantities of the other two. Mono- and polyunsaturated fats contain less hydrogen and are higher in high density lipoproteins (HDL), which protect arteries because they carry cholesterol away. Olive oil is a stable monounsaturated fat and the best choice for cooking. See Glossary, page 262, for information on essential fatty acids.	Eliminate or restrict use of whole milk, butter, cream, cream cheese, sour cream and fried foods. Eliminate or restrict intake of saturated fats — particularly animal fats (butter, lard, fats in meats), palm and coconut oils. Use olive oil for cooking and unrefined, extra-virgin, cold-pressed hemp, sunflower, safflower, soybean or corn oil for salad dressings. Good sources of essential fatty acids include salmon and other cold water fish, avocados, flax seeds, nuts and seeds.

What	Why	How
4. Drink plenty of pure **water**, fruit juices and herbal teas daily.	Water is necessary for the functioning of the body and its systems.	Drink 8 glasses of water each day. Raw fresh juices contain 80 to 90% water and may be substituted for water.
5. Avoid the following:		
• white sugar and flour...	rob the body of nutrients, deplete immune system	Eat whole grain foods and substitute stevia where possible or small amounts of maple syrup, honey or molasses for sugar.
• red meat...	fat content deposits on blood vessel walls	Eat soy products, vegetable protein in combinations (see #2, above, or entry for Protein in Glossary, page 264).
• meat products (such as beef burgers, ham, bacon, sausages, processed meats and offal)...	cause fat deposits and are high in salt and other additives	Eat only organic chicken and fish.
• shellfish...	often contain concentrated toxins from contaminates	Eat shellfish only rarely.
• excess salt...	causes fluid retention and hypertension	Eat celery and other high-potassium vegetables; use herbs as salt substitutes.
• coffee, strong tea...	see entry for coffee on pages 224 to 225	Use coffee substitutes, fresh juices and herbal teas.
• excess* alcohol... * moderate alcohol consumption allows for one glass of beer or wine with meals once or twice per week.	acts as a depressant and robs the body of nutrients.	Substitute fresh juices; eat macrobiotically to reduce cravings.

[1] Rohé, Fred, *The Complete Book of Natural Foods,* Shambhala Publications, 1983, p 31

JUICE MACHINES

Juice is simply the water (up to 90%) and nutrients that have been separated from the indigestible fiber contained in fruits, vegetables and herbs. For this process, a juice machine is essential. Juicing produces a lot of pulp that can be used in other recipes (see Roughies pages 181 to 187).

To make more than half the recipes in this book, you do not need to use a juice machine. To process the flesh of fruits and vegetables — alone or with herbs, nuts, seeds, whole grains or other ingredients — a blender, liquifier or food processor will suffice. This process is referred to in this book as pulping. Retaining and drinking the pulp has the added boost of all the nutrients, fiber, pith and flesh along with the juice.

Types of Juice Machines

There are two basic types of machines:

Masticating. With this type of machine, fruits and vegetables are squeezed through gears that crush them and force them through a fine stainless steel strainer. The pulp is continuously extracted. This type generally extracts more nutrients in the juice; also, because it generates less heat and friction, more enzymes are preserved.

Centrifugal. This type of juicer uses a spinning basket that shreds the fruit and vegetables and forces the juice through a fine stainless steel strainer by centrifugal force. Depending on the make of juicer, pulp can be continuously extracted or collected in the basket. Centrifugal juicers cause oxidation of the nutrients by introducing air into the juice.

Criteria for Choosing a Juice Machine

Ease of use. If a juice machine is easy to use and clean, it will be used more often.

Yield. The goal is to extract the most juice from the fruit or vegetable as possible. Juicers that eject the pulp outside the machine yield less juice than juicers that keep the pulp in the basket.

Type. See above.

Reliability. Look for a 5- to 10-year warranty on motor and parts. Look for companies that supply replacement parts at reasonable cost.

PULPING MACHINES

Most people use a blender, Vitamix® or food processor in addition to a juice machine because there are some fruits and vegetables that do not juice well. Also there are some ingredients — such as flax seeds, dry herbs and wheat germ — that are easier to add to blended drinks than juices.

Even the best juice machine will leave some nutrients in the pulp. Pulping machines cut the food into tiny pieces, making it possible to drink the pulp along with the juice.

Blenders are better at pulping than food processors. The Vitamix® is the best since it reduces foods (even seeds) to microscopic particles. Most blended drinks or smoothies call for some juice and it is best if fresh, raw fruits or vegetables are first juiced using a juice extractor, then added to a pulping machine to complete the recipe.

Extracted juices and blended or pulped drinks all have their place in in a whole food diet.

CLEANING YOUR JUICE MACHINE

Use a stiff brush and hot running water immediately after use to thoroughly clean blades and sieves, ensuring that all bits of vegetable matter are removed. Over time, the strong natural pigments of the raw foods will stain the plastic parts of most juicing and pulping equipment. To remove stains, soak in a sink full of warm water to which 2 tbsp (25 mL) of bleach has been added. (Note that some manufacturers recommend that bleach not be used with their products; check your user's manual.) Most juicer parts are safe in the top shelf of an automatic dishwasher; and the bleach in dishwasher detergent will remove tough stains.

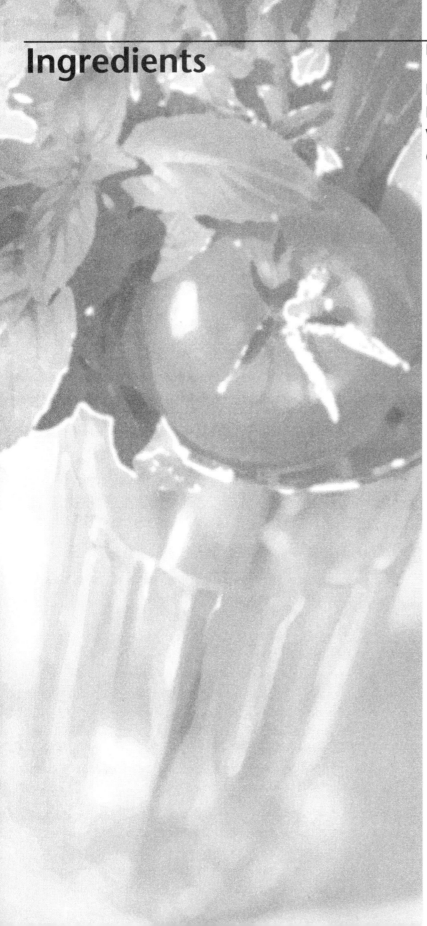

Ingredients

FOODS FOR YOUR JUICER

BUY FRESH

When choosing fruits and vegetables, make sure they are firm and ripe. Herbs should show no signs of wilting, yellowing or rust. Buy only what you plan to use in the next day or two; longer storage will destroy the live enzymes in the plants. Ideally you should shop daily for the fresh fruits, vegetables and herbs you need to make the recipes in this book. If this is impractical, store in the refrigerator for no more than 2 days.

As a rule of thumb, 1 lb (500 g) produce yields roughly 1 to 1 1/2 cups (250 to 375 mL) fresh juice.

BUY ORGANIC

Organic agriculture is a holistic method of farming based on ecological principles with the primary goal of creating a sustainable agricultural system. The USDA National Organic Program defines this goal as, "optimizing the health and productivity of interdependent communities of soil life, plants, animals, and people. Management practices are carefully selected with an intent to restore and then maintain ecological harmony on the farm, its surrounding environment and ultimately the whole planetary ecosystem."

Organic farmers use the principles of recycling, interdependency and diversity in their farm design and farming practices. Organic agriculture is about much more than growing food without synthetic fertilizers and chemical biocides. Organic agriculture uses practices that benefit the planet as well as our bodies.

Because juicing uses fresh fruits, vegetables and herbs almost exclusively, organic produce is clearly the best choice.

For more information: www.organicfood.com

WASH WELL

All fruits, vegetables and herbs — even if organic — should be washed, scrubbed or soaked in a tub of cool water to which 2 tbsp (25 mL) of food-grade peroxide or vinegar has been added. This will remove any soil, as well as bacteria that may have developed during transportation and handling. Spinach and leeks should be soaked to remove grit. In most cases, organic produce can be juiced with the skin on. Exceptions are noted below.

If you can't find organically grown produce, you can use the conventional variety, but only if you wash as directed above and remove the peel. However, because pesticide concentrations are particularly high in non-organic apples, Chilean grapes, cucumbers, peaches, strawberries and apricots, you might consider refraining from using them in juices.

A WORD ABOUT HERBS

Some herbal practitioners recommend using whole fresh herbs for juicing. This is because, as with fruits and vegetables, only the whole fresh juice, taken immediately, captures the entire synergistic complex of healing ingredients locked within the cellular structure of the living plant. (Sigfried Gursche, *Healing with Herbal Juices*, Alive Books, 1993.)

Most herbalists work with the dried form of herbs for medicinal teas because dried herbs are the most widely available and are the easiest to store, transport and work with. For the same reasons, with some exceptions, dried herbs are recommended for use in the tea recipes and some of the juice recipes here. However, if fresh herbs are available, be sure to use them.

For each measure of dried herbs called for in a recipe, use 3 times the quantity of fresh.

Most of the herbs profiled in the following section are available dried from health/alternative stores. Many can be grown in pots or in your garden and some can be wildcrafted (gathered from the wild). See the Sources section (pages 268 to 270) for information on how to obtain herbs by mail.

For the greatest medicinal value, dried herbs should be as fresh as possible. Purchase organic dried herbs from a farm or health/alternative store in small quantities and store for up to 8 or 10 months. If you store your herbs and spices for longer periods, you may not experience the desired effect from them.

Alfalfa
Medicago sativa

A hardy perennial easily grown in most parts of North America.

PARTS USED
Leaves, flowers and sprouted seeds.

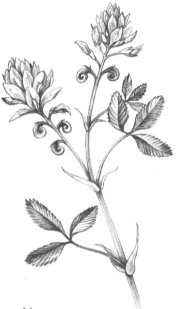

HEALING PROPERTIES
Actions: tonic, nutritive, anti-cholesterol, anti-anemia

Uses: Alfalfa is a cell nutritive and overall tonic for the body, promotes strong teeth, bones and connective tissue. Alfalfa is one of the best sources of chlorophyll, which has the ability to stimulate new skin growth, heal wounds and burns, diminish the symptoms of arthritis, gout and rheumatism, lower cholesterol levels, reduce inflammation and improve the body's resistance to cancer.

AVAILABILITY
Whole or cut dried leaf, available in alternative/health stores. Sprouted seeds readily available.

HOW TO USE IN JUICING
Whole fresh sprigs: Roll in a ball and feed through tube along with other ingredients. Use about 6 sprigs for each 1 cup (250 mL) juice.

Dried leaf and flowers: Crush to a fine powder, then whisk into fresh juice or add to ingredients in blended drinks. Use 1 tbsp (15 mL) for each 1 cup (250 mL) juice.

Infusion: Pour 1/4 cup (50 mL) boiling water over 2 tbsp (25 mL) fresh or 2 tsp (10 mL) dried cut or powdered leaf; allow to steep 10 minutes. Strain, discard herb, and add liquid to 1 cup (250 mL) juice.

Tincture: Add 1 tsp (5 mL) tincture to 1 cup (250 mL) juice.

FOLKLORE
Humanity's oldest crop, to the ancient Arabs, alfalfa was the "father of all foods" (al-fal-fa) and they used it as a nutritive staple.

Astragalus
Astragalus membranaceus

A hardy, shrub-like perennial native to eastern Asia but grown in temperate regions.

PARTS USED
Root.

HEALING PROPERTIES
Actions: immunostimulant, antimicrobial, cardiotonic, diuretic, promotes tissue regeneration

Uses: Throughout the Orient,

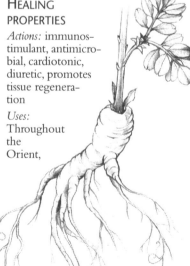

astragalus is used as a tonic, providing powerful stimulation to virtually every phase of immune system activity. It also has been shown to alleviate the adverse effects of steroids and chemotherapy on the immune system and can be used during traditional cancer treatment.

AVAILABILITY
While more and more North American herb farms are growing this exceptional medicinal herb, the most reliable sources for the dried, sliced root are oriental herb stores centered in large urban areas. However, health/alternative stores do carry cut or powdered astragalus and the tincture form.

HOW TO USE IN JUICING
Powder: Add 1 tsp (5 mL) dried powder to 1 cup (250 mL) juice or add to ingredients in blended drinks.

Decoction: In a small saucepan, combine 1/4 cup (50 mL) boiling water and 1 dried root stick or 1 tsp (5 mL) dried chopped root. Simmer with lid on 10 minutes, allow to steep 10 minutes. Strain, discard herb, and add liquid to 1 cup (250 mL) juice.

Tincture: Add 10 to 20 drops to 1 cup (250 mL) juice.

FOLKLORE
The Chinese call astragalus *huang-qi* and add the roots to nourishing soups for the very young and the very old.

Basil
Oscimum basilicum

A bushy annual with large, waxy, deep-green leaves and small tubular flowers in long spikes.

PARTS USED
Leaves and flowering tops.

HEALING PROPERTIES
Actions: antispasmodic, soothing digestive, antibacterial, anti-depressant, adrenal stimulant

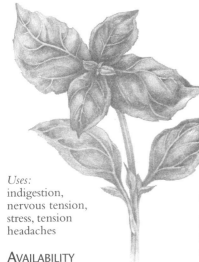

Uses:
indigestion,
nervous tension,
stress, tension
headaches

AVAILABILITY

Fresh sprigs sold in sea-
son at farmers' markets. Cut and
sifted dried leaves available at
health/alternative stores.

HOW TO USE IN JUICING

Whole fresh sprigs: Roll in a ball
and feed through tube along with
other ingredients. Use about
6 sprigs for each 1 cup (250 mL)
juice.

Black Cohosh
Cimicifuga racemosa

A tall, wild woodland perennial,
native to North America with
broadly ovate leaves and spikes of
fragrant white flowers.

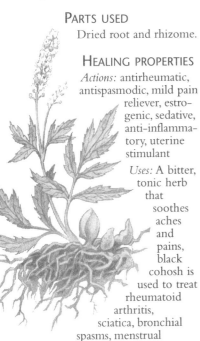

PARTS USED
Dried root and rhizome.

HEALING PROPERTIES
Actions: antirheumatic,
antispasmodic, mild pain
reliever, estro-
genic, sedative,
anti-inflamma-
tory, uterine
stimulant

Uses: A bitter,
tonic herb
that
soothes
aches
and
pains,
black
cohosh is
used to treat
rheumatoid
arthritis,
sciatica, bronchial
spasms, menstrual
cramps, menopausal problems, labor
and postpartum pains.

CAUTION

Avoid in pregnancy and breast-
feeding unless advised otherwise
by your medical practitioner.
Excess dosages can cause
headache.

AVAILABILITY

Seeds, rootlets and plants available from nurseries for growing.
Dried roots and tincture available
at alternative/health stores.

HOW TO USE IN JUICING

Do not add to juice more often
than once daily.

Decoction: In a small saucepan,
combine 1/4 cup (50 mL) boiling
water and 1/2 tsp (2 mL) dried cut
or powdered root. Simmer with lid
on 10 minutes; allow to steep 10
minutes. Strain, discard herb, and
add liquid to 1 cup (250 mL) juice.

Tincture: Add 8 drops to 1 cup
(250 mL) juice.

Borage
Borago officinalis

A self-seeding annual with a
branching, hollow stem that supports long, oval, alternate leaves.
Small blue star-shaped flowers
hang in wide, drooping clusters.
The whole plant is covered with
prickly, silver hairs.

PARTS USED
Leaves and flowering tops.

HEALING PROPERTIES

Actions: adrenal gland restorative,
expectorant, increases milk in
breast-feeding

Uses: coughs, depression, stress, to
strengthen adrenal glands after
medical treatment with corticos-
teroid drugs

AVAILABILITY

Easy to grow in containers or
gardens but not readily available to
purchase. Dried leaves sometimes
available in health/alternative
stores.

HOW TO USE IN JUICING

Whole fresh sprigs: Roll in a ball
and feed through tube along with
other ingredients. Use about
4 sprigs for each 1 cup (250 mL)
juice.

Dried leaf and flowers: Crush to a
fine powder, then whisk into fresh
juice or add to ingredients in
blended drinks. Use 1 tbsp
(15 mL) for each 1 cup (250 mL)
juice.

Infusion: In a teapot, pour 1/4 cup
(50 mL) boiling water over 1 tbsp
(15 mL) fresh or 1 tsp (5 mL)
dried

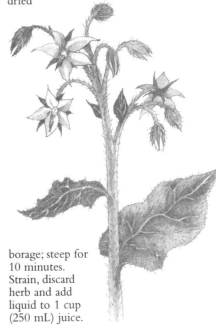

borage; steep for
10 minutes.
Strain, discard
herb and add
liquid to 1 cup
(250 mL) juice.

FOLKLORE

Ego Borago gaudia semper ago
("I, Borage, bring always courage.")
Borage was given to those leaving
to fight in the Crusades.

Buchu
Barosma betulina

A small, green shrub native to
South Africa. Plants in this genus
have attractive flowers and bright
green, ovate, aromatic leaves that
make them popular as ornamentals.

PARTS USED
Leaves.

HEALING PROPERTIES

Actions: diuretic, urinary antiseptic

Uses: Used to treat urinary disorders such as painful urination,
cystitis, prostatitis and urethritis.
Research indicates buchu contains
properties that block ultraviolet
light that could be helpful in skin
preparations.

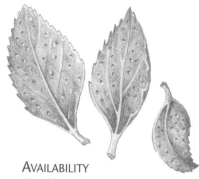

AVAILABILITY

Dried leaves and tincture available in health/alternative stores.

HOW TO USE IN JUICING

Dried leaves: Whisk 1 tsp (5 mL) powdered dried leaves into juices or add to ingredients before blending smoothies or shakes.

Infusion: Pour 1/4 cup (50 mL) boiling water over 1 tsp (5 mL) dried cut or powdered leaf; allow to steep 10 minutes. Strain, discard herb, and add liquid to 1 cup (250 mL) juice.

Tincture: Add 20 to 40 drops tincture to 1 cup (250 mL) juice.

Burdock Leaf
Arctium lappa

A hardy biennial that produces fruiting heads covered with hooked burrs that catch on clothing and the fur of animals. Grows wild extensively in North America.

PARTS USED
Root, stalk, leaves and seeds.

HEALING PROPERTIES

Actions: mild laxative, diuretic

Uses: Leaves may be used in the same way as roots, although they are less effective than the root.

AVAILABILITY

Widely available in rural and urban waste areas, burdock can be easily foraged. Avoid collecting from roadsides, ditches or streams close to field run-off and other areas of pollution. Cut dried leaves and tincture available in alternative/health stores.

HOW TO USE IN JUICING

Whole fresh leaves: Roll in a ball and feed through tube along with other ingredients. Use one leaf for each 1 cup (250 mL) juice.

Dried leaf: Crush to a fine powder, then whisk into fresh juice or add to ingredients in blended drinks. Use 1 to 2 tsp (5 to 10 mL) for each 1 cup (250 mL) of juice.

Infusion: Pour 1/4 cup (50 mL) boiling water over 1 tbsp (15 mL) fresh or 1 tsp (5 mL) dried cut or powdered leaf; allow to steep 10 minutes. Strain, discard herb, and add liquid to 1 cup (250 mL) juice.

Tincture: Add 10 to 40 drops tincture to 1 cup (250 mL) juice.

FOLKLORE

Native American tribes, particularly the Cherokee and Chippewa valued burdock as a medicine.

Burdock Root
Arctium lappa

See Burdock Leaf.

PARTS USED

Root, stalk, leaves and seeds.

HEALING PROPERTIES

Actions: mild laxative, antirheumatic, antibiotic, diaphoretic, diuretic, alterative; a skin and blood cleanser, burdock stimulates urine flow and sweating. Root and seeds are a soothing demulcent, tonic, used to soothe kidneys and relieve lymphatics

Uses: Burdock root is used as a cleansing, eliminative remedy. It helps to remove toxins causing skin problems (including eczema, acne, rashes, boils), digestive sluggishness, or arthritic pains. It supports the liver, lymphatic glands and digestive system.

AVAILABILITY

Dig roots from the wild in the fall. Cut dried root and tincture available in alternative/health stores.

HOW TO USE IN JUICING

Whole fresh root: Scrub and feed through tube along with other ingredients. Use 2 to 3 inches (5 to 7.5 cm) fresh root per 1 cup (250 mL) juice.

Dried root: Crush to a fine powder, then whisk into fresh juice or add to smoothie ingredients. Use 1 tsp (5 mL) for each 1 cup (250 mL) juice.

Decoction: Gently simmer 1 tsp (5 mL) dried root in 1/4 cup (50 mL) water for 15 minutes. Strain, discard herb, and add liquid to 1 cup (250 mL) juice.

Tincture: Add 10 to 20 drops tincture to 1 cup (250 mL) juice.

Burdock Seeds
Arctium lappa

See Burdock Leaf.

PARTS USED
Root, stalk, leaves and seeds.

HEALING PROPERTIES

Actions: prevents fever, anti-inflammatory, anti-bacterial, reduces blood sugar levels

Uses: Burdock root and seeds are a soothing demulcent tonic, used to soothe kidneys and relieve lymphatics.

AVAILABILITY

Seeds gathered from the wild. Not always readily available at health/alternative stores. Burdock tincture available at health/alternative stores.

HOW TO USE IN JUICING

Infusion: In a teapot, pour 1/4 cup (50 mL) boiling water over 1 tsp (5 mL) bruised fresh or dried seeds; steep with lid on for 10 minutes. Strain, discard herb and add liquid to 1 cup (250 mL) juice.

Tincture: Add 10 to 40 drops to 1 cup (250 mL) juice.

Calendula
Calendula officinalis

A prolific annual easily grown from seed (common name: pot marigold).

PARTS USED
Petals.

HEALING PROPERTIES
Actions: astringent, antiseptic, antifungal, anti-inflammatory, heals wounds, menstrual regulator, stimulates bile production

Uses: Calendula acts as an aid to digestion and as a general tonic. It is taken to ease menopausal problems, period pain, gastritis, peptic ulcers, gall bladder problems, indigestion and fungal infections.

AVAILABILITY
Whole dried flowerheads available in alternative/health stores.

HOW TO USE IN JUICING
Infusion: Pour 1/4 cup (50 mL) boiling water over 1 tbsp (15 mL) fresh or 1 tsp (5 mL) dried petals; let steep 10 minutes if using dried, 15 minutes if using fresh petals. Strain, discard herb, and add liquid to 1 cup (250 mL) juice.

Tincture: Add 5 to 20 drops tincture to 1 cup (250 mL) juice.

FOLKLORE
Legend claims that the Romans took marigold from India, where it originated, as a cheaper and more easily obtained substitute for saffron.

Cardamom
Elettaria cardamomum

Originally from Indian rainforests, cardamom is a rhizomatous perennial with large lanceolate leaves. For centuries it has been exported to Europe mainly for its fragrance. When coaxed into blooming, the flowers are white with a dark pink-striped lip.

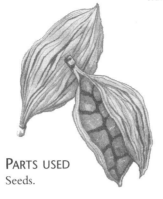

PARTS USED
Seeds.

HEALING PROPERTIES
Actions: antispasmodic, carminative, digestive stimulant, expectorant

Uses: A pungent herb with stimulating, tonic effects that work best on the digestive system, cardamom relaxes spasms, stimulates appetite and relieves flatulence.

AVAILABILITY
Whole dried seeds widely available in supermarkets and alternative/health stores.

HOW TO USE IN JUICING
Dried seeds: Whisk 1 tsp (5 mL) ground cardamom seeds into 1 cup (250 mL) juice or add to smoothie ingredients.

Infusion: In a teapot, pour 1/4 cup (50 mL) boiling water over 1 tsp (5 mL) lightly crushed seeds. Steep with lid on 10 minutes. Strain, discard herb, and add liquid to 1 cup (250 mL) juice.

Catnip
Nepeta cataria

A hardy perennial, favorite of cats, the erect, branched stems bear gray-green, ovate toothed leaves and whorls of white tubular flowers.

PARTS USED
Leaves, stems and flowers.

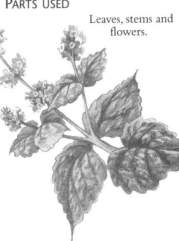

HEALING PROPERTIES
Actions: antispasmodic, astringent, carminative, promotes sweating, cooling, sedative

Uses: Catnip lowers fever, relaxes spasms, increases perspiration, and is often taken at night to ensure sleep. It is also used for diarrhea, stomach upsets, colic, colds, flu, inflammation, pain and convulsions. It is especially useful in children's fevers.

AVAILABILITY
Easily grown in North America. Dried leaves, stems and flowers are available in health/alternative stores.

HOW TO USE IN JUICING
Whole fresh sprigs: Roll in a ball and feed through tube along with other ingredients. Use about 4 sprigs for each 1 cup (250 mL) juice.

Dried leaf and flowers: Crush to a fine powder, then whisk into fresh juice or ingredients in blended drinks. Use 1 tsp (5 mL) for each 1 cup (250 mL) juice.

Infusion: Pour 1/4 cup (50 mL) boiling water over 1 tbsp (15 mL) fresh or 1 tsp (5 mL) dried cut or powdered catnip, allow to steep 10 minutes. Strain, discard herb, and add liquid to 1 cup (250 mL) juice.

Cayenne
Capsicum annum and *Capsicum frutescens*

Tropical perennial, grown as an annual in temperate zones.

PARTS USED
Red pepper fruit.

HEALING PROPERTIES
Actions: stimulant, tonic, carminative, diaphoretic, rubefacient, antiseptic, anti-bacterial

Uses: Cayenne stimulates blood circulation, purifies the blood, promotes fluid elimination and sweat, and is often used as a stimulating nerve tonic. Applied externally, over-the-counter creams and ointments containing the active capsaicin extract are often effective in relieving the pain of osteoarthritis and rheumatoid arthritis, shingles infection, as well as the burning pain in the toes, feet, and legs of diabetic neuropathy and fibromyalgia. *See also* Chile Pepper, page 49.

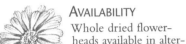

CAUTION

Some natural health practitioners advise that capsicum should not be used internally in cases of chronic inflammation of the intestinal tract, such as in Irritable Bowel Syndrome, ulcerative colitis and Crohn's disease.

AVAILABILITY

Fresh, whole chile peppers available in some ethnic markets, supermarkets and alternative/health stores. Dried whole chiles, and powdered cayenne pepper are widely available.

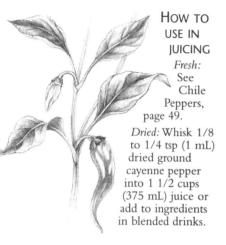

HOW TO USE IN JUICING

Fresh: See Chile Peppers, page 49.

Dried: Whisk 1/8 to 1/4 tsp (1 mL) dried ground cayenne pepper into 1 1/2 cups (375 mL) juice or add to ingredients in blended drinks.

Celery
Apium graveolens

A biennial with a bulbous, fleshy root, and thick, grooved stems. Leaves are pinnately divided. Umbels of tiny green-white flowers are followed by small gray-brown seeds. For medicinal purposes, seeds are taken from wild celery.

PARTS USED

Stem, leaves, roots and seeds.

HEALING PROPERTIES

Actions: anti-inflammatory, antioxidant, carminative, reduces blood pressure, sedative, urinary antiseptic (seeds)

Uses: Celery is an aromatic, tonic herb that is used to treat gout, inflammation of the urinary tract, cystitis, osteoarthritis and rheumatoid arthritis.

CAUTION

Do not use seeds in pregnancy.

AVAILABILITY

Fresh celery is widely available. Seeds should be purchased only from herbalists or health/alternative stores.

HOW TO USE IN JUICING

Whole fresh stalks and leaves: See Celery, page 49.

Dried seeds: Crush to a fine powder, then whisk into fresh juice or add to ingredients in blended drinks. Use 1/4 tsp (1 mL) for each 1 cup (250 mL) of juice.

Infusion: In a teapot, pour 1/4 cup (50 mL) boiling water over 1/4 tsp (1 mL) dried lightly crushed seeds; steep 10 minutes. Strain, discard herb, and add liquid to 1 cup (250 mL) juice.

Chamomile
See German Chamomile

Chickweed
Stellaria media

Found in most parts of North America, chickweed is a low spreading annual with diffusely branched stems, ovate leaves and star-shaped, white flowers.

PARTS USED

Leaves, flowers, roots, stems.

HEALING PROPERTIES

Actions: anti-cancer, anti-inflammatory, antirheumatic, astringent, heals wounds, demulcent

Uses: Chickweed is used to treat rheumatism, constipation, mucus in the lungs, coughs, colds, tumors and blood disorders. Externally used on eczema, psoriasis and other skin conditions.

AVAILABILITY

A common weed, chickweed can be wildcrafted from summer through fall. Dried aerial parts and roots are available in health/alternative stores.

HOW TO USE IN JUICING

Whole fresh sprigs: Roll in a ball and feed through tube along with other ingredients. Use about 6 sprigs for each 1 cup (250 mL) juice.

Dried leaf and flowers: Crush to a fine powder, then whisk into fresh juice or add to ingredients in blended drinks. Use 2 tsp (10 mL) for each 1 cup (250 mL) juice.

Infusion: In a teapot, pour 1/4 cup (50 mL) boiling water over 2 tbsp (25 mL) fresh or 2 tsp (10 mL) dried cut or powdered chickweed; steep 10 minutes. Strain, discard herb, and add liquid to 1 cup (250 mL) juice.

Cinnamon
Cinnamomum zeylanicum

The dried, smooth inner bark of a cultivated laurel-like tree that grows in hot, wet tropical regions of India, Brazil, East and West Indies and Indian Ocean islands.

PARTS USED

Bark.

HEALING PROPERTIES

Actions: carminative, diaphoretic, astringent, stimulant, antimicrobial

Uses: Cinnamon is a warming carminative used to promote digestion and relieve nausea, vomiting, and diarrhea. It is used for upset stomach and Irritable Bowel Syndrome. Recent research has shown that cinnamon helps the body use insulin more efficiently.

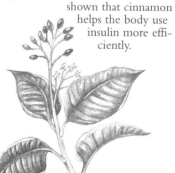

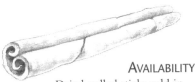

AVAILABILITY

Dried, rolled sticks sold in 2- to 18-inch (5 to 45 cm) lengths. Ground cinnamon and cinnamon powder are widely available.

HOW TO USE IN JUICING

Powder: Whisk 1/4 tsp (1 mL) powdered cinnamon into 1 cup (250 mL) juice or add to ingredients for blended drinks.

Infusion: In a teapot, pour 1/4 cup (50 mL) boiling water over a 1-inch (2.5 cm) stick of cinnamon, broken in pieces; steep with lid on 5 minutes. Strain, discard herb, and add liquid to 1 cup (250 mL) juice.

Clove
Syzygium aromaticus

The pink, unopened flower buds of an evergreen tree native to Indonesia, now grown in Zanzibar, Madagascar, West Indies, Brazil, India and Sri Lanka.

PARTS USED
Dried buds.

HEALING PROPERTIES

Actions: antioxidant, anesthetic, antiseptic, anti-inflammatory, anodyne, antispasmodic, carminative, stimulant, prevents vomiting, antihistamine, warming

Uses: Used for asthma, bronchitis, nausea, vomiting, flatulence, diarrhea, hypothermia. Some studies indicate that cloves may have anticoagulant properties and stimulate the production of enzymes that fight cancer. Clove oil which

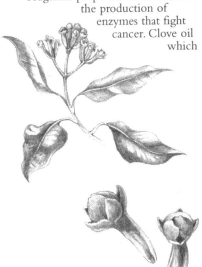

is 60 to 90% eugenol, is the active ingredient in some mouthwashes, toothpastes, soaps, insect repellents, perfumes, foods, veterinary medications and many over-the-counter toothache medications.

AVAILABILITY

Whole, dried buds and powdered cloves are widely available.

HOW TO USE IN JUICING

Powder: Whisk 1/4 tsp (1 mL) powdered cloves into 1 cup (250 mL) juice or add to ingredients in blended drinks.

Infusion: In a teapot, pour 1/4 cup (50 mL) boiling water over 1/4 tsp (1 mL) lightly crushed cloves; steep with lid on 10 minutes. Strain, discard herb and add liquid to 1 cup (250 mL) juice.

Coriander Seeds
Coriandrum sativum

A hardy annual with slender, erect, branched stems that bear pinnate, parsley-like aromatic leaves. Small, flat umbels of tiny white to pale mauve flowers yield round green berries (seeds) that ripen to a brownish yellow.

PARTS USED
Seeds.

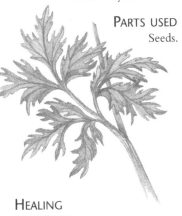

HEALING PROPERTIES

Actions: soothing digestive, stimulates appetite, improves digestion and absorption

Uses: digestive problems, flatulence

AVAILABILITY

Dried seeds readily available in health/alternative stores and ethnic Indian markets.

HOW TO USE IN JUICING
Dried seeds: Crush to a powder; whisk 1/2 tsp (2 mL) into 1 cup

(250 mL) juice or add to ingredients in blended drinks.

Infusion: In a teapot, pour 1/4 cup (50 mL) boiling water over 1 tsp (5 mL) lightly crushed seeds; steep with lid on 10 minutes. Strain, discard herb, and add liquid to 1 cup (250 mL) juice.

Cumin
Cuminum cyminum

Found wild from the Mediterranean to the Sudan and central Asia, the plant is a slender annual with dark green leaves, umbels of tiny white or pink flowers followed by bristly, oval seeds.

PARTS USED
Seeds.

HEALING PROPERTIES

Actions: stimulant, soothing digestive, antispasmodic, diuretic, increases milk in breastfeeding

Uses: indigestion, flatulence

AVAILABILITY

Dried seeds readily available in health/alternative stores and ethnic Indian markets.

HOW TO USE IN JUICING

Dried Seeds: Crush to a powder, whisk 1/2 tsp (2 mL) powder into 1 cup (250 mL) juice or add to ingredients in blended drinks.

Infusion: In a teapot, pour 1/4 cup (50 mL) boiling water over 1/2 tsp (2 mL) lightly crushed seeds. Steep with lid on 10 minutes. Strain, discard herb and add liquid to 1 cup (250 mL) juice.

Dandelion Leaf
Taraxacum officinalis

A hardy, herbaceous perennial, commonly found throughout most parts of North America.

Parts Used

Roots, stem, leaves, flowers.

Healing Properties

Actions: diuretic, liver and digestive tonic

Uses: Dandelion is used for liver, gall bladder, kidney, and bladder ailments, including hepatitis and jaundice, and to promote the flow of urine. The leaf is used specifically to support kidney function.

Availability

Whole plant is easily foraged spring through fall. Fresh leaves in some supermarkets, farmers' markets, health/alternative stores; chopped, dried leaf in health/alternative stores.

How to Use in Juicing

Whole fresh leaves: Roll in a ball and feed through tube along with other ingredients. Use 4 to 6 leaves for each 1 cup (250 mL) juice.

Dried leaf: Whisk 1 tsp (5 mL) chopped, dried leaf into 1 cup (250 mL) juice or add to ingredients in blended drinks.

Infusion: In a teapot, pour 1/4 cup (50 mL) boiling water over 1 tbsp (15 mL) fresh or 1 tsp (5 mL) dried dandelion leaf; steep for 10 minutes. Strain, discard herb, and add liquid to 1 cup (250 mL) juice.

Dandelion Root

Taraxacum officinalis

See Dandelion Leaf.

Parts Used

Roots, stem, leaves, flowers.

Healing Properties

Actions: liver tonic, promotes bile flow, diuretic, mildly laxative, antirheumatic

Uses: See Dandelion Leaf. Root is used specifically to support the liver.

Availability

Dig fresh roots in the fall. Chopped, dried root and tincture is available in health/alternative stores.

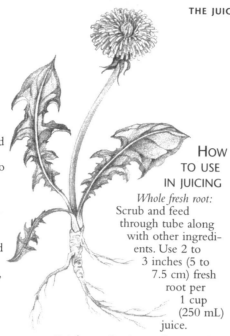

How to Use in Juicing

Whole fresh root: Scrub and feed through tube along with other ingredients. Use 2 to 3 inches (5 to 7.5 cm) fresh root per 1 cup (250 mL) juice.

Dried root: Crush to a fine powder, then whisk into fresh juice or add to smoothie ingredients. Use 1 tsp (5 mL) for each 1 cup (250 mL) juice.

Decoction: Gently simmer 1 tsp (5 mL) chopped dried root in 1/4 cup (50 mL) water for 10 minutes. Strain, discard herb, and add liquid to 1 cup (250 mL) juice.

Tincture: Add 1 tsp (5 mL) to 1 cup (250 mL) juice.

Dill

Anethum graveolens

A tall annual, top-heavy with a long hollow stem growing out of a spindly taproot. Terminal flowers appear in a wide, flat umbel with numerous yellow flowers. Branches along the stem support feathery blue-green leaflets.

Parts Used

Seeds.

Healing Properties

Actions: soothing digestive, anti-spasmodic, increases milk in breast-feeding

Uses: flatulence, infant's colic, bad breath

Availability

Easy to grow. Harvest seeds late summer to early fall. Dried seeds readily available in health/alternative stores and supermarkets.

How to Use in Juicing

Dried seeds: Crush to a powder; whisk 1/2 tsp (2 mL) into 1 cup (250 mL) juice or add to ingredients in blended drinks.

Infusion: In a teapot, pour 1/4 cup (50 mL) boiling water over 1 tsp (5 mL) lightly crushed seeds; steep with lid on 10 minutes. Strain, discard herb, and add liquid to 1 cup (250 mL) juice.

Echinacea

Echinacea angustifolia or E. purpurea

A hardy perennial native to North America with bright purple petals surrounding a brown cone (common name: purple coneflower).

Parts Used

Root (most powerful) and petals.

Healing Properties

Actions: immune stimulating, anti-inflammatory, antibiotic, anti-microbial, antiseptic, analgesic, anti-allergenic, lymphatic tonic

Uses: Echinacea works effectively at the first sign of cold or flu, taken in 4 to 6 doses daily for 10 days. It has interferon-like actions, helping prevent and control viral infections. It hastens the healing of tissue by stimulating the fibroblasts that form new connective tissue. It fights viruses and *candida*.

Availability

Whole or cut, dried root, and dried stems and leaves available in alternative/health stores. Echinacea is also available in tincture and tablet form.

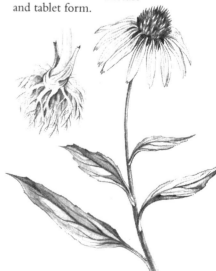

HOW TO USE IN JUICING

Decoction: Gently simmer 1 tsp (5 mL) chopped dried root in 1/4 cup (50 mL) water for 10 minutes. Strain and add to 1 cup (250 mL) juice.

Tincture: Add 1/2 tsp (2 mL) of tincture to 1 cup (250 mL) juice.

FOLKLORE

Native Americans used the fresh juice of *E. angustifolia* to desensitize their feet before walking over hot coals during ceremonies and rituals.

Elder

Sambucus nigra

A fast-growing, hardy perennial shrub, common in many parts of North America.

PARTS USED

Bark, flowers, berries.

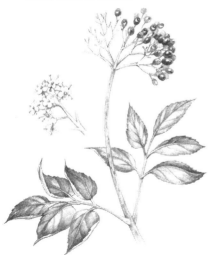

HEALING PROPERTIES

Actions: (flowers) Expectorant, reduce phlegm, circulatory stimulant, promote sweating, diuretic, topically anti-inflammatory. *(berries)* Promote sweating, diuretic, laxative. *(bark)* Purgative, large doses promote vomiting, diuretic.

Uses: Elderberry supports detoxification by promoting bowel movements, urination, sweating and secretion of mucus. Elderberry is effective in combating viruses including colds and flu.

Elderflowers are taken early in the season to strengthen upper respiratory tract and help prevent hay fever.

AVAILABILITY

Dried flowers, fresh or dried berries are available in alternative/health stores. Elder tincture is also available in alternative/health stores.

HOW TO USE IN JUICING

Infusion, flowers: In a teapot, pour 1/4 cup (50 mL) boiling water over 1 tbsp (15 mL) fresh or dried flowers; steep 10 minutes if using dried flowers, 15 minutes if using fresh flowers. Strain and add to 1 cup (250 mL) juice.

Fresh berries: Add up to 1/4 cup (50 mL) fresh berries to other fruits in juicer.

Infusion, berries: Pour 1/4 cup (50 mL) boiling water over 1 tbsp (15 mL) fresh or 1 tsp (5 mL) lightly crushed dried berries; steep 10 minutes. Strain, discard herb, and add liquid to 1 cup (250 mL) juice.

Tincture: Add 1 tsp (5 mL) of tincture to 1 cup (250 mL) juice.

Evening Primrose

Oenotbera biennis

An erect biennial with a rosette of basal leaves. In summer, yellow flowers open at night. Blooms are followed by downy pods containing tiny black seeds.

PARTS USED

Seed oil.

HEALING PROPERTIES

Actions: anticoagulant, anti-inflammatory, improves blood circulation, nutritive; the essential fatty acids in the seed oil help to repair body tissue

Uses: acne, anxiety, arthritis, asthma, breast tenderness, diabetes, dry skin, eczema, hangover, inflammations, high blood pressure, hyperactivity in children, migraines, multiple sclerosis, premenstrual syndrome

AVAILABILITY

Evening primrose oil is available at health/alternative stores.

HOW TO USE IN JUICING

Oil: Whisk 1 tsp (5 mL) oil into 1 cup (250 mL) juice or add to ingredients in blended drinks.

Fennel

Foeniculum vulgare

Fennel looks like a larger version of dill. Stout, solid stems support bright yellow, large umbel clusters of flowers. Thread-like and feathery green leaves alternately branch out from joints of the stem. Flowers appear in summer, followed by gray-brown seeds.

PARTS USED

Seeds.

HEALING PROPERTIES

Actions: soothing diuretic, anti-inflammatory, anti-spasmodic, soothing digestive, promotes milk flow, mild expectorant

Uses: indigestion, flatulence, increasing milk flow in breastfeeding, relieves colic in babies when taken by nursing mother; also used directly for colic, coughs

CAUTION

Fennel is a uterine stimulant, so avoid high doses during pregnancy.

AVAILABILITY

Fennel grows wild throughout Europe and Asia and has naturalized in many other parts of the world, where the fleshy bulb is harvested and used as a vegetable. Easy to grow; harvest seeds in late summer, early fall. Dried seeds readily available in health/alternative stores and supermarkets.

HOW TO USE IN JUICING

Fresh bulb: See Fennel, page 49.

Dried seeds: Crush to a powder; whisk 1/4 tsp (1 mL) into 1 cup (250 mL) juice or add to ingredients in blended drinks.

Infusion: In a teapot, pour 1/4 cup (50 mL) boiling water over 1/4 to 1/2 tsp (1 to 2 mL) lightly crushed seeds; steep with lid on 15 minutes. Strain, discard herb, and add liquid to 1 cup (250 mL) juice.

Fenugreek
Trigonella foenum-graecum

Grown as a fodder crop in southern and central Europe, fenugreek is widely naturalized from the Mediterranean to southern Africa and Australia. This annual has aromatic trifoliate leaves and solitary or paired yellow–white flowers, followed by beaked pods with yellow-brown seeds.

PARTS USED
Aerial parts and seeds.

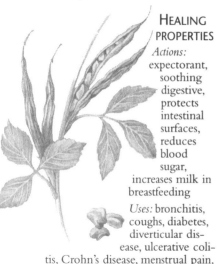

HEALING PROPERTIES
Actions: expectorant, soothing digestive, protects intestinal surfaces, reduces blood sugar, increases milk in breastfeeding

Uses: bronchitis, coughs, diabetes, diverticular disease, ulcerative colitis, Crohn's disease, menstrual pain, peptic ulcer, stomach upsets

CAUTION
Avoid in pregnancy, since fenugreek stimulates the uterus.

AVAILABILITY
Dried seeds from health/alternative stores.

HOW TO USE IN JUICING
Decoction: Simmer gently for 10 minutes 1 to 2 tsp (5 to 10 mL) crushed seeds for each 1 cup (250 mL) water. Strain, discard herb, and add liquid to 1 cup (250 mL) juice.

Feverfew
Tanacetum parthenium

A perennial that ranges throughout northern temperate regions, feverfew is in the same genus as tansy. The oblong, bright green leaves contain pungent volatile oils that may cause unpleasant reactions if handled or consumed in excess. Flowers are small and daisy-like.

PARTS USED
Leaves.

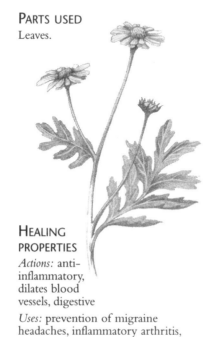

HEALING PROPERTIES
Actions: anti-inflammatory, dilates blood vessels, digestive

Uses: prevention of migraine headaches, inflammatory arthritis, menstrual pain

CAUTION
Avoid in pregnancy, since feverfew stimulates the uterus. Fresh leaves may cause mouth ulcers in sensitive people.

AVAILABILITY
Easily grown, fresh leaves can be harvested from June through late fall. Dried cut leaves available at health/alternative stores.

HOW TO USE IN JUICING
Whole fresh leaves: Roll in a ball and feed through tube along with other ingredients. Use 1 or 2 large leaves for each 1 cup (250 mL) juice.

Dried leaf: Crush to a fine powder, then whisk into fresh juice. Use 1 tsp (5 mL) for each cup (250 mL) juice.

Tincture: Add 5 to 20 drops of tincture to 1 cup (250 mL) juice.

Garlic
Allium sativum

A hardy perennial with an onion-like bulb, easily grown in North America.

PARTS USED
Bulb or "bud" at the root of the plant.

HEALING PROPERTIES
Actions: anti-microbial, antibiotic, cardio-protective, hypotensive, anti-carcinogen, promotes sweating, reduces blood pressure, anti-coagulant, lowers blood cholesterol levels, lowers blood sugar levels, expectorant, digestive stimulant, diuretic, anti-histaminic, antiparasitic

Uses: Research has shown that garlic inhibits cancer cell formation and proliferation. It lowers serum total and low density lipoprotein cholesterol in humans and it reduces the tendency of the blood to clot, thereby reducing the risk of blocked arteries and heart disease. Garlic is an antioxidant and helps stimulate the immune system. It has strong antibiotic and anti-inflammatory properties, making it a good wound medicine. Garlic protects organs from damage induced by synthetic drugs, chemical pollutants and the effects of radiation.

AVAILABILITY
Fresh whole bulbs at farmers' markets, food stores and supermarkets.

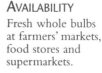

HOW TO USE IN JUICING
Only the fresh cloves have medicinal value. Add one or two fresh cloves to other vegetables when juicing.

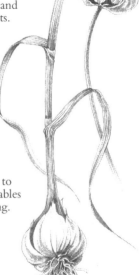

German Chamomile
Matricaria recutita

A low-growing hardy annual. Flowers have daisy-like petals surrounding yellow centers. Easily grown in North America.

PARTS USED
Flowerheads and petals.

HEALING PROPERTIES
Actions: gentle sedative, anti-inflammatory, mild antiseptic, prevents vomiting, anti-spasmodic, carminative, nervine, emmenagogue, mild pain reliever

Uses: anxiety, insomnia, indigestion, peptic ulcer, travel sickness and inflammations (such as gastritis) and menstrual cramps; also reduces flatulence and pain caused by gas

AVAILABILITY
Whole dried flower heads and tincture available in alternative/health stores.

HOW TO USE IN JUICING
Infusion: In a teapot, pour 1/4 cup (50 mL) boiling water over 1 tbsp (15 mL) fresh or 1 tsp (5 mL) dried flower heads; steep for 10 minutes. Strain, discard herb, and add liquid to 1 cup (250 mL) juice.

Tincture: Add 1 tsp (5 mL) of tincture to 1 cup (250 mL) juice.

FOLKLORE
Known as the "ginseng of Europe," chamomile can be found in 18 different medicinal preparations on pharmacy shelves throughout West Germany.

Ginger
Zingeber officinalis

A tender perennial with an edible rhizome, native to Southeast Asia.

PARTS USED
Root.

HEALING PROPERTIES
Actions: anti-nausea, relieves headaches and arthritis, anti-inflammatory, circulatory stimulant, expectorant, antispasmodic, antiseptic, diaphoretic, guards against blood clots, peripheral vasodilator, prevents vomiting, carminative, antioxidant

Uses: Ginger root calms nausea and morning sickness and prevents vomiting. It is a cleansing herb with warming effects. Ginger is used to stimulate blood flow to the digestive system and to increase absorption of nutrients and it increases the action of the gall bladder, while protecting the liver against toxins and preventing the formation of ulcers. Studies show ginger giving some relief from the pain and swelling of arthritis without side effects. Ginger is also used for flatulence, circulation problems, impotence, prevention of nausea after chemotherapy.

CAUTION
Ginger can be irritating to the intestinal mucosa, and should be taken with or after meals. Ginger is contraindicated in kidney disease.

AVAILABILITY
Fresh ginger root and dried powdered ginger are widely available in supermarkets, Asian and Indian markets and health/alternative stores.

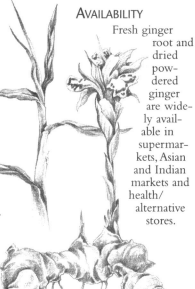

HOW TO USE IN JUICING
Fresh root: Add 1/2- to 1-inch (1 to 3 cm) piece to fruits or vegetables when juicing. Leave peel on if organic.

Infusion: In a teapot, pour 1/4 cup (50 mL) boiling water over 1 tsp (5 mL) grated fresh ginger; steep for 10 minutes. Strain, discard herb, and add liquid to 1 cup (250 mL) juice.

Dried powder: Whisk 1 tsp (5 mL) powdered ginger into 1 cup (250 mL) juice or add to ingredients in blended drinks.

Ginkgo
Ginkgo biloba

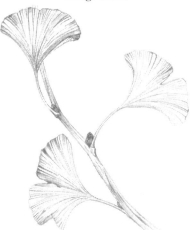

A deciduous tree, one of the oldest species to survive to present day, ginkgo originated in central China but is grown as an ornamental in central North America. Light green, fan-shaped leaves with two lobes turn yellow in autumn.

PARTS USED
Leaves.

HEALING PROPERTIES
Actions: antioxidant, circulatory stimulant, increases blood flow to the brain, relieves bronchial spasms

Uses: asthma, tinnitus, cold hands and feet, varicose veins, hemorrhoids, headache, hangover, age-related memory impairment, hearing loss and eyesight changes; Alzheimer's disease, Raynaud's disease, retinopathy, impotence

AVAILABILITY
Leaves are gathered when yellow, in autumn. Dried ginkgo leaves are available in health/alternative stores.

HOW TO USE IN JUICING

Dried leaf: Crush to a fine powder, then whisk into fresh juice or add to ingredients in blended drinks. Use 1 tsp (5 mL) for each 1 cup (250 mL) juice.

Infusion: In a teapot, pour 1/4 cup (50 mL) boiling water over 1 tbsp (15 mL) fresh or 1 tsp (5 mL) dried leaves; steep for 10 minutes. Strain, discard herb, and add liquid to 1 cup (250 mL) juice.

Liquid extract: Add 40 drops to 1 cup (250 mL) juice.

Ginseng

Siberian: *Eleutherococcus senticosis,*
North American: *Panax quinquefolius,*
Asian: *Panax ginseng*

A hardy perennial, native to cool, wooded areas of eastern and central North America.

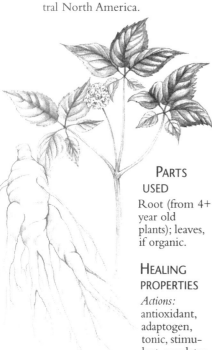

PARTS USED

Root (from 4+ year old plants); leaves, if organic.

HEALING PROPERTIES

Actions: antioxidant, adaptogen, tonic, stimulant, regulates blood sugar and cholesterol levels, stimulates the immune system

Uses: Ginseng helps the body better resist and adapt to stress. It is a mild stimulant and as a tonic, it promotes long-term overall health. Along with increasing resistance to diabetes, cancer, heart disease and various infections, the medical literature on ginseng claims that it can improve memory, increase fertility, protect the liver against many toxins, and protect the body from

radiation. It is also used in impotence and depression.

CAUTION

As a rule, avoid ginseng if you have a fever, asthma, bronchitis, emphysema, high blood pressure or cardiac arrhythmia. Avoid in pregnancy and with hyperactivity in children. Do not take with coffee.

AVAILABILITY

Dried root (whole or chopped), tea, powder and tincture are all found in health/alternative stores and Asian grocery stores. While native to North American woodlands, ginseng has been harvested to near extinction. Please do not collect from the wild or purchase wildcrafted North American ginseng.

HOW TO USE IN JUICING

Fresh root: Add 2- to 3-inch (5 to 7.5 cm) piece to juicing ingredients. Only use organic ginseng and leave peel on.

Dried root: Grate finely and whisk 1/4 tsp (1 mL) powder into 1 cup (250 mL) juice or add to ingredients in blended drinks.

Decoction: Gently simmer 1 tsp (5 mL) chopped dried root in 1/4 cup (50 mL) water for 10 minutes. Strain and add to 1 cup (250 mL) juice.

Tincture: Add 10 to 20 drops of tincture to 1 cup (250 mL) juice.

Goldenrod
Solidago virgaurea

Long used by native people in North America, goldenrod is a perennial with upright stems, oval leaves and yellow flowers that appear in late summer.

PARTS USED
Aerial parts.

HEALING PROPERTIES

Actions: anti-catarrhal, anti-inflammatory, antiseptic to mucous membranes, urinary antiseptic, diuretic, promotes sweating

Uses: bronchitis, coughs, respiratory congestion, urethritis, tonsillitis, prostatitis, kidney and bladder problems

AVAILABILITY

Widely available in the wild and in waste lands, harvest from July through fall. Dried cut leaves, stems and flowers available in health/alternative stores.

HOW TO USE IN JUICING

Whole fresh sprigs: Roll in a ball and feed through tube along with other ingredients. Use 2 to 4 sprigs for each 1 cup (250 mL) juice.

Dried leaf and flowers: Crush to a fine powder, then whisk into fresh juice or add to ingredients in blended drinks. Use 1/4 to 1/2 tsp (1 to 2 mL) for each 1 cup (250 mL) juice.

Infusion: In a teapot, pour 1/4 cup (50 mL) boiling water over 1 tbsp (15 mL) fresh or 1 tsp (5 mL) dried goldenrod; steep for 10 minutes. Strain, discard herb, and add liquid to 1 cup (250 mL) juice.

Gotu Kola
Hydrocotyle asiatica

A small, creeping tropical perennial, this plant has been used for centuries in India for its rejuvenating properties.

PARTS USED
Aerial parts.

HEALING PROPERTIES

Actions: blood tonic, digestive, central nervous system relaxant, laxative, strengthens adrenal glands

Uses: exhaustion, age-related memory loss, nervous disorders, Parkinson's disease, stress

CAUTION

Gotu Kola is not to be used in pregnancy or epilepsy. Do not use for longer than 6 weeks without a break. May aggravate itching. In large doses, may cause headache.

AVAILABILITY

Dried aerial parts may

be available at health/alternative stores. Tincture is available where tablets are sold.

HOW TO USE IN JUICING

Dried leaf and flowers: Crush to a fine powder, then whisk into fresh juice or add to ingredients in blended drinks, use 1/2 tsp (2 mL) for each 1 cup (250 mL) juice.

Infusion: In a teapot, pour 1/4 cup (50 mL) boiling water over 1/2 tsp (2 mL) gotu kola; steep for 10 minutes. Strain, discard herb, and add liquid to 1 cup (250 mL) juice.

Tincture: Add 1/2 to 1 tsp (2 to 5 mL) to 1 cup (250 mL) juice.

FOLKLORE

Gotu kola is one of the most important herbs in Ayurvedic medicine, used for longevity, increasing intelligence and memory, strengthening the immune system and purifying the blood in chronic skin diseases.

Green Tea
Camellia sinensis

Green and black tea comes from a shrub or small tree indigenous to the wet forests of Asia and cultivated commercially in Asia, Africa, South America and in North Carolina.

PARTS USED
Leaves.

HEALING PROPERTIES

Actions: antioxidant, diuretic, recently found to have anti-cancer properties

Uses: Protection against cancer; protection against radiation if taken daily at least a week before exposure.

CAUTION
Green tea contains caffeine, so should be minimized in cases where caffeine aggravates a health condition.

AVAILABILITY

Available dried, in bulk, in Oriental markets and alternative/health stores; sold individually wrapped in supermarkets.

HOW TO USE IN JUICING

Dried leaf: Crush to a fine powder, then whisk into fresh juice or add to ingredients in blended drinks, use 1 tsp (5 mL) for each 1 cup (250 mL) juice.

Infusion: In a teapot, pour 1/4 cup (50 mL) boiling water over 1 tsp (5 mL) dried green tea; steep for 10 minutes. Strain, discard herb, and add liquid to 1 cup (250 mL) juice.

Hawthorn
Crataegus monogyna and *C. oxyacanthoides*

A thorny shrub found throughout northern temperate regions, hawthorn grows wild in hedgerows in Europe and northeastern United States and Canada. Scented white flowers bear dark red, oval fruit with a stony seed.

PARTS USED
Flowering tops, fruit.

HEALING PROPERTIES

Actions: heart tonic, improves coronary circulation

Uses: angina, hypertension, poor circulation

CAUTION

Consult your medical practitioner before taking Hawthorn while taking other heart medication.

AVAILABILITY

Harvest flowering tops in the spring and fresh fruit in late summer and dry for medicinal use.

Dried hawthorn 'berries' are available in health/alternative stores.

HOW TO USE IN JUICING

Fresh berries: For a wonderful heart tonic, add 1/4 to 1/2 cup (50 to 125 mL) fresh berries to any fresh berry or other fruit juice recipe.

Infusion: In a teapot, pour 1/4 cup (50 mL) boiling water over 1 to 2 tsp (5 to 10 mL) bruised fresh or dried hawthorn blossoms or lightly crushed fresh or dried berries. Steep with lid on 10 minutes, strain, discard herb, add liquid to 1 cup (250 mL) juice.

Tincture: Add 10 to 20 drops to 1 cup (250 mL) juice.

Horse Chestnut
Aesculus hippocastanum

A large tree common in North America and southeastern Europe, horse chestnut has palmate leaves and long spikes of white flowers appearing in the spring. Globular, green-brown, spiny fruits replace flowers in summer.

PARTS USED
Bark and seeds (peeled fruit).

HEALING PROPERTIES

Actions: astringent, anti-inflammatory, circulatory tonic, strengthens and tones veins

Uses: varicose veins, hemorrhoids, phlebitis; a tea can be used externally for bruises and leg ulcers

AVAILABILITY

Dried bark and seeds available at health/alternative stores.

HOW TO USE IN JUICING

Infusion: In a teapot, pour 1/4 cup (50 mL) boiling water over 1/2 tsp (2 mL) lightly crushed bark and seeds; steep with lid on 15 minutes. Strain, discard herb, and add liquid to 1 cup (250 mL) juice.

Tincture: Add 30 drops to 1 cup (250 mL) juice.

Hyssop
Hyssopus officinalis

A bushy evergreen perennial with woody stems, hyssop is native to central and southern Europe, western Asia and northern Africa. The upright stem bears linear, opposite leaves and purple flowers in whorls from the dense spikes at the top of the stems.

PARTS USED
Leaves and flowering tops.

HEALING PROPERTIES
Actions: antispasmodic, expectorant, promotes sweating, mild pain killer, diuretic, antiviral against herpes simplex, reduces phlegm, soothing digestive

Uses: asthma, bronchitis, colds, coughs, influenza, fevers, flatulence

AVAILABILITY
Hyssop is easy to grow and is harvested from May through fall in central and northern North America. Dried leaves are available from health/alternative stores.

HOW TO USE IN JUICING
Whole fresh sprigs: Roll in a ball and feed through tube along with other ingredients. Use 4 to 6 sprigs for each 1 cup (250 mL) juice.

Dried leaf and flowers: Crush to a fine powder, then whisk into fresh juice or add to ingredients in blended drinks. Use 1 tsp (5 mL) for each 1 cup (250 mL) juice.

Kava Kava
Piper methysticum

Grown and used in Polynesia, kava kava is an evergreen shrub that belongs to the pepper genus.

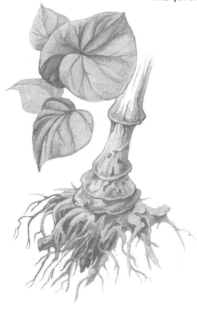

PARTS USED
Root and rhizome.

HEALING PROPERTIES
Actions: antimicrobial (especially to the genito-urinary system), antispasmodic, nerve and muscle relaxant, diuretic, stimulant

Uses: stress, anxiety, chronic fatigue syndrome, fibromyalgia, insomnia, infections of the kidney, bladder, vagina, prostate, urethra

CAUTION
Kava kava is not to be used in pregnancy or breastfeeding. Consult with your medical practitioner before taking with other drugs that act on the nervous system. Do not take for a period longer than 3 months unless advised by your medical practitioner. Do not drive or operate heavy machinery while taking kava kava.

AVAILABILITY
Dried root and liquid extract available from health/alternative stores.

HOW TO USE IN JUICING
Decoction: In a small saucepan, combine 1/2 cup (125 mL) boiling water with 1 tsp (5 mL) dried root; simmer with lid on 10 minutes or until decoction is colored light brown. Strain, discard herb, and add liquid to 1 cup (250 mL) juice.

Liquid extract: Add 1/2 to 1 tsp (2 to 5 mL) to 1 cup (250 mL) juice.

Lavender
Lavandula spp

A shrub-like plant with dense, woody stems from which linear, pine-like, gray-green leaves grow. The tiny flowers grow in whorls on spikes from long stems.

PARTS USED
Leaves, stems and flowering tops.

HEALING PROPERTIES
Actions: relaxant, antispasmodic, anti-depressive, nervous system tonic, circulatory stimulant, antibacterial, antiseptic, carminative, promotes bile flow

Uses: colic, depression, exhaustion, indigestion, insomnia, stress, tension headaches

CAUTION
Avoid high doses in pregnancy; lavender is a uterine stimulant.

AVAILABILITY
Easily grown in temperate climates. Harvest from June through fall. Dried flower buds are available at health/alternative stores.

HOW TO USE IN JUICING
Whole fresh flowers: Feed through tube along with other ingredients. Use 2 to 4 sprigs for each 1 cup (250 mL) juice.

Dried flowers: Crush to a fine powder, then whisk into fresh juice or add to ingredients in blended drinks. Use 1 tsp (5 mL) for each 1 cup (250 mL) juice.

Infusion: In a teapot, pour 1/4 cup (50 mL) boiling water over 1 tbsp (15 mL) fresh or 1 tsp (5 mL) dried flower buds; steep for 15 minutes. Strain, discard herb, and add liquid to 1 cup (250 mL) juice.

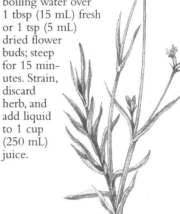

Lemon balm
Melissa officinalis

Opposite, oval, strongly lemon-scented leaves grow on thin, square stems. Flowers are tubular, white or yellow, growing in clusters at the base of the leaves.

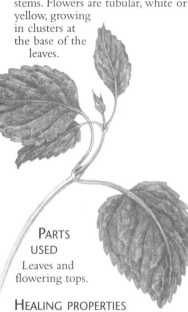

PARTS USED
Leaves and flowering tops.

HEALING PROPERTIES
Actions: antioxidant, anti-histamine, carminative, anti-spasmodic, anti-viral, anti-bacterial, nerve relaxant, anti-depressive, stimulates bile flow, lowers blood pressure

Uses: anxiety, depression, stress, flatulence, indigestion, insomnia

AVAILABILITY
An easily grown perennial; harvest leaves and flowers from June through autumn. Dried leaves available in health/alternative stores.

HOW TO USE IN JUICING
Whole fresh sprigs: Roll in a ball and feed through tube along with other ingredients. Use 4 to 6 sprigs for each 1 cup (250 mL) juice.

Dried leaf and flowers: Crush to a fine powder, then whisk into fresh juice or add to blended drinks, use 1 tsp (5 mL) for each 1 cup (250 mL) juice.

Infusion: In a teapot, pour 1/4 cup (50 mL) boiling water over 1 tbsp (15 mL) fresh or 1 tsp (5 mL) dried lemon balm; steep for 10 minutes. Strain, discard herb, and add liquid to 1 cup (250 mL) juice.

Lemon Verbena
Aloysia triphylla

A fast-growing, deciduous shrub, native to South America. Can grow as tall as 6 feet (2 m). Long, pointed green leaves grow on erect stems that extend from green or brown bark, and turn woody with maturity. Lavender-colored flowers are tiny and grow in spikes.

PARTS USED
Leaves.

HEALING PROPERTIES
Actions: antispasmodic, digestive

Uses: indigestion, flatulence

AVAILABILITY
Dried leaves may be available in health/alternative stores.

HOW TO USE IN JUICING
Whole fresh sprigs: Roll in a ball and feed through tube along with other ingredients. Use 4 to 6 sprigs for each 1 cup (250 mL) juice.

Dried leaf: Crush to a fine powder, then whisk into fresh juice or add to ingredients in blended drinks. Use 1 tsp (5 mL) for each 1 cup (250 mL) juice.

Infusion: In a teapot, pour 1/4 cup (50 mL) boiling water over 1 tsp (5 mL) dried or 1 tbsp (15 mL) fresh, bruised leaves; steep for 10 minutes. Strain, discard herb, and add liquid to 1 cup (250 mL) juice.

Licorice
Glycyrrhiza glabra

A tender perennial, native to the Mediterranean region and southwest Asia.

PARTS USED
Root.

HEALING PROPERTIES
Actions: gentle laxative, tonic, anti-inflammatory, anti-bacterial, anti-arthritic, soothes gastric and intestinal mucous membranes, expectorant

Uses: Licorice root is considered to be one of the best tonic herbs because it provides nutrients to almost all body systems. It detoxifies, regulates blood sugar levels and recharges depleted adrenal glands. It has been shown to heal peptic ulcers and is used to soothe irritated membranes and loosen and expel phlegm in the upper respiratory tract. It is also used to treat sore throat, urinary tract infections, coughs, bronchitis, gastritis, and constipation.

CAUTION
Large amounts taken over long periods of time may cause fluid retention and a reduction in blood potassium levels. Avoid or use sparingly in high blood pressure.

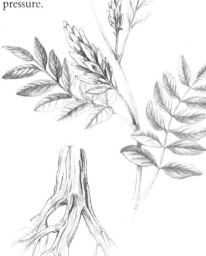

AVAILABILITY
Whole or powdered, dried root available in alternative/health stores. Extracts also often sold, but lack the tonic action.

HOW TO USE IN JUICING
Decoction: Gently simmer 1 tsp (5 mL) chopped dried root in 1/4 cup (50 mL) water for 10 minutes. Strain and add to 1 cup (250 mL) juice.

Linden Flower
(Lime Flowers)
Tilia cordata or *T. eurpoea*

Found throughout northern temperate regions, common linden is a deciduous tree with dark green, shiny, heart-shaped leaves and yellow-white flowers that appear in mid-summer. It is often grown as an ornamental in North America.

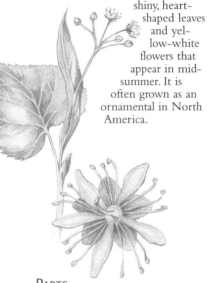

PARTS USED
Flowering tops.

HEALING PROPERTIES
Actions: antispasmodic, promotes sweating (hot tea), diuretic (warm tea), lowers blood pressure, relaxant, mild astringent

Uses: Linden flower tea is a pleasant-tasting, relaxing remedy for stress, anxiety, tension headache and insomnia. It relaxes and nourishes blood vessels, making it useful in high blood pressure and heart disease. In promoting sweating, it is useful in colds, flus and fevers. The tea can be given to children as a calming remedy or to reduce fevers.

AVAILABILITY
Harvest flowering tops in mid-June. Dried flowering tops are available in health/alternative stores. Linden tea in bags is often found in supermarkets.

HOW TO USE IN JUICING
Dried leaf and flowers: Part of linden's actions are due to its essential oils, which are only released with heat. For this reason, dried or fresh linden is not added to juices except as a cooled tea.

Infusion: In a teapot, pour 1/4 cup (50 mL) boiling water over 1 tbsp (15 mL) fresh or dried flowering tops; steep for 10 minutes. Strain, discard herb, and add liquid to 1 cup (250 mL) juice.

Marshmallow
Althaea officinalis

Partial to wet ground, marshmallow is a robust perennial with fleshy taproot and upright stems bearing oval, toothed leaves and pale pink flowers. It is often found in the wild in the Unites States and southern Canada, as well as western Europe to central Asia and north Africa. Hollyhock (*A. rosea*) is in the same genus.

PARTS USED
Flowers, leaves and root.

HEALING PROPERTIES
Actions (root): soothes mucous membranes, diuretic, expectorant, soothes, cleanses and heals external wounds (*leaf*): soothes mucous membranes, diuretic, expectorant, soothes, cleanses and heals external wounds (*flower*): expectorant

Uses: The high mucilage content of marshmallow root makes it useful for soothing inflammation along the digestive tract, the kidneys and the bladder, in peptic ulcer, ulcerative colitis, Crohn's disease, urethritis, hiatus hernia, cystitis, diarrhea and gastritis. The leaf is used for bronchial inflammations such as bronchitis, and in teas for internal ulcerative conditions. The flower is used in expectorant syrups for coughs.

AVAILABILITY
Gather aerial parts from mid-June through autumn and harvest the root in the fall. Dried root is available in health/alternative stores.

HOW TO USE IN JUICING
Whole fresh sprigs: Roll in a ball and feed through tube along with other ingredients. Use 4 to 6 sprigs for each 1 cup (250 mL) juice.

Dried leaf and flowers: Crush to a fine powder, then whisk into fresh juice or add to ingredients in blended drinks. Use 1 tsp (5 mL) for each 1 cup (250 mL) juice.

Infusion: In a teapot, pour 1/4 cup (50 mL) boiling water over 1 tbsp (15 mL) fresh or 1 tsp (5 mL) dried aerial parts; steep for 10 minutes. Strain, discard herb, and add liquid to 1 cup (250 mL) juice.

Whole fresh root: Feed through tube along with other ingredients. Use a 2- to 3-inch (5 to 7.5 cm) piece for each 1 cup (250 mL) juice.

Decoction: In a small saucepan, pour 1/4 cup (50 mL) water over 1 tsp (5 mL) chopped dried root; let stand overnight. Strain, discard herb, and add liquid to 1 cup (250 mL) juice.

Tincture: Add 10 to 20 drops to 1 cup (250 mL) juice.

Meadowsweet
Filipendula ulmaria

A hardy herbaceous perennial found in moist or boggy soils throughout Europe, North America and temperate Asia. Toothed, pinnate leaves grow on upright stems. Creamy white, almond-scented flowers are borne from midsummer to early autumn.

PARTS USED
Aerial parts.

HEALING PROPERTIES
Actions: antacid, anti-inflammatory, anticoagulant, astringent, anti-rheumatic, diuretic, liver supportive, promotes sweating

Uses: The anti-inflammatory and antacid actions of meadowsweet are useful in rheumatoid arthritis, cystitis, peptic ulcer, hyperacidity and gastric reflux. As an astringent, it is used in some types of diarrhea. Meadowsweet protects the mucous membranes of the digestive tract, so it does not produce the stomach bleeding side-effect that is caused by long use of aspirin.

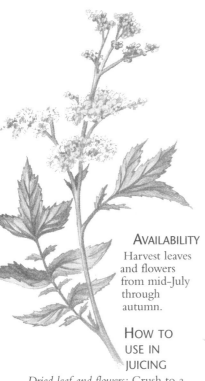

detoxifies, promotes milk flow in breastfeeding

Uses: Milk thistle's strong liver-protective action is important in liver diseases such as alcoholism, cirrhosis and hepatitis, as well as chronic conditions with symptoms of liver congestion such as constipation, bloating and premenstrual syndrome.

AVAILABILITY

Seeds may be collected in mid-summer. Seeds are widely available in health/alternative stores.

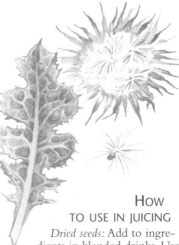

HOW TO USE IN JUICING

Dried seeds: Add to ingredients in blended drinks. Use 1 tsp (5 mL) for each 1 cup (250 mL) juice.

Infusion: In a teapot, pour 1/4 cup (50 mL) boiling water over 1 tsp (5 mL) dried ground seeds; steep for 15 minutes. Strain, discard herb, and add liquid to 1 cup (250 mL) juice.

Tincture: Add 10 to 20 drops to 1 cup (250 mL) juice.

Motherwort
Leonurus cardiaca

A strong-smelling perennial found throughout temperate Europe, Asia and North America. Plamate, deeply lobed leaves grow out of purple stems. Mauve-pink to white flowers grow in whorls from single stems from mid-summer to mid-autumn.

PARTS USED
Aerial parts.

HEALING PROPERTIES
Actions: antispasmodic, nerve and heart sedative, lowers blood pressure, uterine stimulant

Uses: Motherwort has a long history of use in easing menstrual pains. It eases hot flashes and other menopausal symptoms, as well as the anxiety associated with pre-menstrual syndrome. As a heart tonic, motherwort is especially useful in palpitations and other heart conditions where anxiety and tension are involved. Its relaxing actions make it helpful for assisting withdrawal from antidepressant drugs.

CAUTION
Not to be taken in pregnancy or during heavy menstrual bleeding.

FOLKLORE
"Drink motherwort and live to be a continuous source of astonishment and grief to waiting heirs" is an old saying describing its regenerative powers.

AVAILABILITY
Gather aerial parts from mid-summer to mid-autumn. Dried leaves and flowers available in health/alternative stores.

HOW TO USE IN JUICING
Whole fresh sprigs: Roll in a ball and feed through tube along with other ingredients. Use 4 to 6 sprigs for each 1 cup (250 mL) juice.

Dried leaf and flowers: Crush to a fine powder, then whisk into fresh juice or add to ingredients in blended drinks. Use 1 tsp (5 mL) for each 1 cup (250 mL) juice.

Infusion: In a teapot, pour 1/4 cup (50 mL) boiling water over 1 tbsp (15 mL) fresh or 1 tsp (5 mL) dried motherwort; steep for 15 minutes. Strain, discard herb, and add liquid to 1 cup (250 mL) juice.

Tincture: Add 1 tsp (5 mL) to 1 cup (250 mL) juice.

AVAILABILITY
Harvest leaves and flowers from mid-July through autumn.

HOW TO USE IN JUICING
Dried leaf and flowers: Crush to a fine powder, then whisk into fresh juice or add to ingredients in blended drinks. Use 1 tsp (5 mL) for each 1 cup (250 mL) juice.

Infusion: In a teapot, pour 1/4 cup (50 mL) boiling water over 1 tbsp (15 mL) fresh or 1 tsp (5 mL) dried aerial parts; steep for 15 minutes. Strain, discard herb, and add liquid to 1 cup (250 mL) juice.

Tincture: Add 40 drops to 1 cup (250 mL) juice.

Milk Thistle
Silybum marianus

One of two species in the genus (Blessed Thistle being the other), milk thistle is a stout annual or biennial with large, oblong leaves and purple flowers. Black seeds, each bearing a tuft of white hair appear in mid- to late-summer.

PARTS USED
Seeds.

HEALING PROPERTIES
Actions: antioxidant, promotes bile production and bile flow, protects liver by promoting new liver cell development and liver cell repair,

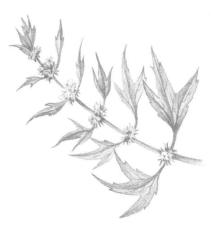

Nutmeg
Myristica fragrans

Native to tropical rainforests in the Moluccas and the Banda Islands, this bushy evergreen tree is grown now commercially in Asia, Australia, Indonesia and Sri Lanka. Pale yellow flowers, produced in axillary clusters, are followed by fleshy, yellow, globe- or pear-shaped fruits (generally called seeds).

PARTS USED
Dried kernel of the nutmeg fruit.

HEALING PROPERTIES
Actions: anti-inflammatory, antispasmodic, carminative, digestive stimulant, sedative

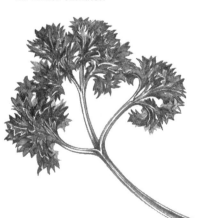

Uses: colic, diarrhea, flatulence, nausea, vomiting, muscle tension

CAUTION
Do not use in pregnancy.

AVAILABILITY
Whole, dried nutmeg seeds are available in health/alternative stores.

HOW TO USE IN JUICING
Dried seeds: Grate to a fine powder, then whisk into juice or add to ingredients in blended drinks. Use 1/4 tsp (1 mL) per serving.

Oats
Avena sativa

This grain is commonly grown throughout North America.

PARTS USED
Seeds and whole plant.

HEALING PROPERTIES
Actions: antioxidant, nerve restorative, antidepressant, nourishes brain and nerves, improves stamina, taken regularly can increase libido

Uses: anxiety, depression, stress, withdrawal from alcohol and antidepressant drugs

AVAILABILITY
Oat seed, straw and oatmeal are available at health/alternative stores.

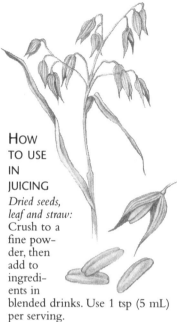

HOW TO USE IN JUICING
Dried seeds, leaf and straw: Crush to a fine powder, then add to ingredients in blended drinks. Use 1 tsp (5 mL) per serving.

Infusion: In a teapot, pour 1/4 cup (50 mL) boiling water over 1 tsp (5 mL) dried oat straw or seed; steep for 15 minutes. Strain, discard herb, and add liquid to 1 cup (250 mL) juice.

Oregon Grape
Berberis aquifolium

Also called mountain grape, *berberis aquifolium* is the state flower of Oregon. Its leaves are holly-like, and the flowers are bright yellow, maturing into grape-like berry clusters. It grows in the mountainous regions of the west coast United States and southern British Columbia.

PARTS USED
Root and rhizome.

HEALING PROPERTIES
Actions: laxative, increases bile secretion, liver stimulant, digestive, antimicrobial for digestive tract, stimulates salivary and stomach secretions including hydrochloric acid

Uses: eczema, psoriasis, constipation, indigestion, blood tonic, liver and gall bladder problems, gum and teeth problems

AVAILABILITY
Dried roots are available from health food stores or by mail order.

HOW TO USE IN JUICING
Powder: Whisk 1/4 to 1/2 tsp (1 to 2 mL) powdered, dried root into 1 cup (250 mL) juice or add to ingredients in blended drinks.

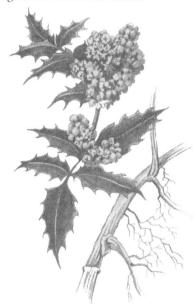

Decoction: In a small saucepan, combine 1/4 cup (50 mL) boiling water and 1 dried root stick or 1/4 to 1/2 tsp (1 to 2 mL) dried chopped root; simmer with lid on 20 minutes, then allow to steep 10 minutes. Strain, discard herb, and add liquid to 1 cup (250 mL) juice.

Parsley
Petroselinum crispum

A hardy biennial, native to the Mediterranean, grown as an annual in colder climates.

PARTS USED

Leaves, stems and roots.

HEALING PROPERTIES

Actions: antioxidant, tonic, digestive, diuretic

Uses: As a diuretic, parsley helps the body expel excess water (by flushing the kidneys). (Note: Always look for and treat underlying causes of water retention.) As a nutrient, it is one of the richest food sources of vitamin C.

CAUTION

Parsley should not be used in high doses during pregnancy because it stimulates the womb. Parsley is contraindicated in cases of kidney inflammation.

AVAILABILITY

Fresh sprigs are available in most supermarkets throughout the year.

HOW TO USE IN JUICING

Whole fresh leaves: Roll in a ball and feed through tube along with other ingredients. Use 6 sprigs for each 1 cup (250 mL) juice.

Dried leaf: Whisk 1 tsp (5 mL) powdered, dried leaf into 1 cup (250 mL) juice or add to ingredients in blended drinks.

Infusion: In a teapot, pour 1/4 cup (50 mL) boiling water over 1 tbsp (15 mL) fresh or 1 tsp (5 mL) dried parsley; steep for 10 minutes. Strain, discard herb, and add liquid to 1 cup (250 mL) juice.

Passionflower
Passiflora incarnata

A perennial climbing vine with deeply lobed leaves and showy fragrant white-to-purple flowers. Some 350 species of passionflower are native to the southern United States and Mexico, with other species growing in tropical Asia and Australia.

PARTS USED

Leaves and flowers.

HEALING PROPERTIES

Actions: antispasmodic, mild sedative, mild pain-reliever, central nervous system relaxant

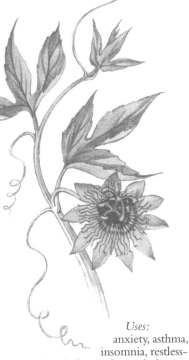

Uses: anxiety, asthma, insomnia, restlessness, headache, Parkinson's disease, antidepressant drug withdrawal, and alcohol withdrawal

AVAILABILITY

Passionflower can be harvested May through July from the wild or from cultivated gardens. Dried passionflower can be purchased in health/alternative stores or by mail order.

HOW TO USE IN JUICING

Dried leaf and flowers: Crush to a fine powder, then whisk into fresh juice. Use 1/4 tsp (1 mL) for each 1 cup (250 mL) juice.

Infusion: In a teapot, pour 1/4 cup (50 mL) boiling water over 1 tbsp (15 mL) fresh or 1/2 tsp (2 mL) dried passionflower; steep for 15 minutes. Strain, discard herb, and add liquid to 1 cup (250 mL) juice.

Tincture: Add 40 drops to 1 cup (250 mL) juice.

FOLKLORE

The distinct flower is said to symbolize the passion of Christ by representing the elements of the crucifixion.

Peppermint
Mentha piperita

An invasive, hardy perennial, native to Europe and Asia but easily grown in North America, peppermint supports bright green, oval aromatic leaves on purple stems. Small pink, white or purple flowers form elongated conical spikes at the tops of the stems.

PARTS USED

Leaves and flowers.

HEALING PROPERTIES

Actions: antispasmodic, digestive tonic, prevents vomiting, carminative, peripheral vasodilator, promotes sweating, promotes bile flow, analgesic

Uses: Taking peppermint before eating helps stimulate liver and gall bladder function by increasing bile flow to the liver and intestines. It is well known for its ability to quell nausea and vomiting. Peppermint is used in ulcerative colitis, Crohn's disease, diverticular disease, travel sickness, fevers, colds, flu, and to improve the appetite.

CAUTION

Do not use during pregnancy or give to children.

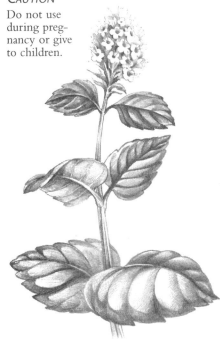

AVAILABILITY

Fresh sprigs in some markets and supermarkets year-round. Dried leaves in alternative/health stores. Teas widely available.

HOW TO USE IN JUICING

Whole fresh leaves: Roll in a ball and feed through tube along with other ingredients. Use 6 sprigs for each 1 cup (250 mL) juice.

Dried leaf: Whisk 1 tsp (5 mL) powdered, dried leaf into 1 cup (250 mL) juice.

Infusion: In a teapot, pour 1/4 cup (50 mL) boiling water over 1 tbsp (15 mL) fresh or 1 tsp (5 mL) dried peppermint; steep for 10 minutes. Strain, discard herb, and add liquid to 1 cup (250 mL) juice.

Plantain

Plantago major and P. lanceolata

Broad-leaved plantain and narrow-leaved plantain are considered common weeds and are found in waste areas throughout North America. Leaves grow in a basal rosette, and flowers top long cylindrical spikes that grow up to 6 inches (15 cm) above leaves.

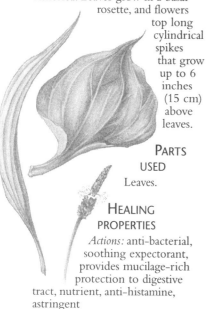

PARTS USED
Leaves.

HEALING PROPERTIES
Actions: anti-bacterial, soothing expectorant, provides mucilage-rich protection to digestive tract, nutrient, anti-histamine, astringent

Uses: coughs, bronchitis, allergies, irritable bowel syndrome, gastric ulcer

AVAILABILITY
The leaves can be collected throughout the summer. Dried leaves are available at health/alternative stores.

HOW TO USE IN JUICING
Whole fresh leaves: Roll in a ball and feed through tube along with other ingredients. Use 2 to 4 leaves for each 1 cup (250 mL) juice.

Infusion: In a teapot, pour 1/4 cup (50 mL) boiling water over 1 tbsp fresh (15 mL) or 1 tsp (5 mL) dried leaves; steep for 15 minutes. Strain, discard herb, and add liquid to 1 cup (250 mL) juice.

FOLKLORE
Fresh plantain leaf is traditionally rubbed on insect bites to soothe inflammation.

Psyllium
Plantago psyllium

The mucilage-rich seeds of *plantago psyllium* (native to the Mediterranean) are similar to those of broad-leaved plantain (*plantago major*), common in Europe and naturalized in North America.

PARTS USED
Seeds.

HEALING PROPERTIES
Actions: soothing, digestive, safe and gentle laxative, cholesterol-lowcring

Uses: Constipation, irritable bowel syndrome, diverticular disease, detoxification, and obesity. The seeds act as a laxative by bulking-up the stool and lubricating the bowel. It is necessary to drink at least one large glass of water when taking 1 to 2 tsp (5 to 10 mL) of the seeds.

AVAILABILITY
Psyllium seeds are widely available in pharmacies and health/alternative stores.

HOW TO USE IN JUICING
Whole seeds: Whisk 1 to 2 tsp (5 to 10 mL) seeds into 1 cup (250 mL) fresh juice or blended drink and drink immediately before they can absorb the moisture. Follow with at least one large glass of water.

Red Clover
Trifolium pratense

A perennial with tubular pink to red flowers throughout the summer, red clover grows in fields throughout North America. It is distinguished by its three long oval leaflets.

PARTS USED
Flowering tops.

HEALING PROPERTIES
Actions: antispasmodic, expectorant, hormone-balancing, nutrient, blood thinning, lymphatic cleanser

Uses: coughs, bronchitis, whooping cough, menstrual problems (because it contributes to blood thinning, don't use red clover in times of heavy menstrual flow)

AVAILABILITY
The flowering tops can be harvested May through September from the wild or cultivated garden. Dried flowers are available in health/alternative stores. Dried clover that has turned brown is of little use; be sure that the flowers are still pink.

HOW TO USE IN JUICING
Whole fresh sprigs: Roll flowering tops in a ball and feed through tube along with other ingredients. Use about 6 sprigs for each 1 cup (250 mL) juice.

Dried leaf and flowers: Crush to a fine powder, then whisk into fresh juice. Use 1 tsp (5 mL) for each 1 cup (250 mL) juice.

Infusion: In a teapot, pour 1/4 cup (50 mL) boiling water over 1 tbsp (15 mL) fresh or 1 tsp (5 mL) dried red clover; steep for 15 minutes. Strain, discard herb, and add liquid to 1 cup (250 mL) juice.

FOLKLORE
Red clover is a folk remedy for prevention and treatment of cancer.

Red Raspberry
Rubus idaeus

A deciduous shrub with prickly stems and pinnately divided leaves, widespread in Europe, Asia and North America. Small white flowers appear in clusters with aromatic, juicy red fruit following in early summer.

PARTS USED
Leaves.

HEALING PROPERTIES

Actions: antispasmodic, astringent, promotes milk in breastfeeding

Uses: Red raspberry leaves have long been used to tone the uterus during pregnancy and labor, resulting in less risk of miscarriage, relief of morning sickness and a safer, easier birth. As an astringent, raspberry leaf is useful in sore throat and diarrhea.

AVAILABILITY

Harvest leaves from early summer through autumn. Dried leaves available in health/alternative stores.

HOW TO USE IN JUICING

Whole fresh leaves: Roll in a ball and feed through tube along with other ingredients. Use about 6 leaves for each 1 cup (250 mL) of juice.

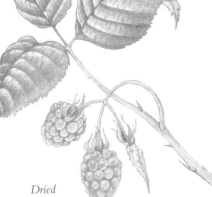

Dried leaf:
Crush to a fine powder, then whisk into fresh juice or add to ingredients in blended drinks, use 1 tsp (5 mL) for each 1 cup (250 mL) juice.

Infusion: In a teapot, pour 1/4 cup (50 mL) boiling water over 1 tbsp (15 mL) fresh or 2 tsp (10 mL) dried bruised leaf, steep for 15 minutes. Strain, discard herb and add liquid to 1 cup (250 mL) juice.

Rose
Rosa

Cultivation of roses dates back thousands of years with *R. rugosa*, *R. gallica*, *R. rubra* and *R. damascena* being among the oldest varieties. *Rosa rugosa* is a deciduous shrub with thorny stems and dark green,

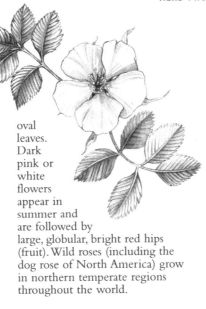

oval leaves. Dark pink or white flowers appear in summer and are followed by large, globular, bright red hips (fruit). Wild roses (including the dog rose of North America) grow in northern temperate regions throughout the world.

PARTS USED

Petals and rose hips.

HEALING PROPERTIES

Actions: Rose hips from *Rosa canina*: nutrient (contain vitamin C), diuretic, astringent, mild laxative. Rose petals from *Rosa gallica, R. damascena, R. centifolia, R. rugosa*: antidepressant, anti-inflammatory, astringent, blood tonic.

Uses (rose hips): Their nutrient value makes them useful in prevention of the common cold and as a tasty addition to herbal teas used to improve immune functioning. As an astringent, they are used in diarrhea. *(rose petals):* Can be added to teas for their relaxing and uplifting fragrance. Used in a bath, they have been known to ease the pains of rheumatoid arthritis.

AVAILABILITY

Harvest petals from mid-summer through autumn and hips in the fall.

HOW TO USE IN JUICING

Dried flowers or hips: Crush to a fine powder, then whisk into fresh juice or add to ingredients in blended drinks. Use 1/2 tsp (2 mL) for each 1 cup (250 mL) juice.

Infusion: In a teapot, pour 1/4 cup (50 mL) boiling water over 1 tbsp (15 mL) fresh petals or chopped fresh hips or 1 tsp (5 mL) dried petals or crushed dried hips; steep for 10 minutes. Strain, discard herb, and add liquid to 1 cup (250 mL) juice.

Rosemary
Rosmarinus officinalis

An evergreen shrub, native to the Mediterranean, rosemary grows to 6 feet (180 cm) in warm climates.

PARTS USED

Leaves and flowers.

HEALING PROPERTIES

Actions: antioxidant, anti-inflammatory, astringent, nervine, carminative, antiseptic, diuretic, diaphoretic, promotes bile flow, anti-depressant, circulatory stimulant, antispasmodic, nervous system and cardiac tonic

Uses: An effective food preservative, rosemary may also be effective in preventing breast cancer. It fights against the deterioration of brain functions (improves memory). It is also useful in treating migraine and tension headaches, nervous tension, flatulence, depression, chronic fatigue syndrome and joint pain.

CAUTION

Avoid large amounts during pregnancy.

AVAILABILITY

Fresh sprigs found in many supermarkets throughout the year. Dried whole and powdered leaf found in supermarkets and health/alternative stores.

HOW TO USE IN JUICING

Whole fresh leaves: Feed through tube along with other ingredients. Use 2 to 3 sprigs for each 1 cup (250 mL) juice.

Infusion: In a teapot, pour 1/4 cup (50 mL) boiling water over 1 tbsp (15 mL) fresh or 1 tsp (5 mL) dried rosemary; steep for 10 minutes. Strain, discard herb, and add liquid to 1 cup (250 mL) juice.

Sage
Salvia officinalis

A hardy, perennial shrub, native to the western United States and Mexico. Tender and hardier varieties of sage are also found in Mexico, the United States and southern Canada. The woody, evergreen shrub has wrinkled, gray-green, oval leaves and purple, pink or white flowers.

PARTS USED
Leaves and flowers.

HEALING PROPERTIES
Actions: antioxidant, antimicrobial, antibiotic, antiseptic, carminative, antispasmodic, anti-inflammatory, circulatory stimulant, estrogenic, peripheral vasodilator, reduces perspiration, uterine stimulant

Uses: Sage's volatile oil kills bacteria and fungi, even those resistant to penicillin. It is very good as a gargle for sore throat, laryngitis and mouth ulcers. Also used to reduce breast milk production, and to relieve night sweats and hot flashes of menopause.

CAUTION
Sage can cause convulsions in very high doses. Do not use where high blood pressure or epilepsy is evident, or during pregnancy.

AVAILABILITY
Fresh sprigs at some supermarkets and farmers' markets. Dried, whole, cut, rubbed or ground widely available.

HOW TO USE IN JUICING
Whole fresh leaves: Roll in a ball and feed through tube along with other ingredients. Use 3 to 4 sprigs for each 1 cup (250 mL) juice.

Dried leaf and flowers: Crush to a fine powder, then whisk into fresh juice or add to ingredients in blended drinks. Use 1/2 tsp (2 mL) for each 1 cup (250 mL) juice.

Infusion: In a teapot, pour 1/4 cup (50 mL) boiling water over 1 tbsp (15 mL) fresh or 1 tsp (5 mL) dried sage; steep for 10 minutes. Strain, discard herb, and add liquid to 1 cup (250 mL) juice.

Saw Palmetto
Seranoa serrulata

Saw palmetto is a clump-forming, evergreen palm with long blue-green leaves and blue-black berries. It grows mainly in the American southeast; forming dense thickets along the Atlantic coasts of Georgia and Florida.

PARTS USED
Berries.

HEALING PROPERTIES
Actions: diuretic, urinary antiseptic, stimulant to the hormone-secreting glands

Uses: benign prostate gland enlargement, lack of sex drive

AVAILABILITY
Berries can be harvested September though January. Dried berries are available in health food stores.

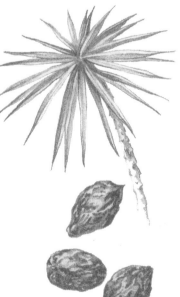

HOW TO USE IN JUICING
Powder: Whisk 1/4 tsp (1 mL) powdered berries into 1 cup (250 mL) juice or add to ingredients in blended drinks.

Infusion: In a teapot, pour 1/4 cup (50 mL) boiling water over 1 tsp (5 mL) fresh or 1/2 tsp (2 mL) dried lightly crushed berries; steep for 10 minutes. Strain, discard herb, and add liquid to 1 cup (250 mL) juice.

Liquid extract: Add 10 to 25 drops to 1 cup (250 mL) juice.

Skullcap
Scutellaria laterifolia

A member of the mint family, this perennial features hooded, violet-blue flowers. It grows in wooded areas in most of the United States and southern Canada except along the west coast.

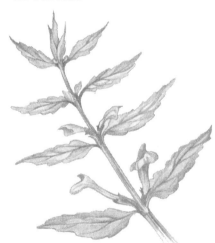

PARTS USED
Stem, leaves and flowers.

HEALING PROPERTIES
Actions: antispasmodic, nourishes central nervous system, relaxing, sedative

Uses: drug addiction withdrawal, premenstrual tension, headache, migraine, mental exhaustion, insomnia, stress

AVAILABILITY
The aerial parts can be collected while the plant is in flower. Dried skullcap is available at health/alternative stores.

HOW TO USE IN JUICING
Whole fresh sprigs: Roll in a ball and feed through tube along with

other ingredients. Use 3 to 4 sprigs for each 1 cup (250 mL) juice.

Dried leaf and flowers: Crush to a fine powder, then whisk into fresh juice in blended drinks. Use 1 tsp (5 mL) for each 1 cup (250 mL) juice.

Infusion: In a teapot, pour 1/4 cup (50 mL) boiling water over 1 tbsp (15 mL) fresh or 1 tsp (5 mL) dried skullcap; steep for 10 minutes. Strain, discard herb, and add liquid to 1 cup (250 mL) juice.

Tincture: Add 40 drops to 1 cup (250 mL) juice.

FOLKLORE

Skullcap is commonly known as "mad-dog" weed, because it was once used as a tea to treat rabies.

Slippery Elm
Ulmus fulva

This deciduous tree is found in damp woodlands in eastern and mid-western United States and in southeastern Canada.

PARTS USED

Dried inner bark.

HEALING PROPERTIES

Actions: soothing digestive, antacid, nutrient, mucilaginous property gives protection to the entire gastrointestinal tract

Uses: peptic ulcer, indigestion, heartburn, hiatus hernia, Crohn's disease, ulcerative colitis, irritable bowel syndrome, diarrhea; a slippery elm bark powder paste is used to soothe and heal wounds and burns; one of the most useful herbs in herbal medicine

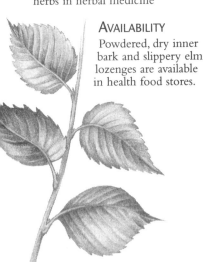

AVAILABILITY

Powdered, dry inner bark and slippery elm lozenges are available in health food stores.

HOW TO USE IN JUICING

Powder: Slippery elm powder does not blend easily into juices. It is best added to ingredients in blended drinks.

Infusion: In a teapot, pour 1/4 cup (50 mL) boiling water over 1 tsp (5 mL) powdered slippery elm; steep for 10 minutes. Add liquid to 1 cup (250 mL) juice.

Spearmint
Mentha spicata

Spearmint is a hardy perennial found in wet soil in most of North America. It is invasive and, like all mints, has a square stem with bright green, lanceolate leaves, and lilac, pink, or white flowers borne in a terminal, cylindrical spike.

PARTS USED

Leaves and flowering tops.

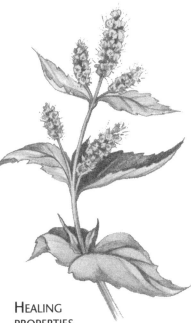

HEALING PROPERTIES

Actions: anti-spasmodic, digestive, induces sweating

Uses: common cold, influenza, indigestion, flatulence, lack of appetite; spearmint is milder than peppermint, so is often used in treating children's colds and flus

AVAILABILITY

Leaves are best harvested just before the flowers open. Dried leaves are available in health food stores.

HOW TO USE IN JUICING

Whole fresh sprigs: Roll in a ball and feed through tube along with other ingredients. Use 4 to 6 sprigs for each 1 cup (250 mL) juice.

Dried leaf and flowers: Crush to a fine powder, then whisk into fresh juice or add to ingredients in blended drinks. Use 1/2 tsp (2 mL) for each 1 cup (250 mL) juice.

Infusion: In a teapot, pour 1/4 cup (50 mL) boiling water over 1 tbsp (15 mL) fresh or 1 tsp (5 mL) dried spearmint; steep for 10 minutes. Strain, discard herb, and add liquid to 1 cup (250 mL) juice.

FOLKLORE

Spearmint is said to repel ants in the home, and to keep mice away from the garden.

St. John's Wort
Hypericum perforatum

Native to woodlands in Europe and temperate Asia, this perennial is also found in temperate areas of the United States and Canada. An upright with straight stems, woody at the base, and 5-petaled, yellow flowers growing from the tips of the branches. When rubbed, the yellow petals stain the fingers red.

PARTS USED

Flowering tops.

HEALING PROPERTIES

Actions: astringent, antiviral, anti-inflammatory, anti-depressant, nervous system tonic, sedative

Uses: St. John's wort is widely used as an anti-depressant, popular because of its effectiveness and rarity of side effects. As a sedative and nervous system tonic, it is useful in neuralgia, shingles, sciatica, tension, anxiety and emotional instability in premenstrual syndrome and menopause.

CAUTION

Recent research studies suggest that St. John's wort increases the metabolising of certain drugs, reducing their level in the blood to the point of being ineffective. If you are taking prescription drugs, consult with your herbalist, doctor or pharmacist before taking St. John's wort.

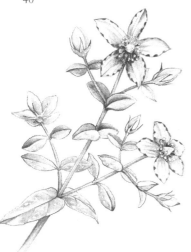

Of particular concern are: oral contraceptives, anti-convulsants, anti-depressants (especially Selective Serotonin Re-uptake Inhibitors), HIV drugs, anticoagulants (Warfarin), cyclosporin (an immunosuppressive drug given after transplants) and digoxin.

AVAILABILITY

Harvest flowering tops for 2 to 3 weeks in mid-summer. Dried aerial parts and tincture available in health/alternative stores.

HOW TO USE IN JUICING

Dried leaf and flowers: Crush to a fine powder, then whisk into fresh juice or add to ingredients in blended drinks. Use 1 tsp (5 mL) for each 1 cup (250 mL) juice.

Infusion: In a teapot, pour 1/4 cup (50 mL) boiling water over 1 tbsp (15 mL) fresh or 1 tsp (5 mL) dried St. John's wort; steep for 15 minutes. Strain, discard herb, and add liquid to 1 cup (250 mL) juice.

Tincture: Add 20 to 40 drops to 1 cup (250 mL) juice.

Stevia
Stevia rebaudiana

A small, tender shrub, native to northeastern Paraguay and adjacent sections of Brazil.

PARTS USED
Leaves.

HEALING PROPERTIES

Actions: energy booster, natural sweetener (without calories), tonic, digestive, diuretic

Uses: Stevia's main benefit is in its use as a safe sweetener and sugar alternative. With its powerfully sweet, licorice taste (stevia is 200 to 300 times sweeter than sugar), stevia prevents cavities and does not trigger a rise in blood sugar. It increases energy and improves digestion by stimulating the pancreas without feeding yeast or fungi.

AVAILABILITY

Dried, cut and powdered leaves and liquid extract are available in health/alternative stores.

HOW TO USE IN JUICING

Whole fresh leaves: Roll in a ball and feed through tube along with other ingredients. Use 2 to 3 leaves for each 1 cup (250 mL) juice.

Dried leaf: Whisk 1/8 tsp (0.5 mL) powdered, dried leaf into 1 cup (250 mL) juice where required.

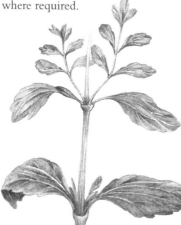

Infusion: In a teapot, pour 1/4 cup (50 mL) boiling water over 1 tsp (5 mL) fresh or 1/4 tsp (1 mL) dried stevia; steep for 10 minutes. Strain, discard herb, and add liquid to 1 cup (250 mL) juice.

Liquid extract: Add 1 to 2 drops to 1 cup (250 mL) juice.

Stinging Nettle
Urtica dioica

Widespread in temperate regions of Europe, North America and Eurasia, this perennial has bristly, stinging hairs on the stem and ovate, toothed leaves that cause minor skin irritation when touched. Small green flowers appear in clusters during the summer.

PARTS USED
Leaves, flowers and root.

HEALING PROPERTIES

Actions (leaves and flowers): astringent, blood tonic, circulatory stimulant, diuretic, eliminates uric acid from the body, nutrient (high in iron, chlorophyll and vitamin C), promotes milk in breastfeeding *(fresh root):* astringent, diuretic

Uses (leaves and flowers): A valuable herb, stinging nettle is useful as a general, everyday, nourishing tonic, as well as specifically in iron-deficiency anemia, gout, arthritis, kidney stones and as a blood tonic in pregnancy, diabetes, poor circulation and chronic skin disease such as eczema. *(fresh root):* The root has a strong action on the urinary system. It is useful in water retention, kidney stones, urinary tract infection, cystitis and prostate inflammation and swelling.

AVAILABILITY

Gather leaves and flowers while plant is flowering in summer, and root in the fall. Dried leaves and flowers available in health/ alternative stores.

HOW TO USE IN JUICING

Infusion: In a teapot, pour 1/4 cup (50 mL) boiling water over 1 tbsp (15 mL) fresh or 1 tsp (5 mL) dried nettles; steep for 15 minutes. Strain, discard herb, and add liquid to 1 cup (250 mL) juice. Note: The sting dissipates when nettles are cooked or infused with boiling water.

Tincture: Add 1 tsp (5 mL) to 1 cup (250 mL) juice.

FOLKLORE

A common remedy for arthritis is flailing the affected joints with fresh nettle leaves. The nettle sting brings the healing blood flow to the affected area.

Thyme
Thymus

A bushy, low growing shrub, easily grown in North America.

PARTS USED
Leaves.

HEALING PROPERTIES
Actions: antioxidant, expectorant, antiseptic, antispasmodic, astringent, tonic, antimicrobial, antibiotic, heals wounds, carminative, calms coughs, nervine

Uses: Thyme is ideal for deep-seated chest infections such as chronic coughs and bronchitis. It is also used for sinusitis, laryngitis, asthma and irritable bowel syndrome.

CAUTION
Avoid in pregnancy. Children under 2 years of age and people with thyroid problems should not take thyme.

AVAILABILITY
Fresh sprigs in farmers' markets in season and most supermarkets year-round. Dried whole leaves in alternative/health stores.

HOW TO USE IN JUICING
Whole fresh leaves: Feed through tube along with other ingredients. Use 6 tender sprigs for each 1 cup (250 mL) juice.

Dried leaf: Whisk 1/2 tsp (2 mL) powdered, dried leaf into 1 cup (250 mL) juice or add to ingredients in blended drinks.

Infusion: In a teapot, pour 1/4 cup (50 mL) boiling water over 1 tbsp (15 mL) fresh or 1 tsp (5 mL) dried thyme; steep for 15 minutes. Strain, discard herb and add liquid to 1 cup (250 mL) juice.

Turmeric
Curcuma longa

A deciduous tender perennial belonging to the ginger family, native to southeast Asia. The long rhizome resembles ginger but is thinner and rounder with brilliant orange flesh.

PARTS USED
Root.

HEALING PROPERTIES
Actions: antioxidant, anti-inflammatory, antimicrobial, anti-bacterial, anti-fungal, antiviral, anticoagulant, analgesic, reduces cholesterol, reduces post-exercise pain, heals wounds, antispasmodic, protects liver cells, increases bile production and flow

Uses: Turmeric appears to inhibit colon and breast cancer and is used in hepatitis, nausea, digestive disturbances, and where gall bladder has been removed. It boosts insulin activity and reduces the risk of stroke. Turmeric is also used in rheumatoid arthritis, cancer, *candida*, AIDS, Crohn's disease, eczema, and digestive problems.

AVAILABILITY
Asian stores stock fresh or frozen whole rhizomes, Oriental markets or natural food stores offer the dried, whole rhizomes, and supermarkets sell ground turmeric.

HOW TO USE IN JUICING
Whole fresh root: Feed through tube along with other ingredients. Use 1/2- to 1-inch (1 to 2.5 cm) pieces for each 1 cup (250 mL) juice. Leave peel on if organic.

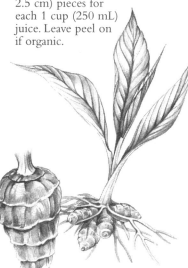

Powder: Whisk 1 tsp (5 mL) powdered, dried root into 1 cup (250 mL) juice or add to ingredients in blended drinks.

Infusion: In a teapot, pour 1/4 cup (50 mL) boiling water over 1 tbsp (15 mL) freshly grated or 1 tsp (5 mL) dried turmeric; steep for 10 minutes. Strain, discard herb, and add liquid to 1 cup (250 mL) juice.

Valerian
Valeriana officinalis

Valerian is a tall, hardy perennial with a strong-smelling white clustered flower. It grows wild in eastern Canada and the northeastern United States.

PARTS USED
Root.

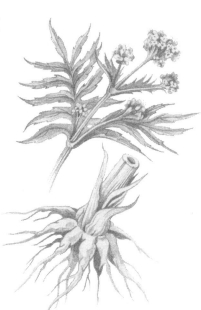

HEALING PROPERTIES
Actions: sedative, relaxant, antispasmodic

Uses: high blood pressure, insomnia, anxiety, tension headaches, muscle cramps, migraine

CAUTION
Some people experience adverse reactions to valerian.

AVAILABILITY
Roots can be harvested in late autumn from the wild or from a cultivated garden. Dried root is available in health food stores. Also available as a tincture.

HOW TO USE IN JUICING

Whole fresh root: Because they're so small, fresh roots are difficult to feed through a juice machine. Instead, make a decoction, and add it to fresh juice.

Decoction: In a small saucepan, combine 1/4 cup (50 mL) boiling water and 1 tbsp (15 mL) fresh chopped root or 1 tsp (5 mL) dried chopped root. Simmer with lid on 10 minutes; steep 10 minutes. Strain, discard herb, and add liquid to 1 cup (250 mL) juice.

Tincture: Add 20 to 40 drops to 1 cup (250 mL) juice.

FOLKLORE

Valerian's botanical name comes from *valere* — "to be strong."

Vitex

(Chaste Tree)

Vitex agnus-castus

A deciduous aromatic shrub or small tree, native to southern Europe. Grown in temperate climates (zones 7 to 10), chaste tree bears palmate leaves, and small, tubular, lilac, scented flowers and fleshy, red-black fruits.

PARTS USED

Berries.

HEALING PROPERTIES

Actions: balances female sex hormones by acting on the anterior pituitary gland

Uses: premenstrual symptoms, painful menstruation, menopausal symptoms

CAUTION

Not to be taken with progesterone drugs.

AVAILABILITY

Dried berries are available in health/alternative stores. Also available as a tincture.

HOW TO USE IN JUICING

Infusion: In a teapot, pour 1/4 cup (50 mL) boiling water over 1 tbsp (15 mL) fresh or 1 tsp (5 mL) dried, lightly crushed berries; steep for 10 minutes. Strain, discard herb, and

add liquid to 1 cup (250 mL) juice.

Tincture: Add 10 to 20 drops to 1 cup (250 mL) juice.

FOLKLORE

With its ability to balance hormones, chasteberry has been used both as an aphrodisiac and an anaphrodisiac.

Wild Lettuce

Lactuca virosa

A tall biennial with lance-shaped leaves and a dandelion-like flower, wild lettuce grows easily from seed.

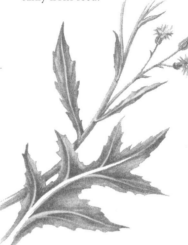

PARTS USED

Dried leaves.

HEALING PROPERTIES

Actions: nerve relaxant, mild sedative, mild pain reliever

Uses: anxiety, insomnia, hyperactivity in children

AVAILABILITY

Leaves can be gathered in June and July.

HOW TO USE IN JUICING

Infusion: Pour 1/4 cup (50 mL) boiling water over 1 tsp (5 mL) dried cut or powdered leaf; steep 10 minutes. Strain, discard herb, and add liquid to 1 cup (250 mL) juice.

FOLKLORE

The milky white latex from the leaves was once sold as "lettuce opium."

Yarrow

Achillea millefolium

A 1- to 3-foot (30 to 90 cm) plant with feathery leaves and a white (occasionally pink) flower, yarrow grows wild throughout North America. This hardy perennial is easily grown in the garden.

PARTS USED

Stems, leaves and flowers.

HEALING PROPERTIES

Actions: anti-inflammatory, bitter, promotes bile flow, promotes sweating, digestive, relaxant, promotes blood circulation, wound healing

Uses: high blood pressure, common cold, fevers, influenza, varicose veins

AVAILABILITY

The above-

ground parts can be harvested while in flower from the wild, June through September. Dried yarrow and tincture is available in health/alternative stores.

HOW TO USE IN JUICING

Dried leaf, stems and flowers: Crush to a fine powder, then whisk into fresh juice or add to ingredients in blended drinks. Use 1 tsp (5 mL) for each 1 cup (250 mL) juice.

Infusion: In a teapot, pour 1/4 cup (50 mL) boiling water over 1 tbsp (15 mL) fresh or 1 tsp (5 mL) dried flowerheads; steep for 10 minutes. Strain, discard herb, and add liquid to 1 cup (250 mL) juice.

Tincture: Add 40 drops to 1 cup (250 mL) juice.

FOLKLORE

Yarrow is said to have been used by Achilles to heal soldiers' wounds during the Trojan war.

Yellow Dock

Rumex crispus

A large perennial with small green (or red) flowers. Yellow dock grows in waste areas throughout North America.

PARTS USED

Root.

HEALING PROPERTIES

Actions: bitter, laxative, lymphatic, increases bile flow

Uses: Roots are high in iron and used in iron-deficiency anemia. Also used to help cleanse the body by supporting liver function and eliminating toxins through the bile. It is an especially helpful cleanser in skin diseases, rheumatoid arthritis, swollen lymph glands and constipation.

AVAILABILITY

Roots can be harvested from the wild in September through November. Dried root is available in health/alternative stores.

HOW TO USE IN JUICING

Whole fresh root: Feed through tube along with other ingredients. Use 3- to 4-inch (7.5 to 10 cm) pieces for each 1 cup (250 mL) of juice. Leave peel on if organic.

Powder: Whisk 1 tsp (5 mL) powdered, dried root into 1 cup (250 mL) juice.

Decoction: In a small saucepan, pour 1/4 cup (50 mL) boiling water over 1 tbsp (15 mL) chopped fresh or 1 tsp (5 mL) chopped dried root. Simmer with lid on 10 minutes; steep for 10 minutes. Strain, discard herb, and add liquid to 1 cup (250 mL) juice.

FOLKLORE

The leaf is rubbed on the skin to relieve the pain of nettle sting.

FRUITS

A WORD ABOUT FRUIT

Fruit supplies the body with natural sugar in the form of fructose that it uses for fuel. The sugar also serves to make some vegetable juices more palatable. The fiber in fresh raw fruit makes it an important food to eat whole in addition to juicing.

CAUTION

Diabetics and people prone to yeast infections and hypoglycemia need to watch how much fruit they use because they cause a rapid rise in blood sugar.

Apples

Actions: tonic, digestive, liver stimulant, diuretic, detoxifying, laxative, antiseptic, lowers cholesterol, anti-rheumatic

Uses: Fresh apples help to cleanse the system, lower cholesterol, keep blood glucose levels up, and aid digestion; the French use the peels in preparations for rheumatism and gout and in urinary tract remedies. Used in cleansing fasts, apples are good sources of vitamin A and also contain vitamins C, B and G. Apples are high in two important phytochemicals: pectin which helps to lower both cholesterol and colon cancer; and boron, thought to help prevent the calcium loss that leads to osteoporosis, boost blood levels of the hormone estrogen (thus assisting menopausal women), and which appears to stimulate the electrical activity

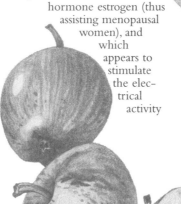

of the brain, increasing the ability to perform tasks quickly and efficiently.

For juicing: Apples are the most versatile fruit for juicing and can be blended with any vegetable juice to give it a natural sweetness. The greener the apple, the sharper its juice. Use the peel (if organic) and core (but not the seeds) when juicing. One pound (500 g), about 4 medium apples, yields about 1 cup (250 mL) juice.

Apricots

Actions: antioxidant, anti-cancer

Uses: Apricots are very high in beta carotene (3 small fresh deliver 2770 IU and 1/2 cup [125 mL] dried contain 8175 IU), the vitamin A precursor which may prevent the formation of plaque deposits in arteries, thus preventing heart disease. Apricots help to normalize blood pressure, heart function and maintain normal body fluid levels. High in potassium, boron, iron, magnesium and fiber with virtually no sodium or fat, fresh or dried apricots are especially recommended for women.

For juicing: Choose firm, fresh, dark yellow to orange apricots. Leave peel on if organic but do not use the pit. Apricot juice blends well with berry juice. One pound (500 g), about 4 apricots, yields about 1 1/2 cups (375 mL) juice.

For pulping: Dried apricots provide extra sweetness to smoothies. Look for sulfate-free dried apricots, especially if allergies exist.

Bananas

Actions: immune booster, lowers cholesterol, anti-ulcer, anti-bacterial

Uses: With their ability to strengthen the surface cells of the stomach lining and protect against acids, bananas are recommended in all cases where ulcers (or the risk of ulcers) is present. High in potassium and vitamin B6, bananas help prevent heart attack, stroke and other heart problems.

For pulping: Often used in fruit smoothies, bananas thicken the mixture and add a fresh fruit flavor. Use one whole banana for every 2 cups (500 mL) of smoothie.

Blackberries

Actions: antioxidant

Uses: An excellent source of vitamin C and fiber and high levels of potassium, iron, calcium and manganese.

For juicing: Use immediately upon picking or purchasing. If necessary, store for 1 day only in the refrigerator. Wash just before using. One pint (2 cups [500 mL]) yields about 3/4 cup (175 mL).

Blackcurrants

Actions: antioxidant, anti-bacterial, immune enhancer, promotes healing, anti-diarrhea, anti-cancer

Uses: Blackcurrant flesh is extremely high in vitamin C (200 mg per 100 g). The skins and outer layers contain anthocyanins, proven to prevent the development of bacteria such as E. coli. Blackcurrants (especially the seeds) are high in gamma linolenic acid (GLA), important for heart health and a number of body functions. For these reasons, whole currants are used in smoothies more often than the extracted juice.

For juicing: Use fresh or frozen red or blackcurrants, including the seeds. The flavor is tart, so blend with other, sweeter juices such as apples, apricots, bananas. Add the pulp to salsas, quick breads, spreads, dips, slaws and fruit pestos. One pint (2 cups [500 mL]) yields about 1/2 cup (125 mL).

For pulping: Use fresh, frozen or dried black or red currants and include the seeds.

Blueberries

Actions: anti-diarrhea, antioxidant, anti-bacterial, antiviral

Uses: Blueberries contain high concentrations of tannins which kill bacteria and viruses, and help prevent or relieve bladder infections. Anthocyanosides protect blood vessels against cholesterol. High in pectin, vitamin C, potassium and natural aspirin, blueberries add extra fiber to smoothies.

For juicing: Use immediately upon picking or purchasing. If necessary, store for 1 day only in the refrigerator. Wash just before using. Flavor can be tart, especially in wild varieties, treat as blackcurrants. To prevent or treat bladder infections, juice at least 1/2 cup (125 mL), add to other ingredients and take daily for a minimum of 3 weeks. One pint (2 cups [500 mL]) yields about 1/2 cup (125 mL).

For pulping: Add 1/4 to 1/2 cup (50 to 125 mL) to smoothies for extra healing benefits.

Cantaloupe

See Melons.

Cherries

Actions: anti-bacterial, antioxidant, anti-cancer

Uses: Cherries are high in ellagic acid, a potent anti-cancer agent, along with vitamins C and A, biotin and potassium. Black cherry juice protects against tooth decay.

For juicing: Do *not* use the seeds One pound (2 cups [500 mL]) yields about 2/3 cup (150 mL).

Citrus Fruits

Oranges, lemons, limes, grapefruit, tangerines

Actions: antioxidant, anti-cancer

Uses: All citrus fruits are high in vitamin C and limonene, thought to inhibit breast cancer. Red grapefruit is high in cancer-fighting lycopene. Oranges are a good source of choline, which improves mental functioning. The combination of carotenoids, flavonoids, terpenes, limonoids and coumarins make citrus fruit a total cancer-fighting package.

For juicing: Remove the peel as it contains bitter elements, but leave as much of the white pith surrounding the sections as possible. The pith contains pectin and bioflavonoids which help the body to absorb vitamin C and are powerful antioxidants, and they strengthen the body's capillaries, assisting circulation and enhancing the skin. If you have a centrifugal extractor, use the seeds; they contain limonoids (protect against cancer), calcium, magnesium and potassium.

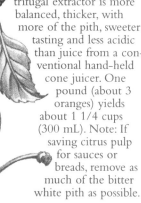

Citrus juice from a centrifugal extractor is more balanced, thicker, with more of the pith, sweeter tasting and less acidic than juice from a conventional hand-held cone juicer. One pound (about 3 oranges) yields about 1 1/4 cups (300 mL). Note: If saving citrus pulp for sauces or breads, remove as much of the bitter white pith as possible.

Cranberries

Actions: anti-bacterial, anti-viral, antioxidant, anti-cancer

Uses:
Extremely useful in urinary and bladder infections, cranberry works in the same way as elderberry to prevent the hooks on the bacteria from attaching to, in this case, the cells of the bladder or urinary tract, rendering them ineffective in causing infection. Best used as a first step in preventing urinary tract and bladder infection, cranberry juice does not take the place of antibiotic drugs which are more effective in eliminating bacteria once an infection has taken hold. High in vitamins C and A, iodine and calcium, cranberries also prevent kidney stones and deodorize the urine.

For juicing: Fresh cranberry juice is much more effective than the commercial variety, which has a high sugar content. In season during the fall, cranberries freeze very well and can be added frozen to smoothies or juiced without thawing. Wash just before using. Flavor is tart, so blend with sweeter juices such as apples, pineapple, apricots, grapes. To prevent or treat bladder infections, juice at least 1/2 cup (125 mL), blend with other juices as desired, and take every day for a minimum of 3 weeks. One pound yields about 3/4 cup (175 mL).

For pulping: Because their flavor is so tart, you may wish to cook cranberries with sugar, honey or stevia and a small amount of water or juice (see **Cranberry Juice,** page 118) before combining with other fruit (such as apples or oranges) and blending for smoothies.

Crenshaw Melon

See Melons.

Figs

Actions: anti-bacterial, anti-cancer, digestive, demulcent, laxative

Uses: The benzaldehyde in figs is an active, cancer-fighting agent. Figs are also high in potassium and naturally sweet.

For juicing: Figs have a low water content and do not juice well.

For pulping: Fresh figs can be found in some supermarkets and most Middle Eastern food markets in summer and early fall. Choose soft, plump figs, remove skin and blend the flesh and seeds.

Use dried or fresh figs or **Fig Milk** (page 216) to sweeten and thicken smoothies.

Grapefruit

See Citrus Fruits.

Grapes

Actions: antioxidant, anti-viral, anti-cancer

Uses: Grapes contain ellagic and caffeic acids, which deactivate carcinogens. Flavonoids in grape juice have heart-protective effects. Grapes are a good source of potassium. Resveratrol, found in red wine and red grape juice, has a protective effect on the cardiovascular system; boron, which helps maintain estrogen levels, may be instrumental in preventing osteoporosis.

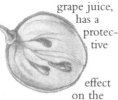

For juicing: Common varieties for juicing include Thompson seedless, concord, red and green seedless grapes. Wash thoroughly and juice whole with skin and seeds intact. Two cups (500 mL) yields about 3/4 cup (175 mL).

For pulping: Use fresh, seedless grapes or raisins in smoothies and blended drinks.

Honeydew Melon

See Melons.

Kiwi

Actions: antioxidant, anti-cancer, aids digestion

Uses: Often used as part of a cleansing regimen or to aid digestion. High in vitamins C and E (one of few fruit to contain vitamin E), which act as antioxidants, protecting cells from damage. Kiwis are also high in potassium and contain some calcium.

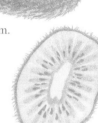

For juicing: Choose ripe fruit that yield to gentle pressure. Peel and feed flesh and seeds through juicer. One pound (about 4 kiwis) yields about 1/3 cup (75 mL).

Lemons

See Citrus Fruits.

Limes

See Citrus Fruits.

Mangoes

Actions: antioxidant, anti-cancer

Uses: Mangoes are high in vitamins A (8000 IU of beta carotene) and C, potassium, niacin, and fiber. They help protect against cancer and atherosclerosis, maintain bowel regularity and assist the body in fighting infection.

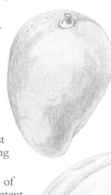

For juicing: Because of their low water content, mangoes do not juice well.

For pulping: Choose large, firm unblemished fruit, yellow to yellow-red in color. Remove peel before using: handle carefully since its sap can irritate the skin.

Melons

Cantaloupe, honeydew, crenshaw, Spanish, musk

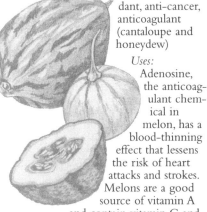

Actions: antioxidant, anti-cancer, anticoagulant (cantaloupe and honeydew)

Uses: Adenosine, the anticoagulant chemical in melon, has a blood-thinning effect that lessens the risk of heart attacks and strokes. Melons are a good source of vitamin A and contain vitamin C and calcium. Melons help reduce the risk of cancer.

For juicing: Choose ripe melons. Peel, cut into chunks, and juice with the seeds. 2 cups (500 mL) melon chunks yields about 2/3 cup (150 mL) juice.

Musk Melon

See Melons

Nectarines

Actions: antioxidant, anti-cancer

Uses: A good source of vitamins A, C, and potassium, nectarines are an original ancient fruit, not a cross between a peach and a plum.

For juicing: Choose fruit that are smooth and tight without soft patches. Cut in half, remove pit, and juice with skin on. Nectarines are sweeter than peaches and can replace them in juicing recipes.

One pound (about 3 nectarines) yields about 1 cup (250 mL) juice.

Oranges

See Citrus Fruits

Papaya

Actions: antioxidant, anti-cancer, aids digestion

Uses: Papaya are high in vitamins A, C and potassium.

For juicing: Because of their low water content, papayas do not juice well.

For pulping: Choose yellow fruit that yields to gentle pressure. Peel, avoiding too much contact with the skin, and cut into pieces. Papayas blend well with other fruits in drinks and serve as a sweet addition that gives a creamy texture to smoothies. Use the seeds, since they contain protein.

Peaches

Actions: antioxidant, anti-cancer

Uses: Rich in vitamin A and potassium, peaches also contain niacin and some iron and vitamin C. Peaches help protect against cancer and heart disease.

For juicing: Choose firm, full-colored fruit that yields to gentle pressure. Cut in half, remove and discard pit and juice with the skin. One pound (about 4 peaches) yields about 2/3 cup (150 mL).

Pears

Actions: protects colon

Uses: Perhaps one of the oldest cultivated fruits, pears are a good source of vitamin C and potassium. Pears are also a sweet source of fiber.

For juicing: Use varieties such as Bartlett, Comice, Seckel and Bosc. Choose firm unblemished pears and juice the whole fruit. One pound (about 3 pears) yields about 1/2 cup (125 mL) juice.

Pineapple

Actions: aids digestion

Uses: A good source of potassium, with some vitamin C and iron, pineapples add a fresh, sweet taste to juices.

For juicing: Heaviness in ripe pineapples indicates juiciness. Choose large, firm fruits. Cut off leaves and rind. Use flesh and core in juices and smoothies. One pound (about 1/3 medium pineapple) yields about 1/2 cup (125 mL) juice.

Plums

Actions: anti-bacterial, antioxidant

Uses: A good source of vitamin A, plums also contain calcium and a small amount of vitamin C.

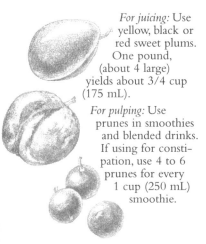

For juicing: Use yellow, black or red sweet plums. One pound, (about 4 large) yields about 3/4 cup (175 mL).

For pulping: Use prunes in smoothies and blended drinks. If using for constipation, use 4 to 6 prunes for every 1 cup (250 mL) smoothie.

Raspberries

Actions: immunity enhancer

Uses: Fruit is rich in potassium and niacin and also contains iron and some vitamin C. (See also Red Raspberry Leaf, pages 36 and 37.)

For juicing: Do not store long. Wash just before juicing. Raspberries blend with other berries in juices and the taste is enhanced with a small amount of citrus juice. One pint (2 cups [500 mL]) yields about 1/2 cup (125 mL) juice.

Rhubarb

Actions: laxative

Uses: Although almost always used as a fruit, rhubarb is actually a vegetable. It is high in potassium and contains a fair amount of iron. The calcium in 1 cup (250 mL) cooked rhubarb is twice that of milk.

For juicing: Use stalks and root, *but not the leaves,* which contain toxic concentrations of oxalic acid. Rhubarb can be juiced

fresh or frozen. To soften its tartness, combine rhubarb with sweeter fruits or juices.

For pulping: Blend chunks with sweeter fruits, or stew it with maple sugar, honey, stevia or sugar, and then use with other fresh fruit in smoothies.

Spanish Melon

See Melons.

Strawberries

Actions: antioxidant, anti-viral, anti-cancer

Uses: Effective against kidney stones, gout, rheumatism and arthritis, strawberries are used in cleansing juices and as a mild tonic for the liver. Strawberries are high in cancer-fighting ellagic acid and vitamin C. They are also a good source of vitamin A and potassium, and contain iron. Both the leaves and the fruit have been used medicinally. A tea from strawberry leaves is used for diarrhea and dysentery.

For juicing: Pick your own or buy brightly colored, firm berries with hulls attached. Do not store long. Wash just before juicing. Strawberries add a sweet and powerful flavor to juices. They are best blended with only one or two other fruits, although they blend well with other berries in juices. The taste is enhanced with a small amount of citrus juice. One pint (2 cups [500 mL]) yields about 1/2 cup (125 mL) juice.

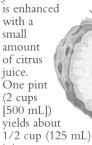

For pulping: Strawberries blend well with banana and other fruit in blended drinks. The traditional smoothie combination includes strawberry, banana and orange juice.

Watermelon

Actions: anti-bacterial, anti-cancer

Uses: Watermelon contains vitamins C and A, iron and potassium.

For juicing: Peel the rind. Use flesh and seeds which contain protein, zinc, vitamin E and essential fatty acids. Watermelon is a refreshing summer juice on its own or blended with other fruits as a thirst quencher. Two cups (500 mL) chunked watermelon yields about 1 cup (250 mL) juice.

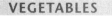

VEGETABLES

Asparagus

Actions: antioxidant, anti-cancer, anti-cataracts, diuretic, promotes healing

Uses: Asparagus is one of only four vegetables high in vitamin E. It is also a source of vitamins C and A, as well as potassium, niacin and some iron.

For juicing: Wash spears (no need to trim them) and feed through tube stalk end first. One pound of asparagus yields about 3/4 cup (175 mL) juice.

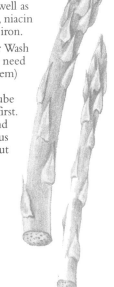

Avocados

Actions: antioxidant

Uses: Avocados contain more potassium than many other fruits and vegetables. While high in essential fatty acids, they contain 17 vitamins and minerals including vitamins A, C, B and E, riboflavin, iron, calcium, copper, phosphorus, zinc, niacin and magnesium as well as more protein than any other fruit. One avocado added to blended drinks adds a creamy texture and exceptional nutrients.

For juicing: Avocados contain little water and do not juice well.

For pulping: Peel and cut in half. Remove pit and cut flesh into pieces. Blend with other fruits or vegetables. Brush with lemon juice to keep flesh from turning brown.

Beans

Green, yellow wax, Italian, snap and string beans; also green peas, snow peas

Actions: helps memory, antioxidant

Uses: Fresh beans and peas are the same botanically as dried beans (also known as legumes or pulses), since they all produce their seeds in pods. A good source of choline, which improves mental functioning, beans contain vitamin A and potassium, along with some protein, iron, calcium and vitamins B and C.

For juicing: Because of their low water content, peas do not juice well.

For pulping: Raw or blanched green peas thicken blended drinks. Wash, shell and add to other fruits or vegetables in the blender in 1/4-cup (50 mL) amounts.

Beets

Actions: anti-bacterial, antioxidant, tonic, cleansing, laxative

Uses: Beet tops (greens) are high in vitamin A and for this reason should always be juiced along with the roots. Beet tops should be used immediately, although the roots can be stored in a cool dark place for up to 2 weeks. Beet roots are high in vitamin A and betaine, an enzyme that nourishes and strengthens the liver and gall bladder. Beets are also an excellent source of potassium. With 8% chlorine, beets are cleansing for the liver, kidney and gall bladder.

For juicing: Scrub roots and, leaving skin on, cut into pieces. Feed tops through juicer by tapping. One pound (2 medium beets with greens) yields about 1 cup (250 mL) juice.

Broccoli

Actions: antioxidant, anti-cancer, anti-cataracts, promotes healing

Uses: Broccoli is one of only four vegetables high in vitamin E. It is also high in cancer-fighting indoles, glucosinolates and dithiolthiones. It has a fair amount of vitamins A, B and C.

For juicing: Use thick stalks and leaves as well as tops. Wash and cut into pieces.

Brussels Sprouts

See Cabbage.

Cabbage

Green, red, savoy, bok choy and Chinese cabbage; also kohlrabi and Brussels sprouts

Actions: immune building, anti-bacterial, anti-cancer, helps memory, antioxidant, promotes healing, anti-cataracts, detoxifying, diuretic, anti-inflammatory, tonic, antiseptic, restorative, anti-ulcer

Uses: High in cancer-fighting endoles and a good source of choline, which improves mental functioning, cabbage is one of only four vegetables high in vitamin E. An excellent remedy for anemia, cabbage has also been used as a nutritive tonic to restore strength during convalescence. Of benefit to the liver, cabbage is also effective in preventing colon cancer and may be of help to diabetics by reducing blood sugar. Cabbage juice is especially effective in preventing and healing ulcers.

For juicing: Wash and cut into chunks, leaving dark green outer leaves on and core intact. Juice Brussels sprouts whole. One pound cabbage (about 1/3 head) yields about 1 cup (250 mL) juice.

Carrots

Actions: antioxidant, anti-cancer, artery-protecting, expectorant, antiseptic, diuretic, immune boosting, anti-bacterial, lowers blood cholesterol, prevents constipation

Uses: Carrots are extremely nutritious and rich in vitamins A, B and C, iron, calcium, potassium and sodium. They have a cleansing effect on the liver and digestive system, help counter the formation of kidney stones and relieve arthritis and gout. Their antioxidant properties from carotenoids (including beta carotene) have been shown to cut cancer risk, protect against arterial and heart disease, and lower blood cholesterol. Carrots enhance mental functioning and decrease the risk of cataracts and macular degeneration.

For juicing: Carrots are the sweetest most versatile vegetable, and can be used in almost any juicing recipe. The deeper the color, the higher the concentration of carotene. Do not use carrot greens for juicing. One pound (about 6 medium) yields approximately 1 cup (250 mL) or more juice.

For pulping: Cooking frees up carotenes (precursors to vitamin A), the anti-cancer agents in carrots. Steam or simmer carrots just until tender, then add to the blender with other fruits or vegetables.

Cauliflower

Actions: antioxidant, anti-cancer

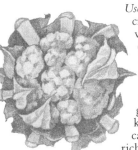

Uses: Like all cruciferous vegetables (cabbage, Brussels sprouts, broccoli, collard greens, kohlrabi), cauliflower is rich in endoles, the cancer preventative chemicals. Contains vitamin C and potassium and some protein and iron.

For juicing: Wash, cut into pieces leaving core and leaves intact. One pound flowerets yields approximately 1 cup (250 mL) juice.

Celery

Actions: anti-bacterial

Uses: Adding celery to vegetable cocktails adds a natural saltiness. Celeriac is also known as celery, the root of a different variety of celery than that used to produce stalks. It adds a stronger celery flavor to juices.

For juicing: Use stalks and leaves. One stalk yields about 1/4 cup (50 mL) juice. Scrub and cut celeriac into pieces.

Celeriac

See Celery.

Chile Peppers

Actions: stimulant, tonic, diaphoretic, rubefacient, antiseptic, anti-bacterial, expectorant, anti-bronchitis, anti-emphysema, decongestant, blood thinner, carminative

Uses: Chiles such as cayenne, jalapeno, ancho/poblano, habanero, morasol, serrano and pasilla (to name only a few), contain the active element capsaicin. High in vitamin A and with some vitamin C, calcium, iron, magnesium, phosphorus and potassium, chili peppers offer important nutrients, along with their characteristic heat, to vegetable juice drinks. Chile peppers help people with bronchitis (and related problems) by irritating the bronchial tubes and sinuses, causing the secretion of fluid that thins the constricting mucus and helps move it out of the body. Capsaicin blocks the pain message from the brain making it an effective painkiller. It also has clot-dissolving properties that make it useful if taken on a consistent basis. *See also* Cayenne, page 21 and types, page 136.

For juicing: Wash peppers and remove stems. Wash hands thoroughly after handling, since capsaicin will irritate skin and is very painful if it contacts the eyes, lips or nasal passages. When first using chile peppers for juicing, juice after all other ingredients have been put through the machine and keep the juice separate. Add it to vegetable juice blends 1 tsp (5 mL) at a time until you reach the level of heat with which you are comfortable. Alternatively, whisk in a drop of hot or jerk sauce (or 1/4 tsp [1 mL] powdered cayenne) to juices and blended drinks.

Collard Greens

See Leafy Greens.

Cucumber

Actions: diuretic

Uses: A moderate source of vitamin A, iron and potassium, cucumber has a very high water content, which makes it a particularly good vegetable for juicing. Shown to contain sterols, which may help the heart by reducing cholesterol.

For juicing: Peel if skin has been waxed. Cut into cubes and leave seeds intact. One pound (about 1 large) yields approximately 1 1/4 cups (300 mL) juice.

Fennel

Actions: antioxidant, seeds are digestive

Uses: A bulb-like vegetable similar to celery, but with a distinctly sweet anise flavor. A good source of vitamin A.

For juicing: Use the leaves if attached to the stalks. Use only one quarter of the bulb (or less) per serving of juice; larger amounts will make the flavor overpowering.

Garlic

See page 26.

Jerusalem Artichoke

Actions: anti-bacterial

Uses: Jerusalem artichokes are the tuberous roots of a plant related to the sunflower (which is why they are often sold as "sunchokes.") Their sweet, nutty flavor blends well in juices. Diabetics easily digest the inulin, a type of carbohydrate found in Jerusalem artichokes. They are also a source of calcium, iron and magnesium.

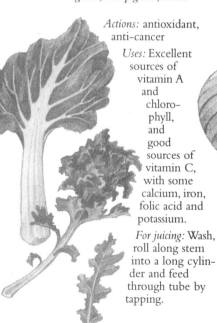

For juicing: Scrub well and cut larger tubers in half. One cup (250 mL) tubers yields about 1/2 cup (125 mL) juice.

Kale

See Leafy Greens.

Kohlrabi

See Cabbage.

Leafy Greens

Kale, Swiss chard, collard greens, mustard greens, turnip greens, lettuce

Actions: antioxidant, anti-cancer

Uses: Excellent sources of vitamin A and chlorophyll, and good sources of vitamin C, with some calcium, iron, folic acid and potassium.

For juicing: Wash, roll along stem into a long cylinder and feed through tube by tapping.

Leeks

Actions: expectorant, diuretic, relaxant, laxative, antiseptic, digestive, hypotensive

Uses: Easily digested, leeks are used in tonics, especially during convalescence from illness. With their warming, expectorant and stimulating qualities, they are blended in toddies for relief from sore throats

For juicing: Leave roots and dark green leaves on, split and wash inner layers well. Feed through tube, one half at a time. Use one half to one leek per serving.

Lettuce

See Leafy Greens.

Mustard Greens

See Leafy Greens.

Onion

Actions: anti-bacterial, anti-cancer, antioxidant, circulatory and digestive stimulant, antiseptic, detoxifying, lowers cholesterol, hypotensive, hypoglycemic, diuretic, heart protective

Uses: Onions help prevent thrombosis, reduce high blood pressure, lower blood sugar, prevent inflammatory responses and inhibit the growth of cancer cells. Shallots, yellow and red onions are the richest dietary source of quercetin, a potent antioxidant and cancer-inhibiting phytochemical.

For juicing: Leave skin on. Cut to fit feed tube. Blend with other juices. One medium onion yields approximately 3 tbsp (45 mL) juice.

Parsnip

Actions: anti-inflammatory, anti-cancer

Uses: Best used fresh, after frost has concentrated the carbohydrate into sugar, making them sweeter for juicing. A good source of vitamin C and E, as well as potassium, with some protein, iron and calcium. Like other root vegetables, parsnips store well and are an excellent winter juicing vegetable.

For juicing: Choose firm, small parsnips. Juice with both ends intact. One pound (500 g), yields approximately 1 cup (250 mL) juice.

Peas

See Beans.

Pepper

Bell or sweet pepper: green, red and yellow

Actions: antioxidant, anti-cancer, heart protective

Uses: High in vitamins C and A and (with some potassium), green, yellow and red peppers make a good addition to vegetable cocktails and blended drinks.

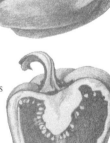

For juicing: Choose thick, fleshy, smooth-skinned peppers. Wash before using. Discard stem, but use seeds. One pound (500 g), yields about 1 1/2 cups (375 mL) juice.

Radish

Red, white and Japanese daikon

Uses: A good source of potassium and iron, radishes lend a pleasantly hot taste to juices.

For juicing: Scrub, leaving root and stem on, but discarding leaves.

Spinach

Actions: anti-cancer, helps memory, antioxidant, anti-cataracts, anti-anemia, promotes healing

Uses: A good source of choline (which improves mental functioning) and folic acid (a heart protector), spinach is one of only four vegetables high in vitamin E. It is also high in cancer-fighting lutein, chlorophyll and vitamins C and A, and is good source of calcium, iron, protein and potassium.

For juicing: Wash well. Roll into a long cylinder along stem and feed through tube by tapping.

Squash

Acorn, butternut, Hubbard, pumpkin, turban

Actions: antioxidant, anti-cancer

Uses: The juice is thick and the yield is not as high as other vegetables, but squash still makes a good winter juicing vegetable.

For juicing: Scrub and remove stem. Use skin (if not too thick or waxed) and juice with seeds (high in cancer-fighting chemicals). One pound (500 g), about half a medium squash, yields about 1/2 cup (125 mL) juice.

Swiss Chard

See Leafy Greens.

Tomato

Actions: antioxidant, anti-cancer

Uses: High in lycopene and glutathione (both powerful antioxidants), raw tomatoes reduce the risk of many cancers. Lycopene is also thought to help maintain mental and physical functioning; it is absorbed by the body more efficiently when tomatoes are juiced. Tomatoes also contain glutamic acid, which is metabolized by the body into gamma-amino butyric acid (GABA), a calming agent, known to be effective for kidney hypertension. Drink tomato juice to relax after a stressful day.

For juicing: Wash. Discard stem and leaves. Use skin and seeds. Twelve ounces (375 g), about 3 small tomatoes, yields 1 cup (250 mL) or more juice.

Turnip

Actions: tonic, decongestant, antibacterial, anti-cancer, diuretic

Uses: Turnip has a beneficial effect on the urinary system, purifies the blood and aids in the elimination of toxins. For this reason, it makes a good addition to cleansing juices. Both the root and the green tops are high in glucosinolates, which are thought to block the development of cancer. Turnips are a good source of calcium, iron and protein.

For juicing: Choose fresh turnips with tops intact. Remove tops; wash, scrub bulbs, cut in half and juice alternately with tops.

Watercress

Actions: antioxidant, diuretic, anti-cancer, tonic, antibiotic, cleansing

Uses: A good source of vitamins C and A, watercress can be found in areas near creeks and streams.

For juicing: Wash well and feed through tube alternately with other vegetables. Watercress adds a bite to juice drinks.

Zucchini

Italian, yellow straightneck, yellow crookneck

Actions: antioxidant

Uses: A good source of vitamins A and C, potassium and niacin, zucchini produce a mild-tasting juice that blends well with stronger-flavored vegetable juices.

For juicing: Choose small, firm zucchini. Scrub well, leaving skin and blossom end on. Ten ounces (300 g), about 1 medium zucchini, yields about 1 cup (250 mL) juice.

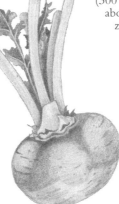

OTHER INGREDIENTS

Blackstrap Molasses

Molasses is a thick syrup by-product of sugar refining, in which the sucrose (sugar) is separated from the liquid and nutrients in the raw cane plant. Several grades of molasses are available. Blackstrap molasses has the least sugar and the most nutrients — iron, 6 of the B vitamins, calcium, phosphorous and potassium.

For juicing: Molasses has a strong flavor, so use sparingly, about 1 to 2 tsp (5 to 10 mL) per 1 cup (250 mL), in juices that require additional sweetening.

Carob

Made from powdered carob beans, carob makes a good substitute for cocoa and chocolate because it has no caffeine, does not need extra sugar, is lower in fat, and provides some calcium and phosphorus. Available in baking chips (used in hot drinks) and in powdered form, which is blended into smoothies and coffee substitutes.

For juicing: To add sweetness to juices; whisk up to 1 tbsp (15 mL) carob into 1 cup (250 mL) juice.

For pulping: Add up to 2 tbsp (25 mL) carob to ingredients before blending.

Cider Vinegar

Juice extracted from certified organic apples and naturally fermented (without heat or the addition of clarifiers, enzymes or preservatives) yields a natural vinegar that contains some pectin, trace minerals and beneficial bacteria and enzymes.

For juicing: For overall health, add 1 tsp (5 mL) natural apple cider vinegar to juice.

Flax Seeds

Flaxseed oil is the best vegetable source for omega-3 fatty acids, which help lubricate the joints and prevent absorption of toxins by stimulating digestion.

For juicing: Whisk in 1 tbsp (15 mL) flaxseed oil for up to 2 cups (500 mL) juice.

For pulping: Add 1 tbsp (15 mL) whole flax seeds to other ingredients before blending.

Grains
Oats, wheat, rye, buckwheat, spelt, amaranth, quinoa

Whole grains are unrefined and therefore they retain all the nutritional value of the bran and germ. They also add fiber and complex carbohydrates to the diet. In all, whole grains offer protein, carbohydrates, phytate, vitamin E, fiber (including lignins), and some B vitamins (thiamin, riboflavin, niacin, folacin), iron, zinc and magnesium.

Actions: anti-cancer, antioxidant, fight heart disease, anti-obesity, lower blood sugar levels

For pulping: Add 2 to 3 tbsp (25 to 45 mL) whole grain flakes to 1 cup (250 mL) blended drinks and milk shakes. Add to roots and nuts for roasted coffee-substitute blends.

Grasses
Wheat, barley

Wheat and barley grass is grown from the seeds (or "berries") of the wheat or barley plant. Harvested when 5 to 6 inches (12.5 to 15 cm) high, the grass is then eaten or juiced fresh or dried and used in powdered form or pressed into pills. High in chlorophyll (a powerful healing agent and infection fighter), beta carotene and vitamins C and E, these green foods are easily added to juices and blended drinks. They are also one of the best plant sources of protein, even better than soy and legumes.

Actions: antioxidant, anti-inflammatory, anti-cancer, antibiotic, blood cleanser, protects against radiation

For juicing: Fresh wheat and barley grasses require a special juicer or attachment to extract their liquid. They have a strong flavor, so mix with water or vegetable juice, not fruit juices. Whisk 1 tbsp (15 mL) powdered wheat or barley grass with 1 to 2 cups (250 to 500 mL) vegetable juice or blended drinks.

CAUTION

Start with small amounts (no more than 2 tbsp [25 mL]) wheatgrass juice daily. Large amounts may cause diarrhea and nausea.

Green Algae
Chlorella, spirulina

Rich in carotenoids and chlorophyll, these microscopic single-celled plants have been shown to be effective in reducing the effects of radiation and may be helpful in cases of HIV infection. Available in capsule or bulk powder.

Actions: Reduces heavy-metal toxicity. Also anti-cancer, immune boosting, lowers blood pressure, antioxidant

For juicing: Add 2 tsp (10 mL) to juice and blended drinks.

Hemp

Hemp seed is high in protein and contains about 30% oil that is high in essential fatty acids — omega-3 and omega-6, as well as GLA. Hempnut, the dehulled seed of the hemp plant, can be used in nut butters, baked products, dips and spreads, as well as incorporated into blended drinks.

For pulping: Add 2 to 3 tbsp (25 to 45 mL) hempnut to blended drinks.

Honey

The sweetness valued of honey is approximately equal to that of invert sugar. The difference is that honey contains small amounts of B vitamins, calcium, iron, zinc, potassium and phosphorous, and has the ability to act as a potent killer of bacteria. Generally, the darker the honey, the higher it is in antioxidants. *See also* page 172.

Actions: antioxidant, anti-bacterial, antimicrobial, calms nerves, anti-diarrhea

For juicing: Use honey as a sweetener for bitter vegetable juices or add to hot toddies and cold remedies to soothe sore throats.

CAUTION

The National Honey Board, along with other health organizations, recommends that honey not be fed to infants under one year of age.

HONEY-RELATED PRODUCTS

Bee pollen is the male seeds of flower blossoms which collect on the legs of the bees as they work. The bees clean it off, mix it with nectar and their own enzymes. It contains proteins, vitamins A, B, C and E, calcium, magnesium, selenium, nucleic acids and lecithin and may be added to blended drinks. Use 1 tbsp (15 mL) bee pollen for up to 2 cups (500 mL) smoothie.

Propolis is a sticky resinous substance collected from coniferous trees, is supportive of the immune system and is used as a tonic. Propolis can be added to blended drinks, 1 tsp (5 mL) for each 1 cup (250 mL) juice or smoothie.

Royal jelly is the milky product fed exclusively to the queen bee. It is known to be rich in the B complex vitamins, as well as vitamins A, C, D and E. Refrigerate fresh royal jelly or purchase freeze-dried for use in juices and blended drinks. Add 1 tbsp (15 mL) royal jelly for up to 2 cups (500 mL) juice or smoothie.

Maple Syrup

The sap from sugar maples *(Acer saccharum)*, red maples *(A. rubrum)* and silver maples *(A. saccharinum)* is collected in the spring when it is flowing from the roots back into the aerial parts of the tree to provide energy for growth. Because the sap is 95 to 97% water, it must be boiled to evaporate the water, leaving a thick, sweet syrup which is composed of 65% sucrose (sugar) with the remaining components being organic acids, minerals (mainly potassium and calcium), and traces of amino compounds and vitamins. One quarter cup (50 mL) maple syrup provides 6% of the recommended daily intake of calcium and thiamin and 2% of magnesium and riboflavin.

For juicing: Stir 1 to 2 tbsp (15 to 25 mL) pure maple syrup (avoid "maple-flavored" syrup, which is primarily corn syrup with artificial flavor) into 1 to 2 cups (250 to 500 mL) juice if a sweetener is required.

Nuts

All nuts are rich in protein, vitamin E, fiber and protease inhibitors, known to block cancer in animal tests. They are also extremely high in fat, but the oil is polyunsaturated and, as such, reduces blood cholesterol. Nuts contain essential fatty acids, which are essential for healthy skin, hair, glands, mucus membranes, nerves, and arteries, as well as being help-ful in preventing cardiovascular disease. Nuts allow a slow steady rise in blood sugar and insulin, making them good foods for diabetics.

Actions: anti-cancer, anti-cholesterol, regulate blood sugar

For juicing: Use ground nuts as a garnish for juices.

For pulping: Add up to 1/4 cup (50 mL) whole nuts or **Nut Milk** (see pages 214 to 215) for blending with other ingredients in smoothies and blended drinks.

CAUTION

Nuts can cause extreme allergic reactions in some people. Also, peanuts and peanut butter may be contaminated by aflatoxin mold, a carcinogen.

Protein Powder

The isoflavones in soy protein (the protein extracted from soybeans) are believed to help reduce the risk of cancers of the breast, endometrium and prostate. Isoflavones also mimic the action of estrogen (thus reducing the symptoms of menopause) and have favorable affects on bone density. Research has shown that soy protein reduces cholesterol levels. Choose raw soy protein powder made from soybeans that are water washed (not in alcohol), organically grown and specifically tested for high isoflavone content.

For pulping: Add up to 3 tbsp (45 mL) to ingredients before blending.

CAUTION

There is growing concern over the prolonged us of soy (see Soy Products, page 54).

Psyllium Seeds

Psyllium seeds act by adding bulk to the stool, causing it to press against the bowel wall, triggering the contractions that lead to a bowel movement. To avoid psyllium seeds causing bowel obstruction, be sure to drink at least 8 glasses of water a day. A diet high in whole fresh fruit and vegetables generally makes it unnecessary to take psylllium seeds.

Dose: Take 1 to 3 tsp (5 to 15 mL) seeds mixed in a little water, followed by a full glass of water, first thing in the morning. Drink another 8 glasses of water throughout the day. Repeat daily for up to 1 week.

CAUTION

Psyllium can cause an allergic reaction in sensitive individuals; discontinue immediately if a reaction develops. It should be avoided by asthmatics. Psyllium must not be taken in cases of bowel obstruction.

Pumpkin Seeds

Pumpkin seeds are beneficial to men because they contain high concentrations of certain amino acids that can reduce the symptoms of prostate enlargement.

For pulping: Add 2 tbsp (25 mL) fresh hulled pumpkin seeds to ingredients for blending.

Ready-to-use Juices

Juice from fresh raw fruits, vegetables and herbs is the best source of nutrients and live energy. Canned or bottled juices have been processed at high heat and may contain added ingredients such as sugar, artificial flavorings, stabilizers, thickeners/thinners, and chemical preservatives. Should you wish to blend ready-to-use juices with fresh juice, choose pure juice with no sugar or additives.

Sea Herbs

Arame, dulse, hijiki, nori, wakame, kelp

Their high concentrations of vitamin A, protein, calcium, iron and other minerals make sea herbs important to overall health. Dried sea herbs are covered in hot water and allowed to soak for 10 to 20 minutes before being used in recipes.

Actions: anti-cancer, diuretic, boosts immune functioning, anti-bacterial

For juicing: Add the soaking water from sea herbs to fresh juices; the salty taste blends well in vegetable juices. Sprinkle powdered or finely cut sea herbs over juice as a garnish.

For pulping: Add 1/4 to 1/2 cup (50 to 125 mL) soaked, simmered sea herbs to other ingredients for smoothies or blended drinks.

Sesame Seeds

A good source of incomplete protein, sesame seeds lend a light nutty taste to juices and blended drinks. Sesame seed oil is exceptionally stable and is a source of vitamin E and co-Q10, an essential coenzyme for metabolism.

Actions: emollient, laxative, antioxidant

For juicing: Sprinkle seeds over juices as a garnish or whisk 1 tsp (5 mL) sesame oil into juices.

For pulping: Add 1 tbsp (15 mL) to other ingredients for blending.

Soy Products

Soybeans are the only known plant source of "complete protein." In other words, they contain all of the necessary amino acids (in the appropriate proportions) essential for cell growth and maintenance. The isoflavones in soy were recently thought to prevent cancers of the prostate, breast, uterus, lungs, colon, stomach, liver, pancreas, bladder and skin. However, new studies have shown conflicting results.

Actions: may be anti-cancer, anticholesterol, immunity boosting

Note: Given the widespread use of genetically modified beans as well as chemicals, pesticides and fertilizers in growing soybeans it is wise to buy fresh or dried beans and soy products from certified organic sources.

Soybeans are available in a whole, raw, dried state and must be reconstituted in the same way as other legumes are soaked and then cooked. After cooking, add 1/2 cup (125 mL) to other ingredients for blending in smoothies.

Tofu, also called "bean curd" or "soy cheese", is easily added to blended drinks. It thickens and smooths the taste. Use the soft variety for drinks. Do not use daily.

Tempeh is a mild, firm white cake made from fermenting cooked soybeans. Usually frozen, 1/4 cup (50 mL) crumbled tempeh may be added to other ingredients for blended drinks. Do not use daily.

Sprouts

High in vitamins B and C, iron, bioflavonoids, and enzymes, sprouts add a green, living, nutritional boost to juices and blended drinks. Alfalfa and bean seeds, grains and herb seeds are easy to grow, sprout well and offer a concentrated blast of the nutrients found in the mature plants.

For juicing: Feed through tube interspersed with firm fruit or vegetables.

For pulping: Add up to 1 cup (250 mL) to blended drinks.

Sunflower Seeds

A good source of vitamin E and zinc, sunflower seeds can be added to other ingredients before blending into smoothies. Use 2 tbsp (25 mL) for up to 2 cups (500 mL) blended drinks.

Tofu

See Soy Products.

Wheat germ

A good source of vitamin E and thiamine, wheat germ can be sprinkled over fresh juices or added to the ingredients before blending into smoothies. Use 2 tbsp (25 mL) for up to 2 cups (500 mL) blended drinks.

Wheat grass

See Grasses.

Yogurt

Yogurt is produced from fermented milk. A beneficial type of bacteria (called lactobacilli) in yogurt restores and maintains a normal microbial balance in the intestinal tract. The acidophilus culture in yogurt helps protect against colon cancer. When buying, check the label to ensure that it "contains active cultures." Yogurt is usually safe for people with milk allergies and is essential to a vegetarian diet.

Actions: anti-bacterial, anti-cancer, anti-ulcer, immune building, lowers blood cholesterol

For juicing: Add up to 1 cup (250 mL) yogurt in blended drinks and stir up to 1/4 cup (50 mL) into fruit or vegetable juices.

To Your Health

Health Conditions

The combined wisdom of common sense, human observation and scientific study all point to the importance of our diet in preventing and controlling disease. General dietary principles are set out in the Guidelines to Good Health (see chart, pages 10 to 11). In this section, we provide recommendations for specific health conditions.

These recommendations are not intended to take the place of consultation with a medical practitioner. For best results, and especially if faced with a serious condition, contact a doctor, medical herbalist or natural health specialist, who can provide you with a diet and lifestyle program suited to your needs. For each condition, the best fruits, vegetables, herbs and other foods are recommended. See the Ingredients section (pages 43 to 54) for information on other ingredients that can be used.

AGING

HEALING FOODS

Fruits and vegetables: apples, blueberries, figs, grapefruit, grapes, melons, oranges, papaya, pears, raspberries, strawberries, beets, broccoli, cabbage, carrots, celery, leafy greens, onions, pumpkin, sweet potatoes, tomatoes

Herbs: cayenne, German chamomile, garlic, ginger, ginkgo, green tea, lemon balm, milk thistle, oregano, parsley, peppermint, rosemary, sage, spearmint, thyme, turmeric

Other: cereal grasses, flax seeds, nuts, olive oil (extra-virgin), pumpkin seeds, sea vegetables, sesame seeds, soy products, sunflower seeds, yogurt with active bacterial cultures

Recent studies show that one of the most important factors contributing to changes in aging is oxidation. Body cells are damaged by "free radicals," the by-products of converting oxygen to energy. The progression of Parkinson's disease and Alzheimer's disease has been linked to oxidative stress. Heart disease, cancer, arthritis and wrinkles are signs of cell damage often caused by free radicals. Antioxidants protect the body from free radical damage.

Several scientific studies show that eating a diet high in nutrients but low in calories helps prevent signs of aging and increases lifespan.

WHAT TO DO

MAXIMIZE	MINIMIZE
• Antioxidants in the diet. Drink anti-oxidant herbal teas	• Animal fats in meat and dairy products. Replace some meat meals with fish and vegetable protein
• Digestion. Remedy digestive problems to improve nutrient absorption (see *Indigestion*, page 84)	**ELIMINATE**
	• Unnecessary calories

HEALING RECIPES

Add 1 tsp (5 mL) herbs and up to 2 tbsp (25 mL) other ingredients recommended (at left) for this condition to the following juices and smoothies.

Juices

Black Pineapple	Blueberry	Allium Antioxidant
Brocco-Carrot	Green Magic	Rust Proofer #1
Moist & Juicy	Grape Heart	Rust Proofer #2

Smoothies

| Beta Blast | Spa Special | Smart Smoothie |

Teas

| Antioxi-T | Green Giant Tea Blend | Raspberry Tea |

Coffee Substitutes

Seed Power Coffee Blend

AIDS
(ACQUIRED IMMUNODEFICIENCY SYNDROME) AND
HIV (HUMAN IMMUNODEFICIENCY VIRUS)

HEALING FOODS

Fruits and vegetables: citrus fruits, peaches, pears, strawberries, asparagus, avocado, broccoli, carrots, cauliflower, leafy greens, onions, squash

Herbs: aloe vera, astragalus, burdock, evening primrose oil, garlic, ginseng, licorice, turmeric

Other: cereal grasses, flax seeds, kelp, legumes, pumpkin seeds, sprouted seeds, soy yogurt, sunflower seeds, tofu, whole grains

There is no known cure for AIDS, and anyone with HIV should be under a doctor's care. But dietary therapy can improve immune function, avoid causes of immune suppression and promote resistance to infections associated with AIDS.

WHAT TO DO

MAXIMIZE	MINIMIZE	ELIMINATE
• Organic vegetables for their high vitamin and mineral content • Shiitake mushrooms strongly support immune system • Garlic guards against opportunistic infections in AIDS	• Sweet foods, including honey and fruit juices, which encourage the growth of molds and yeast	• Refined flour • Fats in meat and dairy products, which decrease immunity • Alcohol increases susceptibility to infection • Food allergies and intolerances (see pages 254 to 255) • Sugar

OTHER RECOMMENDATIONS
- Exercise daily, according to fitness level, to improve circulation and sweat out toxins.
- Practice relaxation exercises such as yoga, tai chi and meditation to increase immunity by decreasing stress.

RECIPES
Add 1 tsp (5 mL) herbs and up to 2 tbsp (25 mL) other ingredients recommended (at left) for this condition to the following juices and smoothies.

Juices

Cauliflower Cocktail	Allium Antioxidant	Brocco-Carrot
C-Green	Leafy Greens	

Green Magic *(use a recommended herb [from list at left] in place of ginkgo)*
Moist & Juicy *(use a recommended herb [from list at left] in place of ginkgo)*

Smoothies

Green Energy *(use a recommended herb [from list at left] in place of ginkgo)*

Teas

Antioxi-T	Immune Regulator

Coffee Substitutes

Immune Blend	Root Coffee Blend

ALLERGIES
(HAY FEVER, ECZEMA AND ASTHMA)

HEALING FOODS

Fruits and vegetables: apples, blueberries, grapes, mangoes, oranges, raspberries, strawberries, asparagus, beets, carrots, onions, red and green peppers, spinach, watercress

The symptoms of allergic reactions in hay fever, eczema and asthma are caused by inflammation, which is the body's normal healing response to injury. In these cases of chronic inflammation, factors such as food intolerances in the diet, stress, and poor digestion can allow a toxin to activate the immune system, causing an inappropriate inflammatory response on the skin, or in the eyes, nose or airways.

Nutrition and herbs can modify this inflammatory response.

continued...

Herbs: astragalus, burdock root*, calendula*, cinnamon, dandelion leaf and root*, elder-flower, garlic, ginger, licorice**, parsley, stinging nettles, thyme, turmeric, yarrow*

Other: flax seeds, nuts (except peanuts), pumpkin seeds, rice, soy products, yogurt with live bacterial cultures, whole grains

* People who are allergic to ragweed are sometimes also allergic to herbs in the same botanical family, (compositae, or daisy). Some of the herbs in this family include burdock, calendula, chamomile, chicory, dandelion, echinacea, feverfew, milk thistle and yarrow.

** Avoid licorice in cases of high blood pressure. Prolonged use not recommended in any circumstances.

WHAT TO DO

MAXIMIZE	ELIMINATE
• Essential fatty acids are anti-inflammatory and reduce the severity of allergies, such as fish, flax seeds, sunflower seeds	• Food allergens and foods of which one is intolerant (see page 256)
• Fruits and vegetables provide flavonoids and antioxidants that reduce allergic reaction	• Sugar, including honey and fruit sugars. Studies have shown that sugars decrease immune functioning by impairing the activity of white blood cells. Sugar also promotes yeast infections, which increase allergic reactions
• Herbs, as required, to optimize digestion (dandelion root) and immunity (astragalus, garlic) and to nourish the nervous system (oat straw, skullcap)	• Alcohol, which depresses immune functioning
	• Mucus forming foods such as dairy products and bananas

OTHER RECOMMENDATIONS

• Stress and high emotion are factors in lowered immunity, which increases susceptibility to allergies. Sleep and relaxation promote the release of immune factors.

• Poor digestive functioning promotes internal toxins and limits the effectiveness of food nutrients. Improving digestion so that food is completely digested often eliminates the allergic reaction. See Food Combining (pages 256 to 257)

• Protein is essential for optimum immune functioning. The best sources are fish such as tuna, salmon, sardines, trout, cod and herring.

RECIPES

Add 1 tsp (5 mL) herbs and up to 2 tbsp (25 mL) other ingredients recommended (at left) for this condition to the following juices and smoothies.

Juices

Berry Fine Cocktail	Citrus Cocktail	Blueberry
Beet	C-Green	Spring Celebration

Grape Power *(use a recommended herb [from list at left] in place of rosemary)*

Smoothies

Green Energy *(use a recommended herb [from list at left] in place of ginkgo)*
Mango Madness *(substitute 1/4 cup (50 mL) yogurt for banana)*

Teas

Aller-free Tea	Immune Regulator	Nettle Tea

HEALING FOODS

Fruits and vegetables: broccoli, cabbage, garlic, onion, spinach

Herbs: ginger, rosemary, stinging nettles

Other: brown rice, eggs, flax seeds, nuts, soy products, sunflower seeds

ALOPECIA

Alopecia, a partial or complete loss of hair, can be caused by severe stress, skin diseases, excessive sunlight, imbalances of thyroid or sex hormones, or by strong chemicals such as those used in cancer treatment or hair treatments, which interfere with nutrition of the hair follicles.

Hair consist largely of protein, which is made from amino acids and minerals, and is thus greatly affected by nutrition.

Rosemary is traditionally used for hair problems. A rosemary tea can be used both internally and externally to stimulate blood circulation to the scalp.

WHAT TO DO	
MAXIMIZE	MINIMIZE
• Antioxidant fruits and vegetables	• Stress. Relaxation exercises such as meditation and yoga can help you deal with the stresses and tensions in your life

INCLUDE IN YOUR DIET

- Foods with a high protein content, such as meat, fish, poultry, eggs, cheese, brown rice, nuts, seeds, soybeans
- Sulfur, found in egg yolk, cauliflower, cabbage, turnips, onions and garlic
- Calcium, found in dairy products, leafy green vegetables and sea herbs

RECIPES

Add 1 tsp (5 mL) herbs and up to 2 tbsp (25 mL) other ingredients recommended (page 59, lower left) for this condition to the following juices and smoothies.

Juices

Allium Antioxidant	Cabbage Cocktail	Cabbage-Rose
Nip of Goodness		

Smoothies

Green Energy

Teas

Circulation Tea

ALZHEIMER'S DISEASE AND DEMENTIA

HEALING FOODS

Fruits and vegetables: blueberries, citrus fruits, grapes, asparagus, broccoli, beets and beet tops, carrots, green peppers, kale, okra, onions, parsley, spinach, sweet potatoes, watercress, yams

Herbs: basil, garlic, German chamomile, ginger, ginkgo, ginseng, gotu kola, dandelion leaves and flowers, lemon balm, licorice root★, stinging nettles, parsley, red clover flowers, rosemary, sage, skullcap, turmeric

Other: Brazil nuts, brown rice, cider vinegar, egg yolks, flax seed, lecithin, legumes, lentils, nuts, oats, extra-virgin olive oil, pumpkin seeds, seaweed, soy products, wheat germ

★ *Avoid licorice in cases of high blood pressure. Prolonged use not recommended in any circumstances.*

Dementia is characterized by impairment of memory, judgement and abstract thinking. It may be caused by stress, impaired circulation resulting from a build-up of fatty deposits in the blood vessels of the brain, or by a degenerative disease such as Alzheimer's. Recognized factors in Alzheimer's disease include acetylcholine deficiency, free radicals, and inflammation of brain tissue. Diet can play a role in prevention by nourishing the brain, by lowering cholesterol that causes fatty deposits in the blood vessels of the brain, and by providing antioxidants to protect against free radicals that cause brain cell damage. Foods that contain choline, a building block of acetylcholine (a brain chemical that plays a key role in cognition and reasoning) may help. These include Brazil nuts, lecithin, dandelion flowers, mung beans, lentils and fava beans.

WHAT TO DO		
MAXIMIZE	MINIMIZE	ELIMINATE
• Fresh fruit and vegetables which provide vitamins and minerals (to feed the brain tissue) and antioxidants to protect against free radicals	• Meat and dairy products	• Refined and processed food
	• Environmental toxins	• Alcohol
• Foods that contain choline, a building block of acetylcholine: Brazil nuts, lecithin, dandelion flowers		• Fatty foods, fried foods and all oils (except extra-virgin olive oil)
• Nuts and seeds, which provide essential fatty acids to nourish the brain		• Aluminum in cookware, foil, deodorants and antacids. There is a suspected relationship between aluminum and Alzheimer's

OTHER RECOMMENDATIONS

- Fatty fish (salmon, sardines, mackerel, herrings) provides essential fatty acids to nourish brain and nerve tissue.
- Rosemary and sage are traditional herbs used to improve memory. Both herbs are rich in antioxidants. Studies show that they contain substances that conserve acetylcholine.
- Ginkgo biloba improves deficient blood flow to the brain.
- Anti-inflammatory herbs (German chamomile, ginseng, licorice, turmeric, white willow bark) may reduce inflammation of brain tissue in Alzheimer's.

RECIPES

Add 1 tsp (5 mL) herbs and up to 2 tbsp (25 mL) "other" ingredients recommended (page 60, lower left) for this condition to the following juices and smoothies.

Juices

Black Pineapple	Blueberry	C-Blend
Grape-Power	Beet	Brocco-Carrot
Leafy Greens	Sea Herb Surprise	Spring Celebration

Smoothies

Smart Smoothie	Sea-Straw Smoothie

Teas

Memory Booster Tea Blend

ANEMIA

HEALING FOODS

Fruits and vegetables: apples, citrus fruit, grapes, peaches, strawberries, beets and beet tops, broccoli, carrots, fennel, green peas, Jerusalem artichoke, leafy greens, watercress

Herbs: burdock root, dandelion leaf and root, nettles, parsley★

Other: almonds, dried apricots, figs, prunes, raisins, black–strap molasses, kelp

★ In pregnancy, limit parsley intake to 1/2 tsp (2 mL) dried herb or a sprig of fresh herb per day. Parsley is not to be taken in kidney inflammation.

Anemia is a deficiency of hemoglobin in the blood, resulting in fatigue and facial pallor. Other symptoms depend on the type of anemia, which can be determined by blood tests. Iron-deficiency anemia is the most common type and may be precipitated by heavy menstrual loss, internal bleeding, dietary deficiency of iron, pregnancy and rheumatoid arthritis. Work to alleviate the underlying cause and to increase absorption of nutrients.

WHAT TO DO

MAXIMIZE	MINIMIZE
• Iron-rich foods such as sea herbs, beets, dried fruit, almonds, spinach, nettles, parsley, watercress • Foods rich in vitamin C; herbal bitters (dandelion root), to improve iron absorption	• Whole wheat bread, which limits iron absorption **ELIMINATE** • Foods that limit iron absorption such as coffee, tea, chocolate, wheat bran

RECIPES

Add 1 tsp (5 mL) herbs and up to 2 tbsp (25 mL) other ingredients recommended (at left) for this condition to the following juices and smoothies.

Juices

Apple-Beet-Pear	Apricot-Peach	Beet and Green Beet
Brocco-Artichoke	Peas Please	Popeye's Power

Smoothies

Sea-Straw

Teas

Dandelion-Parsley	Iron Builder	Nettle Tea

Coffee Substitutes

Easy Root Coffee

ANXIETY STATES
(ANXIETY, STRESS AND PANIC ATTACKS)

Fruits and vegetables:
apricots, bananas, broccoli,
carrots, celery, fennel, leafy
greens, onions, watercress

Herbs: alfalfa, borage, dandelion
greens, garlic, German
chamomile, kava kava, lavender,
lemon balm, parsley*, St. John's
wort, skullcap, valerian**

Other: almond milk, dulse,
honey, kelp, nuts (especially
almonds), tofu, whole grains
(especially oats)

** In pregnancy, limit parsley intake to
1/2 tsp (2 mL) dried herb or a sprig of
fresh herb per day. Parsley is not to be
taken in kidney inflammation.*

*** Valerian has an adverse effect on
some people.*

*Anxiety is characterized by a mood of fear and is often associated with insomnia. Panic
disorders are recurrent attacks of severe anxiety. Causes may include fatigue, stress, nervous disorders, depression or hormone imbalances.*

WHAT TO DO	
MAXIMIZE	**ELIMINATE**
• A diet high in fresh fruit and veg-etable fiber to boost general health level, allowing you to cope better with stress	• Sources of caffeine such as coffee, black and green tea, chocolate and soda drinks
• Foods rich in B vitamins, such as whole grains and leafy green vegeta-bles, to support the nervous system	• Alcohol
	• Refined flour and sugar
	• Chemical food additives
• Foods that are high in calcium and magnesium, such as kelp, dulse, soy products, almonds, kale and pars-ley, to help ease nervous tension	• Foods to which you are allergic or that you find difficult to digest (see pages 254 to 255).
• Herbs that help you to relax and to improve sleep, such as chamomile, lavender or skullcap	
• Meditation and relaxation exercises, to help free nervous energy, allow-ing a more balanced emotional state	

RECIPES

*Add 1 tsp (5 mL) herbs and up to 2 tbsp (25 mL) other ingredients recommended (at left) for
this condition to the following juices and smoothies.*

Juices		
Leafy Greens	C-Green	Popeye's Power
Smoothies		
Almond-Banana-Milk	Brain Builder	
Teas		
Adrenal Support Tea	Calming Cupa Tea Blend	Lavender Tea
Other		
Anxiety Antidote Coffee Substitute		Banana Frappé Shake

ARTHRITIS: RHEUMATOID AND OSTEO

Fruits and vegetables: apples,
cherries, cranberries, grapes,
mango, papaya, asparagus, beets,
broccoli, cauliflower, cabbage,
carrots, celery, Jerusalem artichoke, turnip, onions, watercress

continued...

*Rheumatoid arthritis is the most common chronic inflammatory joint disease. It can
usually be diagnosed by the presence of antibodies (called the "rheumatoid factor") in
the blood. Since it is blood related, rather than wear-and-tear related, it is a disease
that affects the whole system, often with symptoms such as fever, weight-loss, fatigue
and a general decline in health. The joints are usually affected symmetrically. They
include wrists, elbows, ankles, knees, hips, and hand and foot joints, which become
swollen and inflamed. Neck pain and stiffness may result from inflammation of the
spine. Joints can eventually become deformed as the inflammatory fluid in them
impairs the process of tissue repair. Pain and stiffness is usually worse in the morning,
and may wear off during the day.*

Herbs: alfalfa, celery seeds, dandelion root and leaf, fennel seeds, garlic, German chamomile, ginger, lemon balm, licorice★, meadowsweet, parsley★★, rosemary, stinging nettle, turmeric

Other: cereal grasses, dulse, fish oils, kelp, legumes, blackstrap molasses, nuts (especially almonds) olive oil (extra-virgin), soy products, seeds (flax, pumpkin, sesame, sunflower), wheatgerm, whole grains (watch for allergies to wheat and corn), yogurt with active bacterial cultures

★*Avoid licorice in cases of high blood pressure. Prolonged use not recommended in any circumstances.*

★★ *In pregnancy, limit parsley intake to 1/2 tsp (2 mL) dried herb or a sprig of fresh herb per day. Parsley is not to be taken in kidney inflammation.*

Osteoarthritis is a "wear and tear" disorder that usually starts after the age of 50, and is characterized by the degeneration of the cartilage in weight-bearing joints such as hips, knees and spine, as well as joints in the hand. With the degeneration, new bone, cartilage and connective tissues are formed at the joint, leading to limited movement and muscle wasting around the joint. Inflammation is a secondary factor to cartilage degeneration. Pain is usually provoked with movement and disappears with rest, so is typically worse in the evening and better in the morning. Because it is related to the weight on the joints, osteoarthritis improves with weight loss in overweight people. It is often related to an imbalance of minerals in the diet or defective absorption of minerals and can improve with diet change and support for the digestive system.

Arthritis sufferers commonly have poor circulation (signified by cold hands and feet), don't perspire, are constipated, and often overweight. These factors contribute to retention of waste products, which must be addressed first.

WHAT TO DO

MAXIMIZE	ELIMINATE
• Fresh fruits and vegetables	• Food allergies and intolerances. Problem foods often include corn, dairy products, tomatoes, potatoes, eggplant, peppers, cayenne, wheat, eggs, chocolate and peanuts (see pages 254 to 255)
• Fluids, to dilute and wash out toxins	
• Oily fish (salmon, tuna, herring, sardines), which are anti-inflammatory	
• Herbal support for the digestive system (lemon balm, peppermint, chamomile) to improve absorption of nutrients	• Meat, especially red meat (beef, pork and ham), processed meat products (ham, hamburgers, sausages, processed cold meat cuts), which can stimulate inflammation
• Anti-inflammatory herbs (chamomile, ginger, licorice, meadowsweet), to help reduce pain and joint deterioration	• Margarine, shortening and heat processed oils. Replace with extra-virgin olive oil
• Herbal diuretics (dandelion leaf) and lymphatics (red clover flowers), to encourage elimination of waste products	• Shellfish
	• Processed and tinned foods
• Herbal support for the liver (dandelion root, licorice) in its role of eliminating toxins	• Sugar and artificial sweeteners. Replace with honey, maple syrup or stevia
• Herbal circulatory stimulants (ginger, stinging nettle) to improve the blood supply of nutrients to the affected joints	• Citrus fruits, which, in rheumatoid arthritis, often cause allergies
	• All vinegar products (such as pickles) except apple cider vinegar
• Herbal analgesics (chamomile, meadowsweet) for pain relief	• Alcohol
	• Food additives
	• Food contaminants from pesticides
	• Junk food

MINIMIZE
• Refined foods
• Tea, coffee, soda drinks
• Salt and salty food
• Acidic fruits and vegetables, such as rhubarb, cranberry, plums, spinach, chard, beet greens

RECIPES

Add 1 tsp (5 mL) herbs and up to 2 tbsp (25 mL) other ingredients recommended (page 63, lower left) for this condition to the following juices and smoothies.

Juices

Cell Support Cleanser	Crimson Cleanser	Apple Spice Cocktail
Breakfast Cocktail	Cabbage Cocktail	Allium Antioxidant
Brocco-Artichoke	Brocco-Carrot	Carrot-Apple
Cauli-Slaw	Sea Herb Surprise	

Smoothies

Almond-Banana Milk	Calming Chamomile

Teas

Ginger Tea	Gout Buster	Chamomile-Licorice-Ginger

HEALING FOODS

Fruits and vegetables: apples, pears, carrots, beets, broccoli, spinach

Herbs: catnip, cinnamon, German chamomile, lemon balm, parsley*, St. John's wort, stinging nettle

Other: almonds, kelp, sunflower seeds, pumpkin seeds, oats

* In pregnancy, limit parsley intake to 1/2 tsp (2 mL) dried herb or a sprig of fresh herb per day. Parsley is not to be taken in kidney inflammation.

ATTENTION DEFICIT DISORDER

A child may be diagnosed as ADD if he or she is easily distracted, has a short attention span, has difficulty concentrating and impulsively moves from one activity to another. In ADHD (ADD with hyperactivity), there are signs of overactivity. Studies have shown that increasing whole, nutrient-rich food increases the nutrients to the brain, improving mental performance. Other studies show that iron deficiency can cause attention deficits.

Introducing fresh, raw juice to the child's diet is a good way to help the child take more fruits and vegetables. Herbs can help to calm a child's nerves while the diet detoxification process is taking place.

WHAT TO DO

MAXIMIZE	ELIMINATE
• Whole foods (see Guidelines to Good Health, pages 10–11)	• Food additives, coloring, preservatives and sweeteners, which can be toxic to a child's system
• Antioxidant fruits and vegetables	
• Iron-rich foods such as beets, leafy greens, almonds, sea herbs, watercress, and dried fruit such as figs, raisins and apricots	• Sugar and sweet foods and drinks, which deplete the B vitamins necessary for nerve cell function
• Nuts and seeds, to provide zinc, which is necessary for brain function	• Refined foods, including white flour and white sugar products, which deplete the body's supply of zinc
MINIMIZE	• Food allergies are often implicated in ADD. Some of the most common allergens are dairy products, eggs, wheat and oranges. For more on food allergies, see pages 254 to 255. See page 203 for information on milk substitutes.
• Foods that limit iron absorption, such as coffee, tea, chocolate, egg yolk, wheat bran	

RECIPES

Add 1 tsp (5 mL) herbs and up to 2 tbsp (25 mL) other ingredients recommended (at left) for this condition to the following juices and smoothies.

Juices

Autumn Refresher	Pear Pineapple	Brocco-Carrot
Leafy Greens		

Smoothies and Tea

Almond-Banana-Milk	Green Energy *(omit ginkgo)*	Chamomile-Lemon Tea

Milk Shakes

Banana Frappé	Chocolate Shake	Date and Nut Shake

BREASTFEEDING

A nourishing diet, rich in minerals, is essential for the health of mother and baby. To avoid infant colic, use fennel, dill or anise in the breastfeeding mother's food or tea. To reduce breast milk when weaning, drink sage tea.

HEALING FOODS

Fruits and vegetables: bananas, avocado, carrots, green beans, leafy greens, sweet potatoes, watercress

Herbs: alfalfa, borage leaves and flowers, dandelion, fennel seeds, German chamomile, parsley★, red raspberry leaves, stinging nettle

Other: almonds, blackstrap molasses, legumes, sunflower seeds, pumpkin seeds, sea vegetables, wheat germ, whole grains, yogurt with live bacterial culture

★ In pregnancy, limit parsley intake to 1/2 tsp (2 mL) dried herb or a sprig of fresh herb per day. Parsley is not to be taken in kidney inflammation.

WHAT TO DO

MAXIMIZE	MINIMIZE
• Whole foods. (See Guidelines to Good Health, pages 10–11).	• Garlic, onions and hot peppers, which can create gas for the baby
• Foods containing B vitamins (whole grains, leafy green vegetables, sea herbs), which encourage a rich supply of breast milk	• Refined foods, white flour and sugar
• Foods containing calcium to support baby's bone development (leafy greens, sea herbs)	**ELIMINATE** • Food additives, coloring and sweeteners, which can be toxic to a child's system
• Mineral-rich herbal teas such as nettles, red raspberry leaf, alfalfa, red clover flower, dandelion	

RECIPES

Add 1 tsp (5 mL) herbs and up to 2 tbsp (25 mL) other ingredients recommended (at left) for this condition to the following juices and smoothies.

Juices

Kelp	Leafy Greens	Sea Herb Surprise
Folic Plus		

Smoothies

Avocado Pineapple

Teas

Mother's Own	Raspberry Tea

Other

Digestive (Gripe Water)

BRONCHITIS

Bronchitis is an inflammation of the bronchial tubes usually manifested by chest congestion and a persistent cough. Typical causes include bacteria, virus, or exposure to smoke or chemicals. Without treatment, the condition can become chronic.

HEALING FOODS

Fruits and vegetables: apricots, citrus fruit, cranberries, pears, broccoli, cabbage, carrots, leafy greens, onions, red and green peppers, turnips, watercress

Herbs: cayenne, cinnamon, elderberries, fenugreek seeds, garlic, ginger, hyssop, licorice★, marshmallow, nettle leaf, parsley★★, plantain, thyme

Other: legumes, sesame seeds, sunflower seeds, pumpkin seeds, soy products, soy yogurt

★ Avoid licorice in cases of high blood pressure. Prolonged use not recommended in any circumstances.

★★ In pregnancy, limit parsley intake to 1/2 tsp (2 mL) dried herb or a sprig of fresh herb per day. Parsley is not to be taken in kidney inflammation.

WHAT TO DO

MAXIMIZE	MINIMIZE
• Fruits and vegetables, especially those high in vitamin C and beta carotene	• Meat
	• Salt
• Consume raw garlic regularly for its antibiotic effects on the lungs	**ELIMINATE** • Dairy products
	• Sugar
	• Refined flour
	• Alcohol
	• Food allergies and intolerances (see pages 254 to 255)

RECIPES

Add 1 tsp (5 mL) herbs and up to 2 tbsp (25 mL) other ingredients recommended (page 65, lower left) for this condition to the following juices.

Juices

Allium Antioxidant	C-Blitz	Carrot Allium
Gingered Broccoli	Tomato Juice Cocktail	

Teas

Lung Relief

HEALING FOODS

Fruits and vegetables: apples, apricots, blueberries, cherries, citrus fruits, cranberries, figs, grapes, kiwi, mangoes, papaya, peaches, raspberries, strawberries, watermelon, asparagus, beets, broccoli, cabbage, carrots, leafy greens, onions, parsnip, squash, sweet potatoes, tomatoes, watercress

Herbs astragalus, burdock, calendula, cayenne, echinacea, garlic, green tea, licorice*, parsley**, red clover flowers, rosemary, sage, turmeric

Other: extra-virgin olive oil, fish oil, flax seed, legumes, nuts except peanuts, pumpkin seeds, shiitake mushrooms, soy products, spirulina, sunflower seeds, yogurt with live bacterial cultures, wheatgrass, whole grains

*Avoid licorice in cases of high blood pressure. Prolonged use not recommended in any circumstances.

** In pregnancy, limit parsley intake to 1/2 tsp (2 mL) dried herb or a sprig of fresh herb per day. Parsley is not to be taken in kidney inflammation.

CANCER PREVENTION

Risk factors for cancer include the use of tobacco and alcohol, toxins in food, industry and the environment, as well as a family history of cancer. Cancer protection factors include a diet that consists primarily of fresh fruits, vegetables and other whole foods, a healthy active lifestyle, and avoidance of cancer-causing foods and toxins.

WHAT TO DO

MAXIMIZE	ELIMINATE
• Organic foods • Soy products • Antioxidant fruits and vegetables • Nuts and seeds	• Margarine, shortening and cooking oils (except extra-virgin olive oil) • Alcohol, sugar, coffee, salt, pickled and salt-cured foods, fried food • Fried, grilled or barbecued meat, fish and poultry
MINIMIZE	• Smoked or cured meats, including ham, bacon, hot dogs and cold cuts
• Animal protein in meat and dairy products	• Artificial food additives • Refined foods

OTHER RECOMMENDATIONS

• Regular daily exercise

RECIPES

Add 1 tsp (5 mL) herbs and up to 2 tbsp (25 mL) other ingredients recommended (at left) for this condition to the following juices and smoothies.

Juices

Allium Antioxidant	Brocco-Carrot	Cabbage Cocktail
Cauliflower Cocktail	Citrus Cocktail	Immune Juice
Rust Proffer #1 and #2	Tomato Juice Cocktail	

Teas

Antioxi-T	Ginger Tea

CANDIDA

Fruits and vegetables: cranberries, broccoli, cabbage, carrots, cauliflower, celery, leafy greens, onion, squash, sweet potato, sweet red pepper

Herbs: calendula, cloves, dandelion leaf and root, echinacea, garlic, ginger, lemon balm, nettle, parsley*, peppermint, rosemary, thyme

Other: caprylic acid, dulse, kelp, legumes, nuts, extra-virgin olive oil, seeds, soy products, whole grains, plain unsweetened yogurt with active bacterial cultures

* In pregnancy, limit parsley intake to 1/2 tsp (2 mL) dried herb or a sprig of fresh herb per day. Parsley is not to be taken in kidney inflammation.

Candida is a yeast infection that can occur on the external genitalia showing as a discharge in women or a rash in men. It can also occur in the mouth, causing a burning sensation, or in the digestive system, causing bloating. General symptoms can include fatigue, mood changes, depression, poor memory, headaches, sweet cravings, bowel irregularities, muscle and joint problems, and skin problems.

Candida can result from low thyroid function, diabetes, pregnancy, antibiotics, steroids, poor diet, vaginal deodorants and cosmetics or by sexual transmission. Stress, oral contraceptives or hormones and preservatives in food are factors in chronic candida.

Stress can be reduced with nerve-nourishing herbs such as skullcap, vervain or oats.

WHAT TO DO

MAXIMIZE	ELIMINATE
• Antioxidant vegetables	• Any food allergies (see pages 254–5)
• Vegetable protein (soy products or legumes with rice)	• Bananas, citrus fruit, dried fruit, mushrooms
• Fresh, raw garlic; several cloves a day kills the yeast fungus	• Alcohol, coffee, chocolate, tea
• Yogurt with active bacterial cultures, to control yeast growth	• Dairy products, which contain harmful milk sugars and antibiotics. Exception is unsweetened yogurt with active bacterial cultures
MINIMIZE	• Honey, molasses, soy sauce, sugar, sweeteners
• Fruit and fruit juices to reduce excess fruit sugars that encourage the growth of the yeast	• Meat
• High carbohydrate vegetables such as potatoes, corn and parsnips	• Refined foods
	• Vinegar-containing foods such as pickles, mustard, ketchup and salad dressings
	• Yeast (including bakery products with yeast)

RECIPES

Add 1 tsp (5 mL) herbs and up to 2 tbsp (25 mL) other ingredients recommended (at left) for this condition to the following juices.

Juices

C-Blend	C-Green	Green Goddess
Popeye's Power	Rust Proofer #1	Squash Special
Digestive Cocktail Juice		

Teas

Dandelion Tea	Echinacea	Garlic Tea
Ginseng	St. John's wort	

CHRONIC FATIGUE SYNDROME

Fruits and vegetables: apples, bananas, citrus fruit, broccoli, carrots, green beans, green and red peppers, leafy greens, spinach, squash, sweet potatoes, tomatoes, watercress

continued...

Chronic fatigue syndrome, also called myalgic encephalomyelitis and "post viral fatigue," is not well understood. It is characterized by overwhelming fatigue, lack of energy, sleep disturbances and depression, and often features headache, sore throat or swollen glands. It often follows a viral infection, leaving a weakened immune system. Other possible causes include food allergies, poor digestion or absorption of nutrients, antibiotic use and long-term stress.

Herbs: alfalfa, cayenne, dandelion leaf and root, echinacea, evening primrose oil, garlic, ginger, ginseng★, lemon balm, licorice★★, milk thistle, nettle, parsley★★★, St. John's wort

Other: brown rice, cereal grass, dulse, fish oils, flax seed, kelp, legumes, maitake mushrooms, oats, olive oil, pumpkin seeds, sesame seeds, shiitake mushrooms, sunflower seeds, whole grains, yogurt with live bacterial cultures

★ Do not take ginseng in cases of high blood pressure or if you drink coffee. Do not take daily for longer than 4 weeks.

★★ Avoid licorice in cases of high blood pressure. Prolonged use not recommended in any circumstances.

★★★ In pregnancy, limit parsley intake to 1/2 tsp (2 mL) dried herb or a sprig of fresh herb per day. Parsley is not to be taken in kidney inflammation.

WHAT TO DO

MAXIMIZE	ELIMINATE
• Immunity and digestion. See Immune Deficiency, page 82 and Indigestion, page 84. • Antioxidant fruit and vegetables • Nuts and seeds	• Processed and refined foods • Caffeine in coffee, tea, chocolate, soda drinks • Sugar, alcohol, yeast (or foods made with yeast), which can encourage candida infection, often a factor in chronic fatigue • Food allergies and intolerances, commonly dairy products, wheat and corn (see page 256) • Artificial food additives
MINIMIZE	
• Animal protein in meat and dairy products	

OTHER RECOMMENDATIONS
• Regular daily exercise, according to fitness level

RECIPES
Add 1 tsp (5 mL) herbs and up to 2 tbsp (25 mL) other ingredients recommended (at left) for this condition to the following juices.

Juices

C-Blend	Lemon-Lime	Orange Zinger
C-Green	Green Goddess	Popeye's Power
Rust Proofer #1	Squash Special	

Teas
Immune Regulator

Digestive
Digestive Cocktail Juice

HEALING FOODS

COMMON COLD

The common cold is a viral infection of the airways. During cold season, a diet high in fresh fruits, vegetables and garlic is an excellent preventive measure. The severity and duration of the cold can be reduced by promoting elimination through the skin (by sweating) and through the bowel (by consuming plenty of fresh fruit juices, while avoiding slow-digesting meat and dairy products).

Fruits and vegetables: lemon, onions, citrus fruits, carrots

Herbs: astragalus, cayenne pepper, echinacea, elderflowers and elderberries, garlic, ginger, licorice★★, peppermint

Other: honey★★★

★ Sage is not to be taken in high blood pressure, pregnancy or breast-feeding.

★★ Avoid licorice in high blood pressure or for long periods of time

★★★ Honey must not be given to children under one year of age

Help for common cold symptoms:
NAUSEA: tea made from peppermint, German chamomile, ginger or cinnamon
SORE THROAT: gargle or tea made from sage★
COUGHS: tea made from thyme, licorice★★, hyssop, plantain and marshmallow root

WHAT TO DO

MAXIMIZE	ELIMINATE
• Fresh fruits and vegetables and their juices • Hot herbs, such as cayenne and ginger, to promote body heat and discourage the virus • At least 8 cups of water, juices or herbal teas daily	• Animal protein. The high amount of energy required for digestion of meat and dairy products is better used as healing energy.

RECIPES

Add 1 tsp (5 mL) herbs and up to 2 tbsp (25 mL) other ingredients recommended (page 68, lower left) for this condition to the following juices.

Juices

Tomato Juice Cocktail	Lemon-Lime	Allium Antioxidant
C-Blend	C-Blitz	Carrot-Allium
Flaming Antibiotic	Immunity	

Teas

Flu Fighter	Throat Soother	Throat Saver Tea Blend

HEALING FOODS

Fruits and vegetables: apples, pears, prunes, rhubarb, beets, green leafy vegetables, leeks, onions

Herbs: burdock root, German chamomile, cinnamon, dandelion root, fennel seeds, garlic, ginger, lavender, lemon balm, licorice★, peppermint, vervain, yellow dock

Other: dried fruit, flax seeds, legumes, molasses, nuts, psyllium seeds, pumpkin seeds, sesame seeds, yogurt with active bacterial cultures

★ Avoid licorice in cases of high blood pressure. Prolonged use not recommended in any circumstances.

CONSTIPATION

Constipation or failure of bowel elimination, may be caused by diseases such as diverticulitis or anemia, which require treatment (see pages 72 and 61), by nervous stress, lack of exercise, insufficient fiber in the diet, or by taking laxatives, which cause the bowel to be lazy.

Constipation can often be relieved by increasing the amount of fiber in the diet, by regular daily exercise, and by ensuring sufficient daily water intake.

Both over-relaxation and tension can affect the bowel muscles. Stimulation with cayenne or ginger can benefit an over-relaxed person. A relaxing tea of chamomile, lavender, vervain or lemon balm can relax a tense, overstimulated person.

Replacing all dairy products with soy or rice products often relieves constipation in a child.

WHAT TO DO

MAXIMIZE

- Guidelines to Good Health (see pages 10–11)
- Fiber intake by eating fresh, raw fruits and vegetables, legumes, nuts and seeds and whole grains
- Fluids. Drink at least 8 large glasses daily of water, juices or herbal teas
- Bitter herbs (dandelion root, German chamomile, burdock, ginger, fennel, yellow dock), to stimulate digestive juices and gently stimulate the bowel

ELIMINATE

- Refined foods

RECIPES

Add 1 tsp (5 mL) herbs and up to 2 tbsp (25 mL) other ingredients recommended (at left) for this condition to the following juices and smoothies.

Juices

Pear-Fennel	Rhubarb

Smoothies

Prune

Teas

Digestive Tea	Chamomile-Licorice-Ginger	Ginger Tea

Other

Applesauce	Calming Chamomile Tonic	Dandelion Delight Bitter

HEALING FOODS

Fruits and vegetables: black beans, broccoli, carrot, mango, soybeans, spinach, watercress

Herbs: borage, burdock root, cardamom, cayenne, cinnamon, cloves, dandelion root, garlic, German chamomile, ginger, ginkgo, lemon balm, oat seed, parsley*, rosemary, skullcap, St. John's wort, vervain

Other: cereal grasses, evening Primrose oil, flax seed, kelp, nuts, oat bran, oats, pumpkin seeds, sunflower seeds, whole grains

* In pregnancy, limit parsley intake to 1/2 tsp (2 mL) dried herb or a sprig of fresh herb per day. Parsley is not to be taken in kidney inflammation.

DEPRESSION

Depression, a persistently low mood, is often accompanied by headache, insomnia or constant drowsiness, inability to concentrate and low immunity. Although a long-term cure may require counselling support, good nutrition goes a long way in restoring nervous system functioning.

WHAT TO DO

MAXIMIZE
- Guidelines to Good Health (see pages 10–11)
- Foods rich in B vitamins, especially whole grains and leafy green vegetables, to improve nerve function
- Herbs for relaxation, (borage, skullcap, St. John's wort, chamomile, lemon balm), and sleep to counter stress and anxiety
- Liver-supportive herbs (dandelion root, burdock root, rosemary), to stimulate the metabolism and remove toxic wastes that can cause depression
- Nuts and seeds

ELIMINATE
- Food additives, which can contribute to depression

RECIPES

Add 1 tsp (5 mL) herbs and up to 2 tbsp (25 mL) other ingredients recommended (at left) for this condition to the following juices.

Juices		
Brocco-Carrot	C-Green	Leafy Greens

Smoothies	
Green Energy	Smart Smoothie

Teas	
Memory Booster	Spirit Raising Tea

Coffee Substitutes
Seed Power Coffee Blend

HEALING FOODS

Fruits and vegetables: apples, avocado, blueberries, grapefruit, lemon, lime, pears, broccoli, Jerusalem artichoke, leafy greens, onions

Herbs: cinnamon, cloves, coriander, dandelion root and leaf, evening primrose oil, fenugreek seeds, garlic, ginger, ginkgo, linden flowers, stevia, turmeric, yarrow

Other: fish oil, flax seeds, legumes, oats, olive oil (extra-virgin), pumpkin seeds, soy milk, spirulina, tofu, whole grains, yogurt with active bacterial cultures

DIABETES

Diabetes mellitus is an insulin deficiency that results in high blood sugar level. This deficiency affects the metabolism of carbohydrates, protein and fat, which often leads to an increase in the incidence of infections. It is important that a medical practitioner monitor diabetes. If diabetes is not controlled, changes in the blood vessels can lead to high blood pressure and deterioration in circulation, causing kidney, nerve and eye problems.

Type I diabetes begins in childhood, and is controlled by daily insulin injections. The pancreas is unable to produce sufficient insulin.

Type II diabetes usually occurs in adulthood, with obesity being a high risk factor. The pancreas often produces sufficient insulin, but the body is unable to use it efficiently. High blood sugar can be reversed by diet and weight loss. In type II diabetes, diet and herbs can help to regulate blood sugar, improve digestion and intestinal absorption of nutrients, support blood circulation, and improve immunity.

WHAT TO DO		
MAXIMIZE	**MINIMIZE**	**ELIMINATE**
• Fresh organic fruits, vegetables, legumes and unrefined grains, which help to regulate blood sugar and boost the immune system to help resist infection • Omega-3 fatty acids (fish and fish oils, flax seeds, pumpkin seeds and soybean products) which are beneficial to blood circulation	• Animal fats in meat and dairy products. Replace some meat meals with fish and vegetable protein. Replace dairy products with soy alternatives.	• Food allergies and intolerances (see pages 254 to 255) • Dairy products • Potatoes • Dried fruit, sugar, sweeteners (except stevia and small amounts of raw honey) • Fat and oils (except extra-virgin olive oil) • Processed foods • Refined foods • Caffeine in tea, coffee and soda drinks

OTHER RECOMMENDATIONS

• Chronic stress affects sugar levels. Skullcap and oats can help to calm nervous stress.

• Regular daily exercise is important in regulating blood sugar levels.

RECIPES

Add 1 tsp (5 mL) herbs and up to 2 tbsp (25 mL) other ingredients recommended (page 70, lower left) for this condition to the following juices and smoothies.

Juices

Allium Antioxidant	Apple-Beet-Pear	Beta Blast
Brocco-Artichoke		

Smoothies

Blue Cherry	Green Energy	Spa Special

Teas

Circulation Tea	Immune Regulator

Coffee Substitutes

Easy Root Coffee	Seed Power Coffee Blend

DIARRHEA

HEALING FOODS

Fruits and vegetables: cooked apples, bananas, lemon, lime, carrots, potatoes

Herbs: cardamom, German chamomile, fennel seeds, ginger, lemon balm, meadowsweet, nutmeg, raspberry leaves, slippery elm bark

Other: evening primrose oil, flax seed, pumpkin seeds, rice, sunflower seeds, whole grains, yogurt with active bacterial cultures

Diarrhea is an inflammation of the bowel, caused by bacterial or viral infection, food allergies or intolerances, or by malfunctions of the digestive system. Consult a medical practitioner if diarrhea lasts longer than one week.

Diarrhea causes dehydration, which can be life-threatening for small children. In such cases, consult your medical practitioner immediately.

WHAT TO DO		
MAXIMIZE	**MINIMIZE**	**ELIMINATE**
• Intake of water (boiled, then cooled) and herbal teas • Starchy foods (cooked potatoes, carrots, rice)	• Raw fruit, (except bananas), which can promote diarrhea • Raw vegetable fiber, which can irritate an inflamed bowel • Dried fruit	• Alcohol, caffeine, milk, cheese, soda drinks, sugar, sweeteners • Food allergies and intolerances (see pages 254 to 255)

RECIPES

Add 1 tsp (5 mL) herbs and up to 2 tbsp (25 mL) other ingredients recommended (page 71, lower left) for this condition to the following smoothies.

Smoothies

Best Berries (use blueberries)

Teas

Raspberry Ginger

Other

| Applesauce | Apple-Rice Pudding | Banana Frappé Milk Shake |

DIVERTICULAR DISEASE
(DIVERTICULITIS AND DIVERTICULOSIS)

HEALING FOODS

Fruits and vegetables: apples, bananas, grapes, mangoes, pears, prunes, broccoli, cabbage, carrot, celery, leafy greens, watercress

Herbs: cinnamon, fenugreek seeds, garlic, German chamomile, ginger, licorice★, marshmallow leaf and root, peppermint, psyllium seeds, slippery elm bark powder, valerian★★

Other: flax seeds, legumes, oatmeal, spirulina, wheat bran, whole grains, yogurt with live bacterial cultures

★ *Avoid licorice in cases of high blood pressure. Prolonged use not recommended in any circumstances.*

★★ *Valerian has an adverse effect on some people.*

Diverticulosis is characterized by multiple small pouches (diverticula) in the large intestine. Diverticulitis occurs when these pouches become inflamed. It is usually associated with constipation and caused by a lack of fiber in the diet. Symptoms typically include continuous pain in the left abdomen, flatulence, and sometimes diarrhea.

WHAT TO DO	
MAXIMIZE	**ELIMINATE**
• Fruits and vegetables	• Caffeine in tea, coffee, chocolate
• Whole grains and legumes	• Alcohol
• Water (at least 8 large glasses a day)	• Fried foods
	• Pickled foods
MINIMIZE	• Ham and bacon, fatty meat
• Animal protein in meat and dairy products	• Refined and processed foods
	• Spicy foods
	• Sugar
	• Dairy products (except yogurt with active bacterial cultures)
	• Constipation if present. (see page 69 for additional recommendations)

OTHER RECOMMENDATIONS

• Use food combining techniques (see pages 256 to 257).

• Move gradually to a high-fiber diet to avoid digestive problems.

• During periods of inflammation, avoid high-fiber foods (such as raw vegetables, and bran, which can irritate), and maximize healing vegetable juices such as spinach, cabbage, beet, garlic and carrot with soothing slippery elm bark powder.

RECIPES

Add 1 tsp (5 mL) herbs and up to 2 tbsp (25 mL) other ingredients recommended (at left) for this condition to the following juices and smoothies.

Juices

| Cabbage Cocktail | Apple-Pear | Gingered Broccoli |
| Leafy Greens | Popeye's Power | Slippery Beet |

Smoothies

| Mango Madness | Prune Smoothie | Slippery Banana |

Teas

| Digestive Tea | Digestive Stress Soother |

HEALING FOODS

ENDOMETRIOSIS

Endometriosis is a condition in which tissue that is normally found in the uterus wall (endometrium) is found in places outside the uterus, such as the bladder, bowel or fallopian tubes. This tissue responds to the hormonal cycle, shedding blood within these sites. Symptoms can include pain, irregular bleeding, depression and bowel problems.

Fruits and vegetables: apples, apricots, cherries, grapefruit, strawberries, beets, broccoli, cabbage, leafy greens, peas, red and green pepper, squash, sweet potato

Herbs: calendula, chasteberry, dandelion leaf and root, evening primrose oil, German chamomile, meadowsweet, passionflower, rosemary, turmeric, valerian★, vervain

Other: barley, fish oils, legumes, nuts, oats, olive oil (extra-virgin), seeds, tofu, whole grains, soy yogurt with live bacterial cultures

★ *Valerian has an adverse effect on some people.*

WHAT TO DO

MAXIMIZE	MINIMIZE	ELIMINATE
• Antioxidants in the diet (preferably from vegetable sources), help clear up imperfect cells. • Healing essential fatty acids such as fresh nuts, seeds and grains	• Meat and dairy products. Use organic if possible. The hormones in commercial products aggravate the body's hormone balance. • Fruit, which may contribute to blood-sugar problems. Candida is often associated with endometriosis.	• Sugar products • Yeast products (e.g. bread) • Coffee • Alcohol • Junk food • Common food allergens such as dairy products and wheat products. (see pages 254 to 255)

OTHER RECOMMENDATIONS
- Balance hormones with Vitex agnus-castus (chasteberry)
- Analgesics herbs (German chamomile, meadowsweet, passionflower, rosemary, valerian) for pain
- Nervous system tonic: passionflower, valerian, vervain
- Use turmeric for its antimicrobial/antiseptic/anti-inflammatory properties
- Liver-supporting herbs (calendula, dandelion root, rosemary) to metabolize hormones
- Evening primrose oil is an antidepressant and helps clear up abnormal cell growth

RECIPES

Add 1 tsp (5 mL) herbs and up to 2 tbsp (25 mL) other ingredients recommended (at left) for this condition to the following juices.

Juices

Cherry Sunrise	Cabbage Cocktail	Beet
Peas Please	Peppers Please	Squash Special

Teas

Hormone Balancing Tea	Lavender Tea

Coffee Substitutes

Root Coffee	Seed Power Coffee Blend

EYE PROBLEMS
(CATARACTS, GLAUCOMA AND MACULAR DEGENERATION)

HEALING FOODS

Research shows that the risk of cataracts, glaucoma and macular degeneration decreases with a high-antioxidant diet.

Fruits and vegetables: apricots, blackberries, blueberries, citrus fruits, cranberries, grapes, mangoes, peaches, raspberries, strawberries, watermelon, asparagus, avocado, broccoli, cabbage, carrots, green and red peppers, leafy greens, pumpkin, squash, sweet potatoes, tomatoes, watercress   *continued...*

WHAT TO DO

MAXIMIZE	MINIMIZE
• Antioxidant fruits and vegetables, to protect eyes from free radical damage. Carrot juice, spinach and blueberries are especially effective. • Fresh garlic, which is strongly antioxidant	• Fat from meat and dairy products **ELIMINATE** • Refined foods • Fried foods • Sugar and products containing sugar or sweeteners

Herbs: dandelion leaf, garlic, ginger, ginkgo, parsley★, rosemary, turmeric

Other: extra virgin olive oil, nuts, pumpkin seeds, wheat germ, yogurt with active bacterial cultures

★ In pregnancy, limit parsley intake to 1/2 tsp (2 mL) dried herb or a sprig of fresh herb per day. Parsley is not to be taken in kidney inflammation.

RECIPES

Add 1 tsp (5 mL) herbs and up to 2 tbsp (25 mL) other ingredients recommended (at left) for this condition to the following juices and smoothies.

Juices

Cabbage Cocktail	Citrus Cocktail	Tomato Juice Cocktail
Black Pineapple	Blueberry	Blue Water
C-Blend	C-Blitz	Grape Power
Squash Special	Sunrise Supreme	Beta-Carro

Smoothies

Mango Madness	Liquid Gold

Teas

The Green Diablo	Antioxi-T

HEALING FOODS

Fruits and vegetables: bananas, grapes, lime, mangoes, oranges, pineapple, strawberries, broccoli, carrots, leafy greens, onions, spinach, watercress

Herbs: alfalfa, burdock root, cardamom, cayenne, cinnamon, cloves, dandelion leaf and root, garlic, ginger, ginseng★, licorice★★, parsley★★★, peppermint, red raspberry leaves, rose hips, stinging nettles, yellow dock root

Other: almonds, cereal grasses, dates, fish oil, flax seed, oats, pumpkin seeds, sea vegetables, sunflower seeds, whole grains, tofu, wheat germ, yogurt with live bacterial cultures

★ Do not take ginseng in cases of high blood pressure or if you drink coffee. Do not take daily for longer than 4 weeks.

★★ Avoid licorice in cases of high blood pressure. Prolonged use not recommended in any circumstances.

★★★ In pregnancy, limit parsley intake to 1/2 tsp (2 mL) dried herb or a sprig of fresh herb per day. Parsley is not to be taken in kidney inflammation.

FATIGUE

Fatigue is a symptom of many diseases, including anemia, diabetes, hepatitis, low blood sugar, and thyroid disease, which can be determined by blood tests and diagnosed by your doctor. Common non-disease factors include a lack of balance in diet, exercise, work and social life. A balanced diet provides the digestive enzymes required for nutrient processing in the creation of energy from food.

WHAT TO DO

MAXIMIZE	ELIMINATE
• Fresh fruits and vegetables	• Caffeine and sugar, which can cause fatigue
• Whole grains	• Refined flour products, which rob the body of nutrients
• Nuts and seeds	• Canned, pre-packaged and processed foods, which are often low in nutrients and high in chemical additives
• Essential fatty acids (see page 262)	
MINIMIZE	• Margarine, shortening and salad oils (except extra-virgin olive oil)
• Fat in meat and dairy products	
• Fried food	• Alcohol

OTHER RECOMMENDATIONS

- Daily exercise, according to level of fitness.
- Eat smaller meals more often to maintain blood sugar.
- Try using stress-reduction techniques such as yoga, tai chi and meditation. Stress depletes vitality.
- Use liver-supportive herbs (dandelion root, burdock root) to stimulate metabolism and remove toxic wastes that can cause fatigue.

RECIPES

Add 1 tsp (5 mL) herbs and up to 2 tbsp (25 mL) other ingredients recommended (at left) for this condition to the following juices and smoothies.

Juices

Apple Fresh	Brocco-Carrot	Eye Opener
Spiced Carrot	Sunrise Supreme	
Moist & Juicy *(use any recommended herb [at left] in place of ginkgo)*		

Smoothies

B-Vitamin	Brain Builder *(use any recommended herb [at left] in place of ginkgo)*	
Green Energy	Mango Madness	Pineapple-C
Taste of The Tropics		

RECIPES (CONTINUED)
Teas

Adrenal Support Tea	Ginseng	Iron Builder
Mother's Own		

Fruits and vegetables: apples, beets, broccoli, cabbage, cauliflower, celery, fennel, green beans, Jerusalem artichokes, onions, squash, sweet potato, watercress

Herbs: alfalfa, astragalus, burdock root and seeds, calendula, dandelion leaf and root, echinacea, evening primrose oil, garlic, licorice★, milk thistle, parsley★★, passionflower, slippery elm bark powder, St. John's wort, turmeric

Other: barley grass, fish oils, flax seeds, legumes, pumpkin seeds, soy products, sunflower seeds, unsweetened yogurt with live bacterial cultures, whole grains especially brown rice

★ *Avoid licorice in cases of high blood pressure. Prolonged use not recommended in any circumstances.*

★★ *In pregnancy, limit parsley intake to 1/2 tsp (2 mL) dried herb or a sprig of fresh herb per day. Parsley is not to be taken in kidney inflammation.*

FIBROMYALGIA

Fibromyalgia is characterized by tender, aching muscles, joint pain similar to rheumatoid arthritis, fatigue, and sleep disturbances. The areas affected are typically the neck, shoulders, lower back, chest and thighs. It is considered to be a form of chronic fatigue syndrome, with pain rather than fatigue as the dominant feature. Depression is often a feature, aggravated by lack of sleep. The cause can be viral or a build-up of toxins. Food, drugs, allergies and nutritional deficiencies can also be involved. Neither the cause or the cure is well understood, but good nutrition can help recovery.

WHAT TO DO

MAXIMIZE	ELIMINATE
• Antioxidant vegetables	• Sugar and products containing sugar, high-sugar fruits such as dried fruit, bananas, watermelon
• Vegetable protein (see page 53 and Guidelines to Good Health page 10-11)	• Refined flour products, food additives
• Nuts and seeds	• Alcohol
• Legumes	• Food allergies and intolerances, especially gluten (in wheat products) and potatoes, tomatoes, eggplant, peppers
MINIMIZE	• Caffeine in tea, coffee and soda drinks, which decrease mineral absorption and contribute to fibromyalgia
• Fruit intake as excess fruit may contribute to low blood-sugar (see Hypoglycemia)	• Dairy products. Replace with soy products
• Acidic fruit and vegetables (citrus, berries, rhubarb, gooseberries, tomatoes, spinach) which may irritate the condition	• Salty and pickled foods, fried foods
	• Pork, shellfish, fatty meats
	• Artificial food additives

OTHER RECOMMENDATIONS
• Eat oily fish (salmon, trout, cod, halibut, mackerel, herring, tuna), 2 or 3 times a week.

• Practice stress reduction therapies such as tai chi, yoga and meditation.

• Exercise daily, according to fitness level.

RECIPES
Add 1 tsp (5 mL) herbs and up to 2 tbsp (25 mL) other ingredients recommended (at left) for this condition to the following juices.

Juices

Breakfast Cocktail	Cabbage Cocktail	Cauli-Slaw
Beet	Brocco-Artichoke	C-Green
Rust Proofer #2		

Teas

Immune Regulator

Coffee Substitutes

Root Coffee Blend	Easy Root Coffee

FLATULENCE

Fruits and vegetables: apples, kiwi, papaya

Herbs: basil, cardamom, cayenne, German chamomile, cinnamon, cloves, coriander, cumin, dill, fennel seeds, garlic, ginger, mustard seed, peppermint, thyme

Other: yogurt

Gas is a normal result of food breakdown in the digestive system. Beans and other foods high in carbohydrates produce more gas because they are not entirely broken down by digestive enzymes. Bacteria ferment the undigested carbohydrates and gas is released in this process. Other foods produce excess gas when the enzymes normally used for their digestion are not available. The most common example is the unavailability, in some people, of the enzyme needed to digest lactose in dairy products. Artificial sweeteners can also cause gas.

You may experience more gas if you change your diet to one that includes less meat and more beans and other fiber. It is best to make such changes slowly, optimizing your diet in a 4- to 6-week period.

To reduce the "gas effect" of legumes, soak them overnight in lots of water, discard soaking water before cooking, and rinse well before adding them to other dishes. Cook beans, and other foods that give you gas, with herbs that expel gas from the digestive tract (see sidebar).

WHAT TO DO	
MAXIMIZE	**ELIMINATE**
• Digestive herbal teas, taken between meals	• Artificial sweeteners and all foods containing them
• Food combining (see page 256)	• Dairy products (replace with soy products)

RECIPES		
Digestifs		
Before Dinner Mint	Gripe water	James Duke's Carminatea
Pineapple-Ginger	Rosy Peppermint	Spiced Papaya Tea
Gingerade	Tummy Aid	
Teas		
Spiced Papaya	Digestive Tea	

GALLSTONES

Fruits and vegetables: apple, citrus fruit, lemon, pear, asparagus, beets, broccoli, carrots, celery, leafy greens, radish, tomato, watercress

Herbs: dandelion leaf and root, garlic, ginger, milk thistle, parsley*, turmeric

Other: flax seed, lecithin, legumes, oats, olive oil (extra virgin), whole grains

* In pregnancy, limit parsley intake to 1/2 tsp (2 mL) dried herb or a sprig of fresh herb per day. Parsley is not to be taken in kidney inflammation.

Cholesterol from animal fats is a major factor in gallstone formation. Symptoms of gallstones can include indigestion, severe pain in the upper-right abdomen, constipation, flatulence, nausea and vomiting. If a gallstone remains stuck in the bile duct, causing inflammation, it may need to be surgically removed. Diet changes can reduce the risk of gallstone formation. Vegetarians are less likely to develop gallstones.

WHAT TO DO		
MAXIMIZE	**MINIMIZE**	**ELIMINATE**
• Vegetable protein (see page 53 and Guidelines to Good Health, page 10)	• Fatty meats and dairy products	• Sugar
		• Refined food
		• Coffee
• Fruit, vegetables, whole grains and legumes		

OTHER RECOMMENDATIONS
• Fatty fish (salmon, mackerel, sardines, tuna) helps to lower cholesterol levels
• Bitter herbs to increase the bile flow, helping to prevent gallstone formation (see Bitters, pages 207–209)
• Olive oil consumption discourages gallstone formation

RECIPES

Add 1 tsp (5 mL) herbs and up to 2 tbsp (25 mL) other ingredients recommended (page 76, lower left) for this condition to the following juices.

Juices

Lemon Cleanser	Tomato Juice Cocktail	Autumn Refresher
C-Blitz	Apple-Beet-Pear	Brocco-Carrot
Carrot-Apple	C-Green	Dandelion Bitters
Gallstone Solvent	Spring Celebration	Zippy Tomato

Lemon-Lime *(use 1 tsp [5 mL] recommended herb [page 76, lower left] in place of licorice)*

Teas

Ginger

Coffee Substitutes

Root Coffee Blend   Easy Root Coffee

HEALING FOODS

Fruits and vegetables:
avocado, carrot, celery, parsley, bananas, blackberries, cherries, raspberries, strawberries

Herbs: burdock root and seed, celery seed, dandelion leaf, fennel seed, garlic, ginger, licorice★, nettle, parsley★★, turmeric, yarrow, yellow dock

Other: flax seeds

★ *Avoid licorice in cases of high blood pressure. Prolonged use not recommended in any circumstances.*

★★ *In pregnancy, limit parsley intake to 1/2 tsp (2 mL) dried herb or a sprig of fresh herb per day. Parsley is not to be taken in kidney inflammation.*

GOUT

Gout is characterized by increased production of uric acid, which is deposited in the joints, especially fingers and toes. It may be hereditary or may be caused by excess alcohol, meat or starchy food, which increases the production of urates.

Decreasing the production of uric acid and increasing its excretion in the urine helps to control gout.

WHAT TO DO

MAXIMIZE

- Water consumption (at least 8 large glasses daily), to assist in the elimination of urates
- A vegetarian diet
- Herbal teas — celery seed, to dissolve urates; dandelion leaf and stinging nettle to help eliminate urates

MINIMIZE

- Protein (chicken, turkey and white fish are okay in moderation)
- Fat in meat and dairy products
- Salt
- Eggs (from free-range chickens)
- Wheat, which is acid forming. Grains such as brown rice and buckwheat produce less acid.

ELIMINATE

Foods that form acid in the body:

- Pork and beef
- Preserved meats
- Tomatoes
- Spinach
- Vinegar except cider vinegar
- Refined sugar and flour
- Coffee and tea
- Cheese
- Food additives in processed food
- Alcohol

Foods high in purines:

- Organ meats such as kidney and liver
- Shellfish, herring, sardines, anchovies, mackerel
- Peanuts
- Asparagus
- Mushrooms
- Legumes (peas, beans, lentils)

RECIPES

Add 1 tsp (5 mL) herbs and up to 2 tbsp (25 mL) other ingredients recommended (at left) for this condition to the following juices and smoothies.

Juices

Berry Best	Gout Buster	Immune Juice
Celery		

RECIPES (CONTINUED)
Teas

Gout Buster

Coffee Substitutes

Root Coffee Blend

HANGOVER

HEALING FOODS

Fruits and vegetables: apples, bananas, lemon, lime

Herbs: German chamomile, cumin, evening primrose oil, ginger, lavender, meadowsweet, slippery elm bark powder

Other: foods rich in vitamin B vitamins (whole grains and leafy green vegetables)

Alcohol dehydrates the body, creates acidity in the digestive system, causes the loss of potassium and vitamins, and affects the liver and nervous system. Over-consumption can result in symptoms of headache, fatigue, nausea, dizziness and depression. You may get faster relief from these symptoms by using the following recommendations, preferably before retiring.

WHAT TO DO
MAXIMIZE
• Water to rehydrate the body before, during and after drinking
• Juices high in vitamin C
• Herbal tea, to settle the stomach
• Slippery elm bark powder, to protect the stomach from acid

RECIPES
Add 1 tsp (5 mL) herbs and up to 2 tbsp (25 mL) other ingredients recommended (at left) for this condition to the following juice and smoothie recipe.

Juices
Hangover Remedy

Smoothies
Calming Chamomile

Teas
Hangover Rescue

HEADACHES

HEALING FOODS

Fruits and vegetables: apples, bananas, broccoli, leafy greens, watercress

Herbs: cayenne, evening primrose oil, German chamomile, lavender, lemon balm, linden flower, passionflower, rosemary, skullcap, thyme, valerian*, vervain

Other: almonds, legumes, oats, sunflower seeds, tofu, walnuts, wheat germ, whole grains, yogurt with active bacterial cultures

* Valerian has an adverse effect on some people.

Headaches, other than migraines, can be caused by muscular and nervous tension, digestive disorders, blood pressure changes, low blood sugar, withdrawal from caffeine, alcohol or drugs, eye strain, food allergies, a stuffy room, weather changes or posture problems. Avoid foods that are common headache triggers.

WHAT TO DO

MAXIMIZE	ELIMINATE
• Foods high in magnesium (whole grains, legumes, sea herbs, wheat germ, apples, bananas, nuts, seeds, fish). Magnesium relaxes muscles, helping to stop spasms.	• Food allergies and intolerances, commonly dairy products, wheat, corn, oranges and eggs (see pages 254 to 255)
	• Food additives, especially MSG
MINIMIZE	• Nitrate preserved meats, such as bacon, ham, hot dogs
• Salt	• Aspartame sweeteners
• Fatty foods	• Caffeine (from coffee, colas, chocolate) which can cause headaches in some people
	• Cheese and red wine contain substances that cause headaches in some people

OTHER RECOMMENDATIONS

★ Valerian has an adverse effect on some people.

- Lemon balm and meadowsweet tea may be helpful in headaches caused by digestive disorders.
- Skullcap and valerian★ teas can be helpful for stress-related headaches.
- Antispasmodic herbs (cayenne, German chamomile, lemon balm, linden flower, passionflower, skullcap, thyme, valerian★, vervain) can help headaches caused by muscular tension.

RECIPES

Add 1 tsp (5 mL) herbs and up to 2 tbsp (25 mL) other ingredients recommended (page 78, lower left) for this condition to the following juices and smoothies.

Juices

Brocco-Carrot   Cabbage Rose   C-Green
Leafy Greens

Smoothies

Green Energy *(substitute skullcap for ginkgo)*

Teas

Lavender Tea

HEART PROBLEMS
(HIGH CHOLESTEROL, HIGH BLOOD PRESSURE, CARDIOVASCULAR DISEASE, HEART FAILURE AND STROKE)

HEALING FOODS

Fruits and vegetables: apples, apricots, blueberries, blackberries, cranberries, grapefruit★, grapes, kiwi, mangos, melons, oranges, papaya, pineapple, strawberries, asparagus, avocado, broccoli, carrots, celery, leafy greens, lettuce, onions, parsnips, peppers (red and green), peas, squash, watercress

Herbs: cayenne, chicory root, dandelion leaf and root, fenugreek seeds, garlic, ginger, linden flowers, parsley★★, rosemary, stinging nettles, turmeric

Other: almonds, barley, fish oil, kelp, lecithin, legumes, oats, olive oil (extra virgin), seeds (flax, pumpkin, sesame, sunflower), soy products, sprouted seeds and beans, walnuts, whole grains, yogurt with live bacterial cultures

★ Avoid grapefruit if on calcium channel blocker medication

★★ In pregnancy, limit parsley intake to 1/2 tsp (2 mL) dried herb or a sprig of fresh herb per day. Parsley is not to be taken in kidney inflammation.

Family history, cigarette smoking, high alcohol consumption and high "bad" cholesterol intake are major risk factors for high blood pressure, circulation disorders and cardiovascular disease. In most cardiovascular diseases and circulation disorders, cholesterol deposits narrow the arteries, constricting the flow of blood.

Cholesterol is necessary to sustain life. There are two types in human blood: low density lipoprotein (LDL or "bad" cholesterol), which increases the risk of high blood pressure, heart disease and gallstones; and high density lipoprotein (HDL or "good" cholesterol) which reduces the risk of these conditions.

WHAT TO DO

MAXIMIZE	MINIMIZE	ELIMINATE
• Fresh fruits and vegetables, whole grains, nuts and seeds. These help regulate blood pressure, reduce LDLs ("bad" cholesterol) and raise HDLs ("good" cholesterol) • Garlic and onions, to reduce blood pressure and cholesterol • Antioxidant fruit and vegetables, to help prevent cholesterol deposits on artery walls • Red grape juice, to prevent blood clotting	• Alcohol • Coffee • Eggs • Salt and salty foods such as processed food products • Sugar and products containing sugar	• High-fat meats (ham, bacon, pork, steak) and dairy products (except for skimmed milk). • Margarine and salad oils (except extra virgin olive oil) • Fried foods • Pastry • Milk chocolate • Alcohol • Refined sugars and refined flour products • Coconut

OTHER RECOMMENDATIONS

- Supportive therapy for heart problems includes daily exercise (such as walking for 30 minutes a day, depending on level of fitness) and stress-reduction techniques such as yoga, tai chi and meditation
- Eat fatty fish (salmon, mackerel, sardines, tuna) 2 to 3 times a week
- Substitute vegetable protein for some meat meals (see Guidelines to Good Health pages 10–11)
- Use herbs (page 79, lower left) to help lower cholesterol and improve circulation

RECIPES

Add 1 tsp (5 mL) herbs and up to 2 tbsp (25 mL) other ingredients recommended (page 79, lower left) for this condition to the following juices.

Juices

Citrus Cocktail	Melon Morning Cocktail	Eye Opener
Black Pineapple	C–Blitz	C–Blend
Grape-Heart	Grape Power *(use red grapes)*	Allium Antioxidant,
Brocco-Carrot	Peas and Carrots	Spring Celebration
Apple Fresh *(use rosemary in place of ginseng)*		

Teas

Circulation Tea

Coffee Substitutes

Root Coffee Blend   Easy Root Coffee

HEALING FOODS

Fruits and vegetables:
bananas, papaya, beets, cabbage, carrots, celery, cucumber, parsnips

Herbs: calendula, cardamom, German chamomile, dandelion root, dill, fennel, ginger, licorice★, marshmallow root, meadowsweet, parsley★★, slippery elm bark powder

Other: flax seeds

★ Avoid licorice in cases of high blood pressure. Prolonged use not recommended in any circumstances.

★★ In pregnancy, limit parsley intake to 1/2 tsp (2 mL) dried herb or a sprig of fresh herb per day. Parsley is not to be taken in kidney inflammation.

HEARTBURN

Heartburn is a burning sensation in the chest that is related to digestive problems. It may originate from a hiatus hernia, indigestion or inflammation of the stomach. Check with your medical practitioner to determine the cause, especially to eliminate the possibility of heart disease. Relief can be obtained with frequent drinks of therapeutic fruit and vegetable juices, antacid herbs such as dandelion root and meadowsweet, soothing herbs such as marshmallow root and slippery elm bark, and by practising a "food combining" diet (see pages 256 to 257).

WHAT TO DO

MAXIMIZE	ELIMINATE
• Fresh fruits and vegetables	• Coffee, colas, alcohol, chocolate
• Water consumption (between meals only)	• Fried, fatty or spicy foods
• Slippery elm bark powder (especially at night), to protect the stomach from acid	• Citrus fruits and tomatoes
	• Pickled foods
	• Refined flour and sugar
	• Cigarettes
MINIMIZE	• Large meals
• Acid-forming foods such as meat and dairy products	• Antacid and anti-inflammatory drugs, which can irritate stomach lining

RECIPES

Add 1 tsp (5 mL) herbs (see at left) and up to 2 tbsp (25 mL) flax seeds for this condition to the following juices and smoothies.

Juices

Beet	Carrot-Apple	Cabbage Cocktail *(omit garlic)*

Teas

Digestive Stress Soother

Coffee Substitutes

Root Coffee Blend

HERPES SIMPLEX
(GENITAL HERPES AND COLD SORES)

Fruits and vegetables: apple, apricots, berries, grapes, papaya, pears, asparagus, broccoli, cabbage, carrots, leafy greens, onion, squash, watercress

Herbs: astragalus, burdock, calendula, cayenne, cloves, dandelion root, echinacea, elderflowers, garlic, ginseng, lemon balm, parsley*, St. John's wort, yarrow

Other: legumes (except chickpeas), nutritional yeast, seaweeds, sprouted beans, yogurt with active bacterial cultures

In pregnancy, limit parsley intake to 1/2 tsp (2 mL) dried herb or a sprig of fresh herb per day. Parsley is not to be taken in kidney inflammation.

Herpes simplex virus, type 1, can cause cold sores. Genital herpes is caused by the herpes simplex virus, type 2. Once contracted, the virus remains dormant in the nerve endings and may reactivate in a weakened immune system, high stress or with certain foods. Dietary suggestions can complement therapy under a qualified health practitioner for genital herpes. The most effective therapy is to avoid outbreaks by keeping immunity high, managing stress and avoiding foods that trigger the virus. Herbs can help by supporting the immune system and nourishing the nerves, where the virus resides.

WHAT TO DO

MAXIMIZE	MINIMIZE	ELIMINATE
• Antioxidant vegetables	• Fruits	• Nuts, wheat, caffeine, chocolate, carob, bacon, coffee, sugars, tomatoes, eggplant, peppers, mushrooms. These foods are high in arginine, an amino acid that encourages the herpes virus to replicate.
• Fish (salmon, sardines, tuna, halibut), legumes and nutritional yeast. These foods are high in lysine, which appears to inhibit replication of the virus	• Whole grains, seeds, brown rice. While high in argenine (see next column), these foods can be balanced with vegetables that are high in lysine.	
• Antiviral herbs: astragalus, calendula, echinacea, garlic, lemon balm, St. John's wort		• Alcohol, processed foods and unrefined foods, which depress the immune system
• Immune boosting herbs: astragalus, echinacea, burdock		
• Anti-stress herbs: ginseng, St. John's wort, lemon balm		

OTHER RECOMMENDATIONS

• Practice stress reduction techniques such as meditation, yoga and breathing exercises

RECIPES

Add 1 tsp (5 mL) herbs and up to 2 tbsp (25 mL) other ingredients recommended (at left) for this condition to the following juices.

Juices

Breakfast Cocktail	Allium Antioxidant	Brocco-Carrot
C-Green	Cabbage Rose (*use 2 tsp [10 mL] lemon balm instead of rosemary*)	

Teas

Immune Regulator	Cleansing Tea	Herp-eze Tea
Nerve Nourisher		

Tonics

Nerve Support

HYPOGLYCEMIA

see next page...

Hypoglycemia, or low blood sugar, is a disorder characterized by an overproduction of insulin. Symptoms can include aches and pains, constant hunger, dizziness, headache, fatigue, insomnia, digestive disorders, palpitations, tremor, sweating, nausea or nervous tension. You may notice some of these symptoms if you miss a regular meal. Attention to diet can help to control blood sugar levels.

Fruits and vegetables: apples, cherries, grapefruit, plums, raw beets, broccoli, cabbage, cauliflower, raw carrots, Jerusalem artichoke, leafy greens, tomatoes

Herbs: dandelion root, German chamomile, ginseng, licorice★

Other: cereal grasses, flax seeds, kelp, legumes, nuts, seeds, spirulina, whole grains, yogurt with live bacterial cultures

★ *Avoid licorice in cases of high blood pressure. Prolonged use not recommended in any circumstances.*

WHAT TO DO		
MAXIMIZE	**MINIMIZE**	**ELIMINATE**
• Whole grains, vegetables and legumes • Smaller meals eaten more frequently • Eat protein with each meal • Cruciferous vegetables (broccoli, cabbage, cauliflower) help to control blood sugar	• Sweet foods, including fruits, (particularly bananas, watermelon and dried fruit)	• Refined flour and sugar • Black tea, coffee, soda drinks, alcohol • Cigarette smoking, which interferes with blood-sugar mechanisms

RECIPES

Add 1 tsp (5 mL) herbs and up to 2 tbsp (25 mL) other ingredients recommended (at left) for this condition to the following juices.

Juices

Brocco-Artichoke | Cabbage Cocktail | Cauliflower Cocktail
Cherry Sunrise | Leafy Greens | Cruciferous

Teas

Camomile-Licorice★-Ginger | Root Decoction

Coffee Substitutes

Seed Power Coffee Blend

HEALING FOODS

Fruits and vegetables: a variety of highly colored fruit and vegetables

Herbs: astragalus, burdock, cayenne, cloves, echinacea, elder flower and berry, garlic, ginseng, green tea, licorice★, parsley, red clover, rosemary, sage, St. John's wort, thyme, turmeric

Other: cereal grass, legumes, nuts, seeds, shiitake mushrooms, whole grains, yogurt with live bacterial cultures

★ *Avoid licorice in cases of high blood pressure. Prolonged use not recommended in any circumstances.*

IMMUNE DEFICIENCY

A healthy immune system is key to resisting infections, allergies and chronic illness. The immune system protects and defends the body from viruses, bacteria, parasites and fungi. If the immune system is not in top condition, it will not be able to resist these disease-causing agents. Balance in diet, exercise, mental perspective, social life and spiritual life brings and sustains healing.

WHAT TO DO	
MAXIMIZE	**ELIMINATE**
• Whole food diet (see Guidelines to Good Health pages 10–11) • Fresh, raw organic fruits and vegetables, to provide the vitamins, minerals, digestive enzymes and antioxidants necessary for a healthy immune system • Whole grains • Legumes, nuts, seeds and oily fish (salmon, mackerel, herring, sardines), to provide essential fatty acids (EFAs), necessary for cell growth and maintenance • Fluid intake (at least 8 large glasses of water, juices or herbal teas daily)	• Sugar, which depletes vitamins and minerals, impairs the immune system and promotes yeast infections • Refined, processed, preserved foods and soda drinks. These disrupt mineral levels in the body, leading to poor metabolism of essential fatty acids • Food additives, pesticides in non-organic food • Alcohol, which depresses immune functioning • Antibiotics and corticosteroids. While these can be life-saving, overuse can deplete the immune system, causing more complex health problems

WHAT TO DO

MINIMIZE
- Non-organic meat and dairy products – which contain antibiotics and steroid hormones that depress immunity
- Excess fat, which suppresses immunity

ELIMINATE (CONTINUED)
- Margarine, salad dressing and cooking oils (except extra virgin olive oil and some other cold-pressed oils), which inhibit absorption of EFAs, leading to immune dysfunction
- Nitrites in bacon and sausage, which are converted into toxic substances in the body
- Food allergies, commonly dairy products, gluten, corn products, eggs, oranges, strawberries, pork, tomatoes, coffee, tea, peanuts, chocolate (see pages 254 to 255)

OTHER RECOMMENDATIONS
- Protein provides the amino acids necessary for building immune tissue, organs, and for antibody production.
- Optimize digestion to improve availability of nutrients (see Indigestion, page 84).
- Stress depletes the immune system. Practice stress-reduction activities such as yoga, meditation and tai chi.
- Use herbs that are immune system regulators (astragalus, echinacea, garlic, licorice, thyme).
- Use antibiotic herbs (burdock, cayenne, cloves, echinacea, garlic, red clover, thyme).
- Use antiviral herbs (burdock, elder flower and berry, garlic, ginger, lemon balm, licorice, marjoram, St. John's wort, yarrow).
- Use antioxidant herbs (astragalus, ginkgo, green tea, hawthorn, milk thistle, rosemary, sage, turmeric).

RECIPES

Add 1 tsp (5 mL) herbs and up to 2 tbsp (25 mL) other ingredients recommended (page 82, lower left) for this condition to the following juices.

Juices

Berry Fine Cocktail	Melon Morning Cocktail	Eye Opener
Black Pineapple	Allium Antioxidant	Artichoke-Carrot
Blazing Beets	C-Green	Flaming Antibiotic
Rust Proofer #2	Liquid Lunch	Immunity

Teas

Antioxi-T	The Green Diablo	Immune Regulator
Flu Fighter		

IMPOTENCE

HEALING FOODS

Fruits and vegetables: all

Herbs: cinnamon, cayenne, dandelion leaf, evening primrose oil, garlic, ginger, ginkgo, ginseng, nutmeg, saw palmetto, stinging nettles

continued…

Impotence, a man's inability to achieve or maintain an erection, may be caused by stress, insufficient blood supply to the penis (from cholesterol deposits in the blood vessels), excess alcohol, drugs, tobacco, diabetes, prostate enlargement or low testosterone.

A whole food diet helps to provide the vitamins and minerals necessary for sexual health. Herbal circulatory stimulants such as ginger and cayenne are often helpful for impotence caused by deficient circulation. See page 62 for suggestions on alleviating emotional stress.

Other: legumes, fish oil, flax seeds, kelp, nuts, oats, sunflower seeds, pumpkin seeds, soy products, wheat germ

WHAT TO DO

MAXIMIZE
- Fresh fruits and vegetables, whole grains, nuts and seeds. (see Guidelines to Good Health pages 10–11)
- Foods containing vitamin E (whole grain cereals, brown rice, nuts and seeds, wheat germ, soy products, kelp, dandelion leaves, extra virgin olive oil) to protect the arteries to the penis from free radical damage. Recent studies indicate better antioxidant effects when vitamin E comes from food rather than supplements.

ELIMINATE
- Fried foods, junk foods
- Sugar
- Caffeine (coffee, tea, colas)
- White flour products
- Alcohol

MINIMIZE
- Animal protein (except for fish and chicken)

RECIPES

Add 1 tsp (5 mL) herbs and up to 2 tbsp (25 mL) other ingredients recommended (page 83, at left) for this condition to the following juices and smoothies.

Juices
Cajun Cocktail Immune Juice | Blazing Beets | Flaming Antibiotic

Smoothies
B-Vitamin | Green Energy

Teas
Circulation | Adrenal Support | Ginseng

Coffee Substitutes
Seed Power Coffee Blend

INDIGESTION

Fruits and vegetables: apricots, bananas, lemons, mangoes, melons, papaya, pineapple, Jerusalem artichoke, leafy greens, squash, sweet potato

Herbs: cardamom, cayenne, coriander seeds, dandelion root, dill, German chamomile, cinnamon, cumin, fennel, ginger, lemon balm, meadowsweet, peppermint, slippery elm bark powder, turmeric

Other: almonds, barley, cider vinegar, flax seeds, rice, yogurt with active bacterial cultures

Over-eating, irregular eating, excess alcohol or nervous tension may cause occasional indigestion. Symptoms can include abdominal discomfort, nausea or gastric reflux. Chronic indigestion can be caused by irritable bowel syndrome, food intolerances, ulcer or gall bladder disorder. Symptoms of chronic indigestion can include bloating, fatigue, diarrhea or constipation.

WHAT TO DO

MAXIMIZE	MINIMIZE	ELIMINATE
• Relaxed, unhurried meals • Daily intake of yogurt with live bacterial cultures • Antioxidant fruit and vegetables • Food combining (see pages 256 to 257) • Digestive herbal teas, taken regularly between meals	• Alcohol • Tea • Coffee • Dairy products, eggs and meat	• Food allergies and intolerances (see pages 254 to 255) • Sugar and artificial sweeteners • Cold drinks, especially during or after meals • Fruit juices • High-fat foods, fried food • Dairy products (except yogurt) • Salty and spicy food • Refined foods • Heavy meals • Coffee

RECIPES

Add 1 tsp (5 mL) herbs and up to 2 tbsp (25 mL) other ingredients recommended (page 84, lower left) for this condition to the following juices and smoothies.

Juices

Breakfast Cocktail	Pineapple Kiwi	Leafy Greens
Squash Special		

Smoothies

B-Vitamin	Mango Madness

Teas

Digestive Tea	Spiced Papaya

Digestifs

Gripe Water	James Duke's Carminatea	Pineapple-Ginger
Rosy Peppermint	Gingerade	Tummy Aid

INFERTILITY, FEMALE

Some of the factors affecting fertility in women are age, vaginal infections, artificial lubricants, scarring from surgery, ovarian cysts, endometriosis, uterine fibroids, low thyroid function, deficient diet, stress and hormone imbalance.

Most important in ensuring a healthy pregnancy and birth is the mother's health before and during pregnancy. Whole, fresh, natural foods provide the vitamins and minerals necessary for health. For optimal health of the baby, it is worth taking a few months to build the mother's health before pregnancy.

An irregular menstrual cycle is a sign of hormonal imbalance. The herb chasteberry and liver-supportive herbs such as dandelion root may be used for regulating hormone production.

Fruits and vegetables: apricots, oranges, peaches raspberries, asparagus, avocado, beets, broccoli, carrot, leafy greens, sweet potatoes

Herbs: dandelion leaf and root, evening primrose oil, red clover flowers, red raspberry leaf, rosemary, stinging nettle leaf

Other: almonds, adzuki beans, brazil nuts, bulgar, kidney beans, sea herbs, seeds (sunflower, pumpkin, flax, sesame), soy products, wheat germ, yogurt with active bacterial cultures

WHAT TO DO

MAXIMIZE	MINIMIZE	ELIMINATE
• Whole food diet. (see pages 10–11) • Antioxidant fruits and vegetables • Nuts and seeds • Foods containing folic acid (bulgar, orange juice, spinach, beans, sunflower seeds, wheat germ)	• Acid-forming, thus sperm inhibiting, foods (meat, fish, grains, cheese, eggs, tea, coffee, alcohol, cranberries, plums, prunes, lentils, chickpeas, peanuts, walnuts)	• Refined flour • Smoking • Sugar • Artificial food additives

OTHER RECOMMENDATIONS

• For stress, use a tea made from nerve-nourishing herbs such as chamomile, skullcap, oatstraw or vervain, and regularly include relaxing activities such as walking, meditation, yoga or tai chi.

• Balance meat and fish protein (organic if possible) with vegetable proteins, such as soybean products or beans with rice.

RECIPES

Add 1 tsp (5 mL) herbs and up to 2 tbsp (25 mL) other ingredients recommended (page 85, lower left) for this condition to the following juices and smoothies.

Juices

Apricot-Peach	Raspberry Juice	Beet
Brocco-Carrot	Rust Proofer #2	

Smoothies

B-Vitamin	Beta Blast

Teas

Raspberry Tea	Hormone Balancing Tea

INFERTILITY, MALE

HEALING FOODS

Fruits and vegetables:
berries, cantaloupe, grapefruit, kiwi, oranges, strawberries, asparagus, avocado, broccoli, cabbage, cauliflower, leafy greens (especially spinach), peppers

Herbs: astragalus, cayenne, ginger, ginkgo, ginseng, raspberry leaf

Other: bran, fish oils, legumes, nuts, oats, seeds (especially sunflower and pumpkin), soybean products, whole grains

Male infertility is characterized by low sperm count and low sperm motility. The causes can be related to a deficiency in dietary nutrients, hormone imbalance or stress. There is some evidence that suggests the estrogens in pesticides and other chemical pollutants may be a cause of declining sperm counts in the last 50 years.

WHAT TO DO

MAXIMIZE	MINIMIZE
• Antioxidant fruit and vegetables, especially those containing vitamin C. Studies have shown that sperm motility requires a sufficient intake of vitamin C.	• Iodized salt. Excess iodine lowers sperm count.
	• Refined foods such as white rice and white flour products
• Foods containing zinc, required for sperm motility (seafood, legumes, whole grains, sunflower seeds, pumpkin seeds)	• Animal fats in meat and dairy products
	ELIMINATE
• Herbs to improve circulation (cayenne, ginger)	• Alcohol, coffee, tea and cola drinks, which decrease sperm health

OTHER RECOMMENDATIONS

• For stress, use a tea made from the nerve-nourishing herbs such as chamomile, skullcap, oatstraw or vervain, and regularly include relaxing activities such as walking, meditation, yoga or tai chi

RECIPES

Add 1 tsp (5 mL) herbs and up to 2 tbsp (25 mL) other ingredients recommended (at left) for this condition to the following juices.

Juices

Berry Fine Cocktail	Citrus Cocktail	C-Blitz
C-Green	Cauli-Slaw	

Teas

Circulation Tea	Ginseng	Raspberry Tea

Tonics

Stress Tonic

INFLAMMATORY BOWEL DISEASE

HEALING FOODS

see next page...

Crohn's disease and ulcerative colitis are serious diseases. Read all reference information on these diseases and consult with an experienced medical practitioner.

Fruits and vegetables: juice of beets and beet tops, carrot juice and boiled carrots, spinach juice

Herbs: garlic, German chamomile, marshmallow root, slippery elm bark powder, valerian★

Other: ground flax seeds, kelp, psyllium seed, rice

★ Valerian has an adverse effect on some people.

WHAT TO DO

MAXIMIZE	ELIMINATE
• Rice and cooked root vegetables	• Red meat which contributes to inflammation. Substitute with oily fish (salmon, sardines, tuna) and a little white chicken meat
• Beet juice, which provides nutrition, cleanses the blood and supports detoxification in the liver	• All foods that commonly cause bowel irritation: coffee, chocolate, mushrooms, alcohol, soft drinks, all junk food, all artificial coloring and flavoring, fried foods, salt
• Raw garlic daily, to cleanse the bowel of toxins	• Food allergies and intolerances, commonly dairy products, wheat, rye, oats and corn products, citrus fruits, eggs, cruciferous vegetables (broccoli, cabbage, cauliflower, Brussels sprouts), tomatoes, yeast (see page 254 to 255)
• Food Combining, (see pages 257–258) to optimize nutrition and absorption of nutrients	• Sugar and sugar products
• Water and herbal teas between meals	• Cigarettes

RECIPES

Add 1 tsp (5 mL) herbs and up to 2 tbsp (25 mL) other ingredients (at left) recommended for this condition to the following juices.

Juices

Beet	Leafy Greens	Popeye's Power

Teas

Digestive Stress Soother

INFLUENZA

HEALING FOODS

Fruits and vegetables: lemon, oranges, pineapple, broccoli, carrots, Jerusalem artichoke, parsley, strawberries, spinach, watercress

Herbs: boneset, cayenne, cinnamon, echinacea, elder flower and berry, garlic, ginger, licorice★, peppermint, thyme, yarrow

Other: kelp, psyllium seed, well-cooked mushy rice

★ Avoid licorice in cases of high blood pressure. Prolonged use not recommended in any circumstances.

Influenza is a viral infection of the respiratory tract. Symptoms can include chills, fever, cough, headache, achiness, fatigue, and lack of appetite. Treating the flu early can shorten recovery time and avoid more serious disease. Top priorities are rest, to allow the body's energies to focus on healing, and plenty of fluids, to encourage elimination of toxins.

Eating small meals, mainly vegetable juices, reduces the energy required for digestion, allowing more energy to be focussed on healing. "Hot" herbs, such as ginger and cayenne, increase the body temperature, discouraging the influenza virus.

WHAT TO DO

MAXIMIZE	ELIMINATE
• Fresh fruits and vegetables	• Alcohol, sugar and sugar products, which decrease immunity.
• Fluids: at least 8 large glasses a day of water, juices and herbal teas	

RECIPES

Add 1 tsp (5 mL) herbs and up to 2 tbsp (25 mL) other ingredients recommended (at left) for this condition to the following juices.

Juices

Brocco-Artichoke	Brocco-Carrot	Carrot-Allium
Flaming Antibiotic	Pineapple-Citrus	Spring Celebration
Immunity		

Teas

Antioxi-T	Flu Fighter

Mulled Juices

Antibiotic Toddy

INSOMNIA

HEALING FOODS

Fruits and vegetables: apples, bananas, lettuce, leafy greens

Herbs: German chamomile, hops★, lavender, lemon balm, passionflower, skullcap, St. John's wort, valerian★★, wild lettuce leaves

Other: honey, nuts, oats, sunflower seeds, brown rice, yogurt with live bacterial culture

★ *Hops are not to be taken in cases of depression*

★★ *Valerian causes adverse effects in some people.*

The inability to sleep may be caused by low blood sugar levels (see Hypoglycemia, page 81), anxiety, depression, heat or cold, or caffeine ingestion. Foods high in B vitamins, calcium and magnesium supply nutrients that calm the nerves, allowing sleep.

WHAT TO DO	
MAXIMIZE	**ELIMINATE**
• Calming, caffeine-free drinks	• Alcohol
• Foods high in B vitamins (whole grains, leafy green vegetables, broccoli, wheat germ), calcium (yogurt, tofu, broccoli) and magnesium (apples, avocados, black grapes, nuts, brown rice)	• Caffeine in tea, coffee, chocolate, soda drinks
	• Food additives

RECIPES

Add 1 tsp (5 mL) herbs and up to 2 tbsp (25 mL) other ingredients recommended (at left) for this condition to the following juice and smoothie.

Juices

Leafy Greens

Smoothies

Almond-Banana Milk

Teas

| Lavender | Nerve Support | Calming Cupa Tea Blend |

Coffee Substitutes

Anxiety Antidote

IRRITABLE BOWEL

HEALING FOODS

Fruits and vegetables: apples, apricots, kiwi, lemon, papaya, pineapple, broccoli, cabbage, carrot, parsley, spinach, tomato

Herbs: German chamomile, cinnamon, dandelion, fennel, ginger, lemon balm, licorice★, peppermint, slippery elm bark powder

Other: flax seeds, nuts, oat bran, tofu, yogurt with active bacterial cultures

★ *Avoid licorice in cases of high blood pressure. Prolonged use not recommended in any circumstances.*

Bloating, abdominal pain and diarrhea and/or constipation characterize irritable bowel syndrome.

Healing factors include diet, stress management and elimination of allergens. Herbs can be used to soothe the intestine, reduce inflammation, improve digestion, calm the nerves and promote intestinal healing.

WHAT TO DO	
MAXIMIZE	**ELIMINATE**
• Fish and vegetable proteins (nuts, seeds, tofu and beans)	• Alcohol
• Raw fruits and vegetables, to provide immune-boosting vitamins C and E, and to improve bowel function, helping to eliminate toxins	• Coffee
	• Red meat
	• Refined sugar and refined flour
	• Artificial sweeteners
• Flax seed and flax oil, which are soothing and anti-inflammatory, helping to heal the bowel and improve bowel function	• Fats and oils (except extra virgin olive oil)
• Food combining (see pages 256–7)	• Food allergies and intolerances, commonly dairy products, citrus fruit, caffeine, wheat and corn (see pages 254 to 255)

RECIPES

Add 1 tsp (5 mL) herbs and up to 2 tbsp (25 mL) other ingredients recommended (page 88, lower left) for this condition to the following juices.

Juices

Cabbage Cocktail	Cauliflower Cocktail

Teas

Digestive Stress Soother	Pepper-Spice	Ginger Tea

KIDNEY STONES

HEALING FOODS

Fruits and vegetables: apricots, mango, melon, peaches, asparagus, broccoli, celery, corn, fennel, leeks, onions

Herbs: goldenrod, marshmallow leaf and root, plantain, stinging nettles

Other: brown rice, seeds (flax, pumpkin, sesame, sunflower), whole grains

Kidney stones are 60% less common in vegetarian diets. A high-fiber, high-fluid, low-protein diet is the best preventive medicine. Diets high in animal protein encourage stone formation. Kidney stones are usually formed from calcium and oxalic acid. Stones consisting of uric acid and other mineral combinations are less common. Consult your health care practitioner to determine the type of stone and possible causes.

WHAT TO DO

MAXIMIZE	ELIMINATE
• Water intake (at least 2 large glasses of water 4 times a day between meals), to flush out stones and avoid bacterial build-up	• Salt and high-sodium foods such as bacon and processed food
	• Sugar
• Alkaline-forming foods such as oranges, lemons, all vegetables, (for uric acid stones)	• High-oxalate foods such as leafy greens, rhubarb, coffee, tea, chocolate, grapefruit, parsley, peanuts, strawberries, tomatoes (for oxalate stones)
MINIMIZE	
• Animal protein in meat and dairy products	• Seafood (for uric acid stones)
	• Alcohol
	• Refined flour

OTHER RECOMMENDATIONS

• Replace animal protein with soy and other vegetable protein (see Guidelines to Good Health page 10)

• Marshmallow leaf tea is soothing to the urinary system and may help break up stones

RECIPES

Add 1 tsp (5 mL) herbs and up to 2 tbsp (25 mL) other ingredients recommended (at left) for this condition to the following juices and smoothies.

Juices

Apricot-Peach	ABC Juice	Allium Antioxidant

Smoothies

Mango Madness

Teas

Free Flow

Coffee Substitutes

Seed Power Coffee Blend

LARYNGITIS

Fruits and vegetables: all fruit, carrot juice

Herbs: garlic, ginger, sage★, thyme

Other: honey★★

★ Avoid sage in cases of high blood pressure, pregnancy or breast-feeding

★★ Honey must not be given to children under one year

Laryngitis is an inflammation of the vocal cords that may be associated with a cold or other infection, or caused by excessive use of the voice. It is important to rest the voice for a few days. If laryngitis is accompanied by fever and a cough, or lasts longer than 2 days, consult a medical practitioner.

WHAT TO DO
MAXIMIZE
- Fruit and fruit juices
- Herbal teas and gargles

RECIPES
Add 1 tsp (5 mL) herbs and up to 2 tbsp (25 mL) other ingredients recommended (at left) for this condition to the following juices.

Juices		
Apricot-Peach	Beta Blast	C-Blend

Teas	
Antioxi-T	Throat Saver Tea Blend

LIVER PROBLEMS

Fruits and vegetables: apples, blackberries, dark grapes, plums, raspberries, beets, carrots, celery, leafy greens, onions, tomatoes, watercress

Herbs: alfalfa, astragalus, burdock root, cayenne, chicory root, dandelion root, fennel, fenugreek, German chamomile, ginger, dandelion leaf and root, lemon balm, licorice★, garlic, milk thistle, nettle leaf, parsley★★, rosemary, turmeric, yellow dock root

Other: cereal grasses, flax seeds, lecithin, legumes, olive oil (extra virgin), sea herbs, spirulina, whole grains

★ Avoid licorice in cases of high blood pressure. Prolonged use not recommended in any circumstances.

★★ In pregnancy, limit parsley intake to 1/2 tsp (2 mL) dried herb or a sprig of fresh herb per day. Parsley is not to be taken in kidney inflammation.

The liver is responsible for removing toxins that can interfere with nervous system functioning, digestive processing, heart function and circulation. Excess fat, chemicals, intoxicants and refined or processed food disrupt liver processing. Anger, nervous tension, mood swings and depression, skin problems, gall bladder problems, candida, menstrual and menopausal problems can result from poor liver function. The following dietary suggestions can supplement orthodox treatment in liver diseases such as hepatitis.

WHAT TO DO

MAXIMIZE	ELIMINATE
• Fruit and vegetables	• Foods that interfere with liver processing: animal fats, dairy products, eggs, refined foods, margarine, shortening, oils except extra virgin olive oil, alcohol, processed foods
• Legumes and whole grains	
• Bitter foods and herbs (asparagus, citrus peel, dandelion leaf, root and flowers, milk thistle seeds, chamomile flowers), which stimulate liver function	• Fried foods
• Water intake (at least 8 large glasses daily)	• Tobacco
• Dandelion root tea or "coffee"	• Sugar, sweets and junk food
	• Toxins in non-organic food

MINIMIZE
- Animal protein: replace with a little fish and vegetable protein (see Guidelines for Good Health, pages 10–11)

RECIPES
Add 1 tsp (5 mL) herbs and up to 2 tbsp (25 mL) other ingredients recommended (at left) for this condition to the following juices.

Juices			
Cell Support Cleanser	Apple Pear	Apple-Beet-Pear	Beet
Apple Fresh	Carrot-Apple	Popeye's Power	
Tomato Tang	Sunrise Supreme (use blackberries instead of strawberries)		

Teas	
Immune Regulator	Cleansing Tea

Coffee Substitutes
Root Coffee Blend

LOW LIBIDO

HEALING FOODS

Fruits and vegetables: apples, lemons, red grapes, beets, leafy greens, leeks, onions, watercress

Herbs: cayenne, cinnamon, cloves, fennel seeds, garlic, ginger, ginseng, mustard, parsley*, peppermint, rose petals, rosemary, stinging nettles

Other: almonds, Brazil nuts, fish oil, flax seeds, honey, legumes, oats, pumpkin seeds, soy products, grasses, sunflower seeds, walnuts, wheat germ, whole grains

* In pregnancy, limit parsley intake to 1/2 tsp (2 mL) dried herb or a sprig of fresh herb per day. Parsley is not to be taken in kidney inflammation.

Low libido, a lack of sexual interest or energy, can be remedied by nourishing the reproductive organs and improving overall energy levels.

Eat a whole food diet to provide the basic vitamins and minerals required for sexual health. Antioxidant fruits and vegetables improve circulation by preventing cholesterol deposits on blood vessel walls. The essential fatty acids in nuts and seeds are especially important in regulating sexual response.

Where stress is a factor, use nerve-nourishing oats, lemon balm or skullcap.

WHAT TO DO

MAXIMIZE	ELIMINATE
• Antioxidant fruit and vegetables	• Alcohol
• Nuts and seeds	• Coffee
• Whole grains	• Dairy products
• Herbs that stimulate circulation and energy (cayenne, cinnamon, cloves, garlic, ginger, rosemary) as well as the other herbs listed at left, which have been used traditionally as aphrodisiacs	• Refined and processed food
	• Sugar
	MINIMIZE
	• Meat

RECIPES

Add 1 tsp (5 mL) herbs and up to 2 tbsp (25 mL) other ingredients recommended (at left) for this condition to the following juices and smoothies.

Juices

Apple Fresh	Allium Antioxidant	Beet
Blazing Beets	Leafy Greens	

Smoothies

Green Energy

Teas

Ginseng	Circulation Tea

Other

Applesauce

LUPUS

HEALING FOODS

Fruits and vegetables: apples, apricots, blackberries, black currants, blueberries, cantaloupe, cherries, grapes, pineapple, avocado, broccoli, cabbage, carrots, cauliflower, fennel, leafy greens, onion, squash, watercress

continued...

There are two forms of the autoimmune disease lupus erythematosus: "discoid" (DLE), which affects only the skin, and "systemic" (SLE), which affects the connective tissue throughout the body. Early symptoms of SLE are fatigue, weight loss and fever, progressing to arthritis-like joint pains. In later stages, SLE may affect the kidneys and heart. Because this disease attacks the body's immune system, it is important to avoid viral infections, stress and fatigue. Nutrition and herbs can help by providing support and nourishment to the immune system, and to the organs responsible for detoxification. Relaxation exercises and plenty of sleep are important factors in supporting the immune system.

Herbs: burdock root, dandelion root and leaf, echinacea, elder-flower, evening primrose oil, fennel, garlic, ginger, lemon balm, licorice★, meadowsweet, stinging nettles, red clover flower, St. John's wort, thyme, turmeric

Other: cereal grasses, fish oil, flax seeds, legumes, olive oil (extra virgin), seeds, shiitake mushroom, soy products, whole grains, soy yogurt

★ Avoid licorice in cases of high blood pressure. Prolonged use not recommended in any circumstances.

★★ In pregnancy, limit parsley intake to 1/2 tsp (2 mL) dried herb or a sprig of fresh herb per day. Parsley is not to be taken in kidney inflammation.

WHAT TO DO	
MAXIMIZE	**ELIMINATE**
• Antioxidant fruit and vegetables • Water intake (a minimum of 8 glasses daily), to help eliminate toxins • Essential fatty acids in nuts and seeds (especially freshly ground flax seeds), to strengthen the immune system and improve blood flow	• Animal protein from meat and dairy products, which contribute to the progression of lupus. Substitute with vegetable protein soy products, legumes and rice • Food allergies and food intolerances. Keep a diet diary to note symptom changes in relation to food eaten (see pages 254 to 255) • Salad and cooking oils (except extra virgin olive oil), which promote inflammation • Sugar and alcohol, which inhibit immune functioning • Alfalfa seeds and sprouts which can cause inflammation

OTHER RECOMMENDATIONS

• Eat oily fish (salmon, mackerel, sardines, herrings) provides healing omega-6 oils three times a week
• Use anti-inflammatory herbs (German chamomile, elderflower, fennel, ginger, meadowsweet, turmeric)
• Use herbs that help elimination of toxins (burdock, dandelion root and leaf, parsley★★)
• Support the immune system with herbs and foods such as echinacea, garlic, shiitake mushroom, cereal grasses
• Exercise daily, according to fitness level

RECIPES

Add 1 tsp (5 mL) herbs and up to 2 tbsp (25 mL) other ingredients recommended (at left) for this condition to the following juices.

Juices

Apricot-Peach	Black Pineapple	Pine-Berry
Brocco-Carrot	Cauli-Slaw	C-Green
Cruciferous	Blueberry	

Teas

Immune Regulator	Antioxi-T	Nerve Nourisher

Coffee Substitutes

Easy Root Coffee

HEALING FOODS

Fruits and vegetables: apples, avocados, bananas, berries, grapes, peaches, pears, asparagus, carrots, celery, fennel, green bell pepper, leafy greens, tomatoes, watercress

continued...

MENOPAUSE

Menopause occurs when menstruation ceases. Hormonal changes around that time can result in irregular menstruation, hot flashes, mood changes and vaginal dryness. Stress magnifies these symptoms. Regular daily exercise, relaxation and a good diet (see Guidelines to Good Health, pages 10–11) will support a smooth transition and decrease the risk of heart disease and osteoporosis.

Nutritional and herbal support helps to balance hormones, improve blood circulation, support the elimination of toxins and reduce nervous tension.

In addition to the transition-smoothing herbs listed (page 93, upper left), the following herbs can be used for specific conditions and symptoms:
Chasteberry — to balance hormones

Herbs: dandelion root, fennel, garlic, ginseng, lemon balm, licorice★, motherwort, red clover flowers, rosemary, sage

Other: dried fruit, flax seeds, lentils, sea herbs, soy products, sunflower seeds, extra virgin olive oil, pumpkin seeds, wheat germ, whole grains, yogurt with live bacterial cultures

★ *Avoid licorice in cases of high blood pressure. Prolonged use not recommended in any circumstances.*

Ginseng, skullcap, oats or vervain — for stress and nervous tension
Valerian — for insomnia
Black cohosh — for joint pain, hot flashes or depression
Hawthorn berries — where there is a family risk of heart disease.

WHAT TO DO		
MAXIMIZE	**MINIMIZE**	**ELIMINATE**
• Antioxidant fruits and vegetables	• Animal fats	• Caffeine in tea, coffee, cocoa and chocolate
• Nuts and seeds		• Sugar
• Whole grains		• Cigarettes
		• Alcohol

RECIPES
Add 1 tsp (5 mL) herbs and up to 2 tbsp (25 mL) other ingredients recommended (at left) for this condition to the following juices and smoothies.

Juices
Apple Fresh	Grape Power	Leafy Greens
Pear-Fennel	Peppery Tomato Cocktail	Spring Celebration
Bone Builder		

Smoothies
Best Berries	Green Energy *(use ginseng in place of ginkgo)*

Teas
Women's Own	Cleansing Tea

HEALING FOODS

MENSTRUAL DISORDERS

Amenorrhea (absence of menstruation), dysmenorrhea (painful menstruation) and premenstrual syndrome (PMS) are often caused by a hormone imbalance, which is sometimes related to an excess of stress, exercise or animal products in the diet. Other factors can include insufficient blood or lymphatic circulation.

Fruits and vegetables: apricots, blueberries, blackberries, citrus fruit, grapes, strawberries, beets including greens, broccoli, carrots, leafy greens

Herbs: chasteberry, dandelion root and leaf, evening primrose oil, garlic, ginger, parsley★, skullcap, stinging nettles, yarrow

Other: almonds, dulse, fish oil, flax seeds, kelp, lecithin, legumes, nuts, pumpkin seeds, sesame seeds, soy products, sunflower seeds, whole grains

★ *In pregnancy, limit parsley intake to 1/2 tsp (2 mL) dried herb or a sprig of fresh herb per day. Parsley is not to be taken in kidney inflammation.*

The natural approach is to:
* *Balance hormones*
* *Support blood and lymphatic circulation to the pelvic organs*
* *Promote relaxation, regular moderate exercise and nutrition*
* *Improve digestion and elimination to improve nutrient absorption and to help regulate hormones*

WHAT TO DO	
MAXIMIZE	**ELIMINATE**
• Fruits and vegetables, especially those listed at left	• Refined food, which lacks minerals and vitamins
MINIMIZE	• Caffeine in coffee, tea and soda drinks, which depletes calcium and other minerals
• Salt and salty foods	• Sugar and sweeteners
• Alcohol	• Non-organic meat and dairy products, which can contain artificial hormones

OTHER RECOMMENDATIONS
* Balance lean meat or fish protein with vegetable protein (see page 10)
* Ensure sufficient dietary calcium (by eating foods such as yogurt, broccoli, tofu
* Exercise daily, according to fitness level

RECIPES

Add 1 tsp (5 mL) herbs and up to 2 tbsp (25 mL) other ingredients recommended (page 93, lower left) for this condition to the following juices and smoothies.

Juices

Beet	Brocco–Carrot	C–Green
Leafy Greens	Popeye's Power	Sunrise Supreme
Eye Opener *(use blueberries, blackberries or strawberries)*		

Smoothies

Best Berries	Pump It Up

Teas

Ginger Tea	Hormone-Balancing Tea

HEALING FOODS

Fruits and vegetables: beets, blackberries, broccoli, cantaloupe, carrots, celery, leafy greens, onion

Herbs: cayenne, cinnamon, dandelion leaf and root, fever-few, garlic, German chamomile, ginger, lemon balm, parsley★, vervain

Other: brown rice and rice bran, flax seeds, legumes, pumpkin seeds, sunflower seeds, whole grains

★ In pregnancy, limit parsley intake to 1/2 tsp (2 mL) dried herb or a sprig of fresh herb per day. Parsley is not to be taken in kidney inflammation.

MIGRAINE

A migraine headache starts with the constriction of blood vessels in the brain, followed by an expansion, which causes the pain. Warning symptoms — such as vision changes or mood changes — can come with the blood vessel constriction. The pain usually starts on one side, but may spread to both sides, and may be accompanied by nausea or dizziness. Migraine triggers can include strong emotion, hormonal changes, food allergies and some medications, including oral contraceptives.

WHAT TO DO

MAXIMIZE	ELIMINATE
• Vegetable protein (see Guidelines to Good Health, page 10) • Fresh fruit and vegetables	• Caffeine from coffee, colas, chocolate • Food allergies and intolerances associated with migraine. The most common are dairy products, wheat, eggs, oranges, MSG (see pages 254 to 255)
MINIMIZE	• Dietary triggers: red wine, cheese, corn, smoked or pickled fish, sausages, hot dogs and all other pre-served meats, pork, shellfish, walnuts
• Animal fats • Sugar	• Food additives • Alcohol

OTHER RECOMMENDATIONS
• Eat oily fish (cod, salmon, trout, tuna) 2 or 3 times a week
• A leaf or two of fresh feverfew, taken daily can help prevent migraines
• Practice food combining (see page 258)

RECIPES

Add 1 tsp (5 mL) herbs and up to 2 tbsp (25 mL) other ingredients recommended (at left) for this condition to the following juices and smoothies.

Juices

Beet	Brocco–Carrot	C–Green
Liquid Lunch		

Smoothies

Calming Chamomile

Teas

Ginger Tea	Migraine Buster

MULTIPLE SCLEROSIS

Fruits and vegetables: grapes, pineapple, beets, cabbage, cauli-flower, leafy greens

Herbs: astragalus, dandelion root, evening primrose oil, ginger, ginseng, skullcap

Other: flax seeds, fish oil, lecithin, soy milk, cereal grasses, olive oil (extra virgin), brown rice, wheat germ, mung beans, sea vegetables, tofu

Multiple sclerosis is the breakdown of the protective myelin sheaths around the brain and spinal cord. Although the cause is not known, there have been impressive results with the recommendations given below.

WHAT TO DO

MAXIMIZE	ELIMINATE
• Foods low in saturated fat	• Candida infections
• Essential fatty acids (evening primrose oil, flax seed oil, fish oils)	• Allergies and food intolerances from the diet (see pages 254 to 255)
• Foods high in B vitamins (fish, wheat germ and sea herbs) and magnesium (apple, avocado, banana, leafy greens, fish, nuts, soy products, brown rice, wheat germ), to nourish the nerve tissue	• Coffee
	• Red meat, including the dark meat on chicken or turkey
	• Dairy products, eggs
	• Gluten
• Lifestyle quality. Evaluate and reduce stresses in your life, assisted by meditation, yoga, tai chi or taking daily long walks in natural surroundings	• Fats and oils except cold-pressed oils such as extra virgin olive oil
	MINIMIZE
	• Animal fats

RECIPES

Add 1 tsp (5 mL) herbs and up to 2 tbsp (25 mL) other ingredients recommended (at left) for this condition to the following juices and smoothies.

Juices

Beet	Cauli-Slaw	Green Beet
Leafy Greens	Sea Herb Surprise	

Smoothies

Smart Smoothie

Teas

Nerve Nourisher	Immune Regulator

Tonics

Astragalus	Spring Tonic

OSTEOPOROSIS

Fruits and vegetables: pineapple, avocado, broccoli, cabbage, leafy greens, watercress

Herbs: alfalfa, chamomile, dandelion leaf, oat straw parsley*, plantain, stinging nettles

Other: blackstrap molasses, dried fruit, fish and fish oil, legumes, nuts and seeds, feta cheese, sardines, salmon, seaweeds, spirulina, tofu, whole grains, yogurt with active bacterial cultures

Osteoporosis is progressive bone loss and decreased bone density and strength, caused by loss of calcium from the bones. Consumption of calcium-rich foods along with other nutrient-rich food helps to promote bone strength. Calcium absorption requires adequate dietary vitamins and minerals.

Factors in bone loss:
- *Age*
- *Decreased estrogen levels. Estrogen enhances calcium absorption*
- *Weight-bearing exercise increases calcium absorption; inactivity decreases it*
- *Some prescription drugs interfere with calcium absorption*
- *Chronic stress depletes immediate supply and stored levels of calcium*
- *Lack of minerals and vitamins in the diet inhibits calcium absorption*
- *Disease of thyroid or adrenal gland*

In pregnancy, limit parsley intake to 1/2 tsp (2 mL) dried herb or a sprig of fresh herb per day. Parsley is not to be taken in kidney inflammation.

WHAT TO DO

MAXIMIZE	MINIMIZE (CONTINUED)
Foods known to promote calcium absorption:	*Foods known to increase calcium loss:*
• Raw fruits and green vegetables	• High-protein (meat and dairy) diets lead to bone loss through calcium excretion in the urine
• Nuts and seeds	• Fats, which decrease calcium absorption in the stomach
• Legumes	• Refined flour, which is nutrient depleted, causing a deficiency of minerals
MINIMIZE	• Prepared food which contains chemicals that add toxins and deplete minerals
Foods known to increase calcium loss:	• Food grown with non-organic fertilizers cause depletion of minerals
• Sugar, salt, caffeine which cause calcium to be excreted through the urine	• Bran, tomatoes, potatoes, eggplant and peppers
• Alcohol	
• Phosphorus rich foods especially soft drinks	

RECIPES

Add 1 tsp (5 mL) herbs and up to 2 tbsp (25 mL) other ingredients recommended (see left) for this condition to the following juices and smoothies.

Juices

Black Pineapple Bone Builder	Brocco-Carrot	Leafy Greens

Smoothies

Avocado–Pineapple	B-Vitamin	Sea-Straw Smoothie

Teas

Bone Blend	Cleansing Tea	Digestive Tea

Tonics

Astragalus

HEALING FOODS

Fruits and vegetables: apples, blackberries, cherries, citrus fruit, grapes, pineapple, strawberries, watermelon, asparagus, broccoli, cabbage, celery, cucumber, fennel, leafy greens, lettuce, Jerusalem artichokes, radishes, watercress

Herbs: cayenne, chickweed, dandelion leaf and root, evening primrose oil, fennel, garlic, ginger, parsley*, psyllium seeds

Other: cider vinegar, flax seeds, kelp, legumes, soy products, walnuts, whole grains

In pregnancy, limit parsley intake to 1/2 tsp (2 mL) dried herb or a sprig of fresh herb per day. Parsley is not to be taken in kidney inflammation.

OVERWEIGHT

Excessive weight can be caused by insufficient exercise (relative to the amount eaten), hormonal imbalances, and some drugs (including corticosteroids and birth control pills). Long-term weight loss is most effectively achieved by adopting a whole food diet and increased exercise.

WHAT TO DO

MAXIMIZE	MINIMIZE	ELIMINATE
• Fresh fruits and vegetables, which help speed up the metabolism and eliminate toxins	• Refined flour products, fast food and junk foods	• Sugar and artificial sweeteners
• Water intake (at least 8 glasses a day), to help reduce appetite and eliminate toxins	• Fats from meat, dairy and salad oils (except extra virgin olive oil)	• Fried food
	• Starchy food, including breads, corn, parsnips, potatoes, squash, sweet potatoes	• Food additives

OTHER RECOMMENDATIONS

• Eat oily fish (salmon, sardines, mackerel) 2 or 3 times a week to help the body burn excess fat.

• Consider food allergies and intolerances that may affect digestion. Common allergies include milk products, eggs, oranges and gluten (see pages 254–5).

- Eat fruit between meals for optimum digestion and to discourage snacking on junk foods.
- Exercise daily, according to fitness level.
- Drink fresh juices as an alternative to empty-calorie drinks and snacks.

RECIPES

Add 1 tsp (5 mL) herbs and up to 2 tbsp (25 mL) other ingredients recommended (page 96, lower left) for this condition to the following juices and smoothies.

Juices

Citrus Cocktail	Melon Morning Cocktail	Black Pineapple
Cherry Sunrise	Sunrise Supreme	Brocco–Artichoke
C-Green	Popeye's Power	Soft Salad
The Chiller		

Smoothies

B-Vitamin	Sea-Straw Smoothie

Teas

Ginger Tea	Cleansing Tea	Digestive Tea

PARKINSON'S DISEASE

HEALING FOODS

Fruits and vegetables: bananas, blueberries, strawberries, beets, carrots, leafy greens, lettuce, potatoes

Herbs: alfalfa, evening primrose oil, ginger, ginkgo, milk thistle seed, passionflower, St. John's wort

Other: legumes, nuts, oats, olive oil, peanuts, seeds (flax, sesame, sunflower and pumpkin), soy lecithin, spelt flour, whole grains (except wheat)

Parkinson's disease — with its symptoms of muscular rigidity, loss of reflexes, slowness of movement, trembling and shaking — is caused by degeneration of nerve cells within the brain, leading to a deficiency of the neurotransmitter dopamine. While there is no cure for Parkinson's, dietary therapy can help to prevent degeneration of neurons by neurotoxins. Choose food that is high in antioxidants, and avoid free-radical-causing pollutants and heavy metals by choosing fresh, organic foods.

WHAT TO DO

MAXIMIZE	MINIMIZE	ELIMINATE
• Raw, antioxidant, organic fruits and vegetables, to optimize vitamins, minerals and digestive enzymes • Nuts and seeds (especially sunflower seeds), to provide vitamin E, which can slow progression of the disease. Legumes are also a source of vitamin E	• Protein from meat and dairy products, which aggravates Parkinson's symptoms	• Refined and processed foods • Sugar and artificial sweeteners • Alcohol • Wheat and liver contain manganese, which may aggravate the disease • Fatty foods, fried foods, margarine and oils (except extra virgin olive oil)

OTHER RECOMMENDATIONS

- Fava beans (broad beans) contain levodopa, a precursor to dopamine. Eating 1/2 cup (125 mL) a day can decrease the amount of medication required. Discuss with your doctor to avoid overdosing.
- Passionflower herb can help reduce tremors.
- Ginkgo biloba improves blood circulation to the brain, bringing more nutrients to prevent cell damage.
- Avoid aluminum-containing antacids, cookware, deodorants and water. Aluminum may have adverse effects in Parkinson's.
- Ground flax seeds help with constipation and provide essential fatty acids to nourish brain and nerve tissue.
- Fatty fish (salmon, sardines, mackerel, herrings) provides essential fatty acids to nourish brain and nerve tissue.

RECIPES

Add 1 tsp (5 mL) herbs and up to 2 tbsp (25 mL) other ingredients recommended (page 97, lower left) for this condition to the following juices and smoothies.

Juices		
Beet	C-Green	Eye Opener

Smoothies		
Spa Special	Smart Smoothie	Pump It Up *(use flax seeds instead of protein powder)*

Teas		
Ginger Tea	Circulation Tea	Antioxi-T

PEPTIC ULCERS
(GASTRIC ULCER AND DUODENAL ULCER)

HEALING FOODS

Fruits and vegetables: apples, apricots, bananas, blueberries, cantaloupe, cherries, red grapes (with seeds), mangoes, papaya, pears, avocado, cabbage, carrots, cucumber, broccoli, leafy greens, onions, watercress

Herbs: calendula, cinnamon, cloves, dandelion root, echinacea, garlic, German chamomile, ginger, green tea, licorice*, marshmallow root, meadowsweet, parsley**, slippery elm bark powder, tumeric

Other: barley, cereal grass, extra-virgin olive oil, honey, legumes, seeds, oats

* Avoid licorice in cases of high blood pressure. Prolonged use not recommended in any circumstances.

** In pregnancy, limit parsley intake to 1/2 tsp (2 mL) dried herb or a sprig of fresh herb per day. Parsley is not to be taken in kidney inflammation.

Stomach and intestinal ulcers, called peptic ulcers, occur when the protective mucous lining breaks down, usually caused by an infection from heliobacter pylori *bacteria. Food allergies are often connected. Aspirin, steroid medication and non-steroidal anti-inflammatory medications increase acid secretions that break down the protective mucous lining of the intestine. Stress is a factor. Healing involves minimizing acids that erode the stomach and intestinal lining, protecting and soothing the intestinal lining, stimulating the immune system and inhibiting bacteria. Herbs that have anti-inflammatory, anti-bacterial, calming and mucous-protective actions are helpful in healing ulcers.*

WHAT TO DO

MAXIMIZE
- Fruits and vegetables, which provide healing vitamins and protection from infection. Fully ripe, sweet fruit is more soothing than sour fruits
- Slippery elm bark powder which provides a coating to the intestinal tract that protects against acid. It is especially effective taken at bedtime, to provide protection from acids while sleeping.
- Fluid intake (between meals only)

MINIMIZE
- Salt

ELIMINATE
- Caffeine in tea, coffee, chocolate and decaffeinated coffee, which stimulates secretion of stomach acid
- Dairy products, which lead to increased acidity
- Alcohol, soda drinks and refined grains, which promote ulceration
- Refined grains and sugar
- Ulcer-causing drugs such as steroids, aspirin and other non-steroidal anti-inflammatories
- Very hot liquids, which irritate the ulcer
- Cigarette smoking
- Fried foods and oils (except extra virgin olive oil)

OTHER RECOMMENDATIONS
- Eat smaller, more frequent meals and avoid eating late at night
- Seek stress handling techniques such as meditation, yoga and tai chi
- Drink raw cabbage juice daily
- Practice food combining techniques (see pages 256 to 257)

RECIPES

Add 1 tsp (5 mL) herbs and up to 2 tbsp (25 mL) other ingredients recommended (page 98, lower left) for this condition to the following juices and smoothies.

Juices

Cabbage Cocktail	Berry Best	Pear-Fennel

Smoothies

Blue Cherry	Calming Chamomile	Pump It Up

Mango Madness *(use apple juice instead of orange juice)*

Teas

Digestive Stress Soother	Immune Regulator	Chamomile-Licorice-Ginger

Tonics

Stress Tonic

Other

Root Coffee Blend

PREGNANCY

HEALING FOODS

Fruits and vegetables: bananas, cantaloupe, citrus fruit, strawberries, avocados, carrots, leafy greens, peas, sweet potato, watercress

Herbs: alfalfa, dandelion root and leaf, lemon balm, nettles, oatstraw, red raspberry leaf, rose hips

Note: See Herbs to Avoid in Pregnancy, pages 258 to 259.

Other: dulse, flax seeds, kelp, legumes, blackstrap molasses, nuts (especially almonds) olive oil (extra virgin), soy products, seeds (especially sunflower), wheatgerm, whole grains, yogurt with live bacterial cultures

Nutrition is vital to the baby's health during both preconception and in pregnancy. Ideally, nutrients should come from food rather than supplements. Choose natural, unprocessed whole grains, beans, fruit, vegetables, nuts and seeds as the base of your diet, adding sufficient protein in the form of lean meat, fish or soybean products.

WHAT TO DO

MAXIMIZE	MINIMIZE	ELIMINATE
• Fruits and vegetables	*Foods known to increase calcium loss:*	• Alcohol
• Nuts and seeds		• Food additives
• Folic acid (egg yolk, wheat germ, leafy greens, soy beans, asparagus, oranges)	• Sugar and sweeteners	• Food pesticides,
	• Tea, coffee, soda drinks	• Junk food
• Omega-3 oils (flax seeds, walnuts, oily fish [salmon, tuna, mackerel, herring, sardines])	• Fats	
	• Refined flour	
	• Bran, tomatoes, potatoes, eggplant, peppers	

RECIPES

Add 1 tsp (5 mL) herbs and up to 2 tbsp (25 mL) other ingredients recommended (at left) for this condition to the following juices and smoothies.

Juices

Beta Blast	Citrus Cocktail	Folic Plus
Kelp	Leafy Greens	Peas & Carrots

Smoothies

Avocado-Pineapple

Teas

Mother's Own

HEALING FOODS

Fruits and vegetables: apples, citrus fruits, pears, asparagus, beets, broccoli, cauliflower, leafy greens, onions, tomatoes, watercress

Herbs: garlic, ginger, goldenrod, green tea, fresh nettle root, parsley, plantain, saw palmetto berries

Other: almonds, Brazil nuts, cashews, flax seeds, kelp, pecans, pumpkin seeds, sesame seeds, turmeric

PROSTATE ENLARGEMENT, BENIGN

Prostate enlargement commonly occurs in 50% of men age 50, 60% of men age 60, and so on to 100% of men age 100. Enlargement blocks the urinary passage, obstructing the flow of urine.

WHAT TO DO

MAXIMIZE	MINIMIZE
• Antioxidant fruits and vegetables	• Fat in meat and dairy products
• Tomatoes, to reduce risk of prostate cancer	**ELIMINATE**
• Soy foods, which have a prostate-protective effect	• Caffeine in coffee, tea, chocolate and soda drinks, which limits calcium absorption
• Zinc-rich foods (shellfish, brown rice, legumes, leafy greens, dried fruit, onions, sunflower seeds, pumpkin seeds, egg yolk). Zinc has been shown to reduce prostate size	• Alcohol, which flushes zinc out of system
	• Foods containing additives, pesticides or hormones
• Foods containing vitamin C (citrus fruits, berries, leafy greens, parsley, peppers), help zinc absorption	• Margarine and cooking oils (except extra virgin olive oil)
	• Fried foods
• Foods rich in vitamin B6 (bananas, cabbage, egg yolk, leafy greens, legumes, prunes, raisins, soybeans, sunflower seeds), to improve effectiveness of zinc	• Sugar and sugar products

OTHER RECOMMENDATIONS

• Eat oily fish (salmon, mackerel, sardines, tuna) 2 to 3 times a week.

• Ensure sufficient dietary protein to help absorb zinc.

RECIPES

Add 1 tsp (5 mL) herbs and up to 2 tbsp (25 mL) other ingredients recommended (at left) for this condition to the following juices and smoothie recipes.

Juices

Berry Fine Cocktail	C-Blend	C-Blitz
Raspberry Juice	Allium Antioxidant	Kelp
Spring Celebration	Tomato Juice Cocktail	ABC Juice
Beet	C-Green	Leafy Greens
Cruciferous	Strawberry-Orange Lemonade	

Smoothies

B-Vitamin

Teas

Free Flow	Ginger Tea	Saw Palmetto

HEALING FOODS

Fruits and vegetables: apricots, cantaloupe, citrus fruit, mango, pumpkin, strawberry, watermelon, asparagus, broccoli, cabbage, carrots, green beans, leafy greens, papaya, red and green bell pepper

continued...

SINUSITIS

Inflammation of the sinuses can result from colds, influenza, allergies or dental infections. Avoid mucous-forming food in the diet, and look for food allergies.

Herbs: cayenne, dandelion leaf and root, elderflowers, ginger, echinacea, garlic, parsley★

Other: legumes, lentils, pumpkin seeds, sea herbs, sunflower seeds, wheat germ

★ *In pregnancy, limit parsley intake to 1/2 tsp (2 mL) dried herb or a sprig of fresh herb per day. Parsley is not to be taken in kidney inflammation.*

WHAT TO DO

MAXIMIZE	ELIMINATE
• Foods high in vitamin C such as citrus fruit, strawberry, parsley • Foods rich in vitamin E (wheat germ, nuts, seeds, cabbage, soy lecithin, spinach, asparagus) • Beta carotene from foods such as carrots, mango, cantaloupes, apricots, watermelon, red pepper, pumpkin, leafy greens, parsley, papayas • Zinc-rich foods such as pumpkin seeds, fish and sea herbs • Liquids: water and vegetable juices • Fresh, raw garlic daily to reduce and prevent sinus congestion	• Alcohol • Bananas, which are mucous forming • Dairy products (except yogurt with active bacterial cultures) • Eggs • Food allergies and intolerances (see pages 254 to 255) • Refined sugar and flour products
	MINIMIZE • Starchy foods such as grains

RECIPES

Add 1 tsp (5 mL) herbs and up to 2 tbsp (25 mL) other ingredients recommended (at left) for this condition to the following juices.

Juices

Beta Blast	C–Blitz	Brocco–Carrot
Allium Antioxidant	Beta-Carro	

Coffee Substitutes

Seed Power Coffee Blend

SKIN CONDITIONS
(ACNE, DRY SKIN, PSORIASIS, ROSACEA)

HEALING FOODS

Fruits and vegetables: apples, apricots, berries, cantaloupe, grapes, mangoes, papaya, pears, carrots, cucumber, leafy greens, beets and beet greens, pumpkin, squash, watercress

Herbs: burdock root, leaf and seeds, calendula, cleavers, dandelion root and leaf, echinacea, evening primrose oil, licorice★, fennel, red clover flower, stinging nettles, yellow dock root

Other: olive oil (extra virgin), soy products, pumpkin seeds, sesame seeds, sunflower seeds, flax seeds, lentils, oats, seaweeds, spirulina, whole grains, yogurt with active bacterial cultures

★ *Avoid licorice in cases of high blood pressure. Prolonged use not recommended in any circumstances.*

Acne usually responds to the dietary changes and cleansing herbs listed at left. When acne is related to the menstrual cycle, include the hormone-balancing herb Chasteberry (Vitex agnus-castus).

Dry skin. Adding essential fatty acids to your diet helps to nourish dry skin. Food sources include extra virgin olive oil, freshly ground flax seeds, fresh walnuts and hazelnuts and oily fish, such as mackerel, sardine and salmon.

Psoriasis is an increase in proliferation of skin, causing red, scaly plaques. It usually affects the elbows and knees. The cause is unknown, but it is often related to stress and emotional state. Herbs such as chamomile, skullcap, lemon balm can help to provide relaxation. Sunlight and sea bathing are helpful treatments. Relaxation exercises such as meditation, yoga and tai chi can help bring the emotional state into balance. A "healthy skin" diet is also important. Avoid nuts (which can aggravate psoriasis) as well as citrus fruits and tomatoes.

Rosacea. Acne rosacea is a chronic inflammatory skin disease in which too much oil is produced by the glands in the skin. It is often associated with digestive disorders. The dietary suggestions and cleansing herbs listed on the following page are usually effective in clearing this condition.

WHAT TO DO

MAXIMIZE	MINIMIZE	ELIMINATE
• Fresh fruits and vegetables	• Salt	• Red meat
• Foods rich in beta carotene (carrots, broccoli, leafy greens, apricots, papaya)	• Animal protein. Replace with vegetable protein (see Guidelines to Good Health, page 10)	• Shellfish
		• Sugar
		• Fried foods
• Blood-cleansing herbs (dandelion, burdock, yellow dock)		• Oranges
		• Chocolate
		• Refined flour
• Herbal nerve relaxants (chamomile, skullcap, lemon balm, oat seed)		• Coffee, black tea
		• Dairy products
		• Soda drinks
• Seeds (flax, pumpkin, sunflower)		• Artificial food additives including sweeteners
		• Alcohol

OTHER RECOMMENDATIONS

- Drink at least 8 cups water or herb teas a day to flush out toxins
- Eat oily fish (salmon, sardines, mackerel) 2 to 3 times a week to provide skin-nourishing essential fatty acids

RECIPES

Add 1 tsp (5 mL) herbs and up to 2 tbsp (25 mL) other ingredients recommended (page 101, lower left) for this condition to the following juices.

Juices

Crimson Cleanser	Breakfast Cocktail	Beta Blast
Pear-Fennel	Carrot-Apple	Beet
Leafy Greens	Popeye's Power	

Teas

Cleansing Tea

SMOKING (QUITTING)

HEALING FOODS

Fruits and vegetables: cantaloupe, citrus fruit, broccoli, carrots, leafy greens

Herbs: German chamomile, red clover, skullcap

Other: oats, oat bran, pumpkin seeds, sunflower seeds, tofu

As well as being a major cause of heart and lung disease and cancer, smoking contribute to loss of calcium (leading to osteoporosis) and is a risk factor in high blood pressure and ulcers. By constricting the blood vessels, thus decreasing blood circulation to peripheral parts of the body, smoking increases the risk of stroke, impotence in men, and face wrinkles in women.

Studies have shown that, whether you are a smoker or not, fresh fruit and vegetables improve respiratory function and reduce the risk of any kind of cancer.

WHAT TO DO

REDUCE CRAVINGS

- Maintain constant blood sugar by eating 6 meals a day, consisting of fresh fruits, and vegetables, with a little protein and whole grains.
- Ease withdrawal symptoms with a mainly vegetarian diet, which slows down the removal of nicotine from the body.
- Exercise regularly. Walking and breathing exercises are excellent.
- Snack on sunflower seeds and pumpkin seeds – the zinc content may reduce cravings by blocking taste enzymes.
- Eat plenty of oats. Studies show that oats diminish cravings.
- Soothe the nerves by drinking calming herbal teas.

RECIPES

Add 1 tsp (5 mL) herbs and up to 2 tbsp (25 mL) other ingredients recommended (page 102, lower left) for this condition to the following juices and smoothies.

Juices

Beta Blast	C–Blast	Grapefruit
Orange Zinger	Brocco-Carrot	Leafy Greens

Smoothies

Beta Blast	Calming Chamomile	Green Energy

Specialty Drinks

Melon Cocktail

Teas

Calming Cuppa	Nerve Nourisher

URINARY TRACT INFECTIONS

HEALING FOODS

Fruits and vegetables:
blueberry, cranberries, lemon, watermelon, carrot, celery, fennel, onion, parsnip, turnip

Herbs: buchu, cinnamon, coriander, cumin, dandelion leaf, echinacea, fennel seeds, garlic, marshmallow root, nettle, slippery elm bark powder, yarrow★

Other: pumpkin seeds, yogurt with active bacterial cultures, barley

★ *Avoid yarrow in pregnancy.*

Urinary tract infections can be caused by yeast or bacteria. The infection can pass into the bladder, causing cystitis.

Cystitis, inflammation of the bladder, is characterized by frequent, painful urination. Bacteria settle into the irritated tissue of the bladder.

WHAT TO DO

MAXIMIZE

- Water intake. Drink 8 to 10 cups (2 to 2 1/2 L) of water, vegetable juices and herbal teas daily, to dilute and wash out the bacteria
- Unsweetened cranberry and blueberry juices, to prevent bacteria from adhering to the bladder
- Onions and garlic are anti-bacterial. Raw garlic is best. Add garlic to juices and use, freshly squeezed, on salads and vegetables or chop a garlic clove into pieces small enough to swallow
- Barley water. This is an old, soothing remedy for inflammation
- Herbs that are anti-bacterial, soothing to the bladder, and those which promote urination (see recommendations at left)

MINIMIZE

- Meat. Replace with vegetable protein (tofu, or legumes and rice)
- Alcohol, sugar and artificial food additives, which irritate an inflamed bladder
- Refined sugar and flour products
- Dairy products

ELIMINATE

- Caffeine in coffee, tea and soda drinks

Add 1 tsp (5 mL) herbs and up to 2 tbsp (25 mL) other ingredients recommended (at left) for this condition to the following juices and smoothies.

Juices

Blue Water	Cranberry Juice	Celery
Nip of Goodness		

Smoothies

Cran-Orange	Watermelon

Teas and Tonics

Free Flow Tea	Barley Water Tonic

UTERINE FIBROIDS

Fruits and vegetables: apples, beets, carrots, celery, leafy greens, watercress

Herbs: burdock root, chasteberry, cinnamon, dandelion leaf and root, garlic, ginger, red clover, red raspberry leaf, stinging nettle, vervain, yarrow, yellow dock

Other: kelp, tofu, whole grains

Uterine fibroids are benign growths that are stimulated by estrogen. They can cause pain, heavy menstrual bleeding, anemia, and bladder problems. At menopause, when estrogen levels drop, fibroids usually shrink.

Increase pelvic circulation with exercise such as walking, yoga and dancing.

Correct anemia, if present (see Anemia, page 61). Correct constipation, if present (see Constipation page 69)

WHAT TO DO

MAXIMIZE	ELIMINATE
• Sea herbs to reduce tumor growths	• Non-organic meat, poultry and dairy products, which contain estrogen
• Roughage from fresh fruits and vegetables and whole grains, to improve elimination of toxins	• Caffeine, which increases estrogen levels
• Hormone-balancing herbs (chasteberry) and liver-supporting herbs and vegetables (beets, carrots, dandelion root, burdock root, milk thistle seed)	• Fried food, margarine and oils (except extra virgin olive oil)
	• Alcohol
	• Food additives, preservatives and colorings, which contribute to accumulation of toxins and hormone imbalance

RECIPES

Add 1 tsp (5 mL) herbs and up to 2 tbsp (25 mL) other ingredients recommended (at left) for this condition to the following juices.

Juices

Beet *(add 1/2" piece ginger)*	Carrot-Apple	Kelp
Leafy Green		

Teas

Circulation Tea	Relax Tea	Cleansing Tea
Hormone Balancing Tea		

Coffee Substitutes

Easy Root Coffee

VARICOSE VEINS AND HEMORRHOIDS

Fruits and vegetables: berries (blueberries, strawberries, raspberries, blackberries), cherries, citrus fruits, pears, red grapes, broccoli, cabbage, leafy greens, onions, watercress

Herbs: alfalfa, burdock seed and root, cayenne, dandelion leaf and root, garlic, ginger, horse chestnut, parsley*, witch hazel, yarrow

Other: buckwheat, dulse, kelp, legumes, nuts, oats, olive oil (extra virgin), soy products, seeds (flax, sunflower, pumpkin, sesame), wheat germ, whole grains

Varicose veins develop when there is a restriction in blood flow from the legs towards the heart. Blood pools and stretches the veins. Age and genetic predisposition are factors. Possible causes include valve damage, which alters the flow of blood, high blood pressure causing blockage, blood flow restriction from tight clothing, excess weight and lack of exercise. The risk increases in pregnancy and with age. The veins can be kept in good shape with a diet high in whole foods.

Hemorrhoids are varicose veins around the anus.

WHAT TO DO

MAXIMIZE

• Foods high in vitamin E (whole grains, wheat germ, legumes, nuts and seeds, leafy greens, sea herbs, soy), to improve circulation

• Foods high in vitamin C (citrus fruits, red and green peppers, berries, leafy greens), to strengthen blood vessels

* In pregnancy, limit parsley intake to 1/2 tsp (2 mL) dried herb or a sprig of fresh herb per day. Parsley is not to be taken in kidney inflammation.

OTHER RECOMMENDATIONS

- Remedy constipation, which worsens the condition (see Constipation page 69)
- Eat oily fish (salmon, sardines, mackerel, herring) 2 to 3 times a week to provide essential fatty acids helpful for circulation and for maintaining elasticity of veins.
- Exercise daily, according to fitness level.
- Immediately after a hot bath, rinse legs with cold water and astringe the veins with witch hazel water. Or avoid hot baths entirely.
- Do not massage varicose veins.
- Avoid standing for long periods of time.
- Raise feet on a footstool whenever possible.

RECIPES

Add 1 tsp (5 mL) herbs and up to 2 tbsp (25 mL) other ingredients recommended (page 104, lower left) for this condition to the following juices and smoothies.

Juices

Berry Fine Cocktail	Berry Best	C-Blend and C-Blitz
Cherry Juice	Orange Zinger	Raspberry Juice
Sunrise Supreme	Cabbage-Broccoli	C-Green
Green Goddess	Leafy Greens	Strawberry-Orange Lemonade

Smoothies

Blue Cherry *(use 3 tbsp [45 mL] buckwheat instead of banana)*
Sea-Straw Smoothie   Spa Special *(use any recommended herb in place of milk thistle)*

Teas

Varicosi Tea	Circulation Tea	Cleansing Tea

WATER RETENTION/EDEMA

Fruits and vegetables: blueberries, cantaloupe, grapes, strawberries, watermelon, asparagus, beets, broccoli, cabbage, carrots, celery, corn, cucumber, leafy greens, squash, watercress

Herbs: burdock, dandelion leaf and root, garlic, parsley*, stinging nettle

Other: adzuki beans and other legumes, fish oils, whole grains

* In pregnancy, limit parsley intake to 1/2 tsp (2 mL) dried herb or a sprig of fresh herb per day. Parsley is not to be taken in kidney inflammation.

Water retention can be a symptom of serious conditions such as high blood pressure, heart disease, kidney disease and liver disease. Or it may simply be the result of medications, poor circulation, allergies, anemia and protein deficiency. Consult with your medical practitioner to determine the cause. Water retention in the late stages of pregnancy must always be referred to a doctor. Strong diuretics and water-loss diets can reduce water retention in the short term, but can result in kidney damage if used long term. Water retention can result from too much (or too little) dietary protein, insufficient water intake, and as a condition of PMS and menopause. Consult with your medical practitioner in all cases of water retention.

WHAT TO DO

MAXIMIZE	MINIMIZE	ELIMINATE
• Water intake. Drink at least 8 large glasses daily • Raw fruits and vegetables	• Table salt, sea salt, soy sauces and salted snacks which can cause water retention • Tea and coffee, which are strong diuretics that can cause kidney strain if used excessively	• Food allergies and intolerances, (commonly dairy and wheat), which may cause water retention (see pages 254 to 255) • Sugar • Refined flour

OTHER RECOMMENDATIONS

- Exercise daily (according to fitness level) to improve circulation and reduce water retention.

- Use tonic diuretics such as dandelion root, nettles, asparagus, corn, grapes, cantaloupe, cucumber, and watermelon. All can be used regularly.

- Use stronger diuretics such as parsley and celery only occasionally.

RECIPES

Add 1 tsp (5 mL) herbs and up to 2 tbsp (25 mL) other ingredients recommended (page 105, lower left) for this condition to the following juices.

Juices

Berry Best	Blue Water	ABC Juice
Cabbage Cocktail	C-Green	Brocco-Carrot
Green Goddess	Leafy Greens	Liquid Lunch
Popeye's Power		

Teas

Cleansing Tea	Nettle Tea

Coffee Substitutes

Root Coffee Blend	Easy Root Coffee

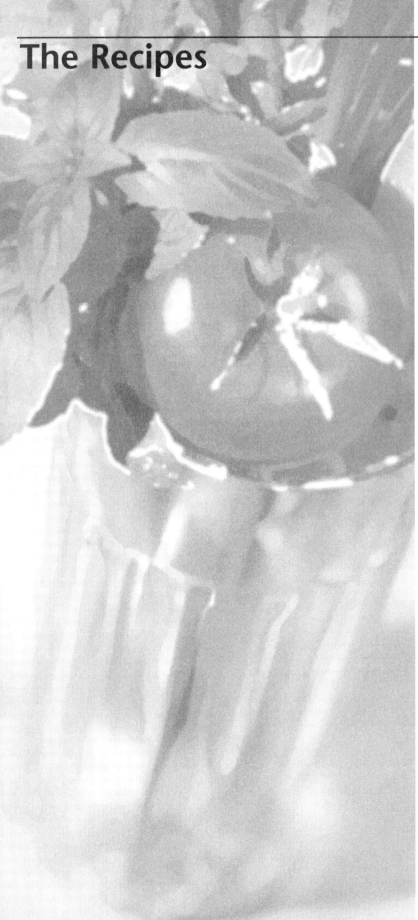

The Recipes

Juicing Guidelines

Taken as part of a healthy diet — and in amounts that are reasonable — juices round out our daily requirement for fresh fruits and vegetables. More importantly, they are the very best way to obtain the nutrients and phytochemicals those foods are meant to contribute to our health and well being.

TASTE

Juices should taste pleasant.

When you begin to juice, unless you have already changed your diet to a *whole foods* way of eating, you may find that the taste of fresh, raw juice is "different" or too strong. But once your taste buds have adjusted, you will notice that both the juice and pulp from fresh, organic fruits and vegetables offer pure bursts of clear, true flavor. Fruit juices are intensely sweet and, depending on individual preferences, may need to be balanced with lemon or beet. Foods like sauces and soups cooked with the pulp are different from the bottled, canned and boxed tastes of convenience foods — they are the taste of health.

A rule of thumb for diluting stronger vegetable juices is to use the ratio of 3 mild ingredients (apples or carrots) to 1 strong ingredient (cabbage, broccoli, leafy dark vegetables).

When you begin juicing, purchase twice as many organic apples as any other single fruit or vegetable and use them in the above ratio. Gradually incorporate more variety and stronger-tasting vegetables such as cabbage, spinach and fresh herbs (leaves and roots). Start taking fresh raw juice slowly — one or two glasses a day for several days — to allow the body time to adjust. Minor discomfort may be experienced in the form of gas and slight abdominal pain. This transitory stage should be short. After that, drink as much raw juice as feels comfortable. It is impossible to overdose on raw juice if common sense is used. Sip slowly and savor each glass!

JUICE FRESH, DRINK IMMEDIATELY

Buy fresh, ripe organic fruits, vegetables and herbs. Juice immediately (or within one or two days) and drink right away. The nutrients in raw juice are highly volatile and will begin to deteriorate as soon as they are exposed to the air. Vitamin C — so important in preventing some types of cancer, cataracts in the eyes, heart disease, bleeding gums, high blood pressure and infertility — is extremely volatile, subject to deterioration by heat, exposure to air and storage. Consequently, when produce is picked, the vitamin C begins to dissipate. The very best way to ensure the maximum amount of vitamin C (and other critical enzymes and phytochemicals) from food is to take fresh, raw juice that has just been made.

STORING FRESH JUICE

To maximize nutrients from the juice of fruits, vegetables and herbs, it is imperative to start with perfectly ripe produce and drink the raw juice immediately once it has been separated from the pulp. Should it be necessary to make juice in advance, keep the following in mind:

• Use glass containers, fill to the top and cap with a tight-fitting lid.

• Juices made at home are not pasteurized and have no "shelf-life." For this reason, they must be kept in the refrigerator and will stay mold- and bacteria-free for up to two days only. However, try to drink fresh juice within 1 to 2 hours.

USING PULP

Pulp is a natural by-product of juicing. While juices contain a concentrated amount of nutrients, the pulp retains the fiber and a substantial amount of nutrients as well. Pulp from fruits and vegetables can be saved for use in many recipes.

To use pulp for frozen desserts, soups, sauces, casseroles, vegetable stocks, dressings, baked goods, salads and many other dishes, cut out the core and seeds and peel the fruit or vegetable before juicing. For best results, blend pulp using blender or food processor before using. Measure 2 cups (500 mL) of the blended pulp and transfer to a freezer bag or covered container. Store in the refrigerator if the pulp will be used within a day, or label and freeze until needed. Versatile fruits or vegetables such as apples, carrots and tomatoes should be juiced first, the pulp collected and kept separate from other juice ingredients, making them easy to add to apple sauce, muffins, cakes or tomato sauces and salsas. For recipes that use pulp, see Frozen Treats (see page 167) and Roughies (see page 182).

Fruit Juices

Apple Fresh

Serves 1

3	apples, washed and cut into pieces	3
1 cup	washed red grapes	250 mL
Half	lemon, peeled	Half
1/2 tsp	powdered ginseng	2 mL

1. Using juicer, process apples, grapes and lemon. Whisk together and pour into a large glass. Whisk in ginseng.

Apple Pear

Serves 1

2	apples, washed and cut into pieces	2
2	pears, washed and cut into pieces	2
1	1/2-inch (1 cm) piece ginger root	1
1/2 cup	washed red or green grapes	125 mL
1/2 tsp	ground cinnamon	2 mL

1. Using juicer, process apples, pears, ginger and grapes. Whisk together and pour into a large glass. Whisk in cinnamon.

Apple-Beet-Pear

Serves 1 or 2

2	apples, washed and cut into pieces	2
1	pear, washed and cut into pieces	1
3	beets, scrubbed and washed (tops and stems intact)	3
Half	lemon, peeled	Half
1	1/2-inch (1 cm) piece ginger root	1

1. Using juicer, process apples, pear, beets (with tops and stems), lemon and ginger. Whisk together and pour into 1 large or 2 smaller glasses.

Apricot-Peach

2	peaches, peeled, pitted and halved	2
2	apricots, peeled, pitted and halved	2
1/2 cup	washed green grapes	125 mL
Quarter	head fennel, washed and cut into pieces	Quarter

1. Using juicer, process peaches, apricots, grapes and fennel. Whisk together and pour into a glass.

Autumn Refresher

If using pulp for Basil-Pear Sherbet (see recipe, page 177), peel and seed pears and apple before juicing; also remove white pith and seeds from the lime.

3	pears, washed and cut into pieces	3
2	peaches, peeled, pitted and halved	2
1	apple, washed and cut into pieces	1
Half	lime, peeled	Half

1. Using juicer, process pears, peaches, apple and lime. Whisk together and pour into a glass.

Berry Best

1 cup	washed blueberries	250 mL
1 cup	washed pitted cherries	250 mL
1/2 cup	washed grapes	125 mL
Quarter	cantaloupe, peeled and cut into pieces	Quarter

1. Using juicer, process blueberries, cherries, grapes and melon. Whisk together and pour into a glass.

Beta Blast

Serves 1

3	carrots, scrubbed	3
2	apricots, peeled, pitted and halved	2
Quarter	cantaloupe, peeled and cut into pieces	Quarter

1. Using juicer, process carrots, apricots and cantaloupe. Whisk together and pour into a glass.

Beta-Carro

Serves 1

3	carrots, scrubbed	3
3	apricots, peeled, pitted and halved	3
3	peaches, peeled, pitted and halved	3

1. Using juicer, process the carrots, apricots and peaches. Whisk together and pour into a glass.

Black Pineapple

Serves 1

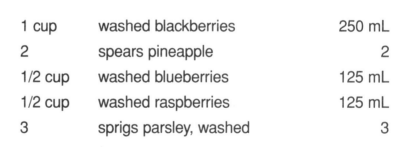

1 cup	washed blackberries	250 mL
2	spears pineapple	2
1/2 cup	washed blueberries	125 mL
1/2 cup	washed raspberries	125 mL
3	sprigs parsley, washed	3

1. Using juicer, process blackberries, pineapple, blueberries, raspberries and parsley. Whisk together and pour into a glass.

Blueberry

1 cup	washed blueberries	250 mL
1 cup	washed pitted cherries	250 mL
1/2 cup	washed red grapes	125 mL
1/2 cup	washed raspberries	125 mL

1. Using juicer, process the blueberries, cherries, grapes and raspberries. Whisk together and pour into glass.

Blue Water

1 cup	washed blueberries	250 mL
1	slice (2 inch [5 cm]) watermelon, cut into pieces	1
1/4 cup	washed cranberries, fresh or frozen	50 mL

1. Using juicer, process blueberries, watermelon and cranberries. Whisk together and pour into a glass.

Carrot Fennel Orange

If using pulp for Carrot Fennel Orange Frappé (see recipe, page 171), remove white pith and seeds from lemon and oranges before juicing.

1	lemon, peeled and halved	1
4	oranges, peeled and quartered	4
3	carrots, scrubbed	3
Quarter	head fennel, washed and cut into pieces	Quarter

1. Using juicer, process lemon, oranges, carrots and fennel. Whisk together and pour into 2 glasses.

C-Blend

Serves 1

2	oranges, peeled and quartered	2
1	grapefruit, peeled and quartered	1
1	lime, peeled and halved	1
1/2 cup	washed cranberries, fresh or frozen	125 mL
1 tbsp	honey (optional)	15 mL

1. Using juicer, process oranges, grapefruit, lime and cranberries. Whisk together and pour into a glass. Whisk in honey, if desired.

C-Blitz

Serves 1 or 2

Parsley packs a whopping amount of vitamin C and is one of the few herbs commonly available fresh throughout the year.

1	grapefruit, peeled and quartered	1
2	oranges, peeled and quartered	2
3	kiwi, peeled and halved	3
6	springs parsley, washed	6

1. Using juicer, process grapefruit, oranges, kiwi and parsley. Whisk together and pour into 1 large or 2 smaller glasses.

Cherry Juice

Serves 1

1 cup	washed pitted cherries	250 mL
Quarter	head fennel, washed and cut into pieces	Quarter
1 cup	washed grapes	250 mL
Half	lime, peeled and halved	Half

1. Using juicer, process cherries, fennel, grapes and lime. Whisk together and pour into a glass.

Cherry Sunrise

Serves 1

1 cup	washed pitted cherries	250 mL
1	grapefruit, peeled and quartered	1
1	apple, washed and cut into pieces	1
1	handful chamomile flowers (optional)	1

1. Using juicer, process cherries, grapefruit, apple and, if using, chamomile. Whisk together and pour into a glass.

Cran-Apple

Serves 1

3/4 cup	washed cranberries	175 mL
3	carrots, scrubbed	3
2	apples, washed and cut into pieces	2

1. Using juicer, process the cranberries, carrots and apples, whisk together. Whisk together and pour into a glass.

Cranberry

Serves 1

1 cup	washed cranberries, fresh or frozen	250 mL
1 cup	washed grapes	250 mL
2	spears pineapple	2

1. Using juicer, process cranberries, grapes and pineapple. Whisk together and pour into a glass.

Cranberry Juice

Serves 3

Cranberries may be (and often are) juiced and blended with sweeter juices, but this recipe provides the tart, original flavor of whole berries. The sugar content of this juice is much lower than that found in commercially prepared products. Omit the cinnamon and nutmeg if you wish. The astragalus adds immune-boosting properties to the juice.

4 cups	washed whole cranberries	1 L
4 cups	water	1 L
2 cups	apple juice	500 mL
2	slices dried astragalus root (optional)	2
2 tbsp	granulated sugar	25 mL
2 tsp	ground stevia	10 mL
1/2 tsp	ground cinnamon	2 mL
1/4 tsp	ground nutmeg	1 mL

1. In a large saucepan, combine cranberries, water, apple juice, astragalus (if using), sugar and stevia; bring to a boil. Reduce heat and let bubble gently for 15 minutes or until berries burst. Remove from heat and strain the mixture, pressing on solids to extract as much juice as possible.

2. When juice has drained through, discard astragalus (pulp may be used in another recipe) and whisk in cinnamon and nutmeg. Cool before drinking or blend with other juices for use in fruit punches or frozen treats.

3. To store: Pour juice into a clean glass container with lid; keep in refrigerator and use within 2 days.

CRANBERRIES (*VACCINIUM MACROCARPON*)

Cranberries are native to North America, but were introduced to Europeans in 1677, when colonists sent King Charles II a gift from the New World consisting of 2 hogsheads of "samp" (Indian corn, broken and boiled), 3,000 codfish and 10 barrels of cranberries.

Cranberry vines grow in marshy ground or bogs, where they typically require 5 years to become established before harvesting. Once mature, like strawberry plants, they grow rapidly, with runners shooting out in all directions. An established plant should yield for more than 100 years.

Although mechanized harvesters are most common, some cranberries are still picked by hand, using a wooden scoop specially designed with wire tines forming a comb-like end that disengages the cranberries from the vines and funnels them into an attached box. Cranberries are sorted according to their bounce and packers have devised several ingenious devices to separate the berries with the most rubbery quality from their less energetic relations.

Eye Opener

Serves 1

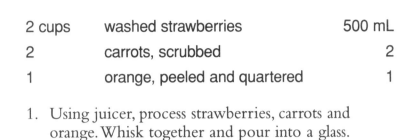

2 cups	washed strawberries	500 mL
2	carrots, scrubbed	2
1	orange, peeled and quartered	1

1. Using juicer, process strawberries, carrots and orange. Whisk together and pour into a glass.

Grapefruit

Serves 1

Use pulp in Grapefruit Frappé (see recipe, page 170). Be sure to remove white pith and seeds before juicing.

1	orange, peeled and quartered	1
2	grapefruits, peeled and quartered	2
1	lemon, peeled and halved	1

1. If using pulp for Grapefruit Frappé, grate zest from orange and set aside to add to pulp. Remove white pith when peeling orange, cut in half and remove seeds.

2. Using juicer, process orange, grapefruits and lemon. Whisk together and pour into a glass.

Grape Heart

Serves 1

2 cups	washed red grapes	500 mL
1	grapefruit, peeled and quartered	1
1 tsp	powdered dried linden flowers	5 mL

1. Using juicer, process the grapes and grapefruit. Whisk together and pour into a glass. Whisk in linden flowers.

Grape Power

Serves 1 or 2

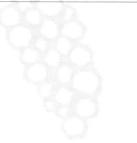

2 cups	washed green grapes	500 mL
1	green pepper, washed and cut into pieces	1
3	sprigs parsley, washed	3
1	sprig rosemary, washed	1

1. Using juicer, process grapes, pepper, parsley and rosemary. Whisk together and pour into 1 large or 2 smaller glasses.

Hangover Remedy

Serves 1

4	apples, washed, cut into pieces	4
1	1/2-inch (1 cm) piece ginger root	1
Half	lemon, peeled and halved	Half
1/2 tsp	crushed lavender buds	2 mL

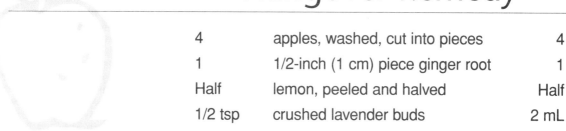

1. Using juicer, process the apples, ginger and lemon. Whisk in lavender and pour into a glass.

Lemon Aid

Serves 2

This juice is quite tart, but very refreshing, so taste before adding the honey.

Use pulp in Lemon Sauce (see recipe, page 185). Before juicing, be sure to remove white pith and seeds from lemons, and peel watermelon and cucumber.

2	lemons, peeled and halved	2
1	2-inch (5 cm) slice watermelon, cut into chunks	1
Half	cucumber, scrubbed and cut into chunks	Half
1 tsp	honey (optional)	5 mL

1. Using juicer, process lemons, watermelon and cucumber. Whisk together and pour into a glass. If desired, whisk in honey.

Lemon-Lime

Serves 1

1	orange, peeled and quartered	1
1	lime, peeled and halved	1
1	lemon, peeled and halved	1
1 tsp	powdered licorice (see note at left)	5 mL

Do not use licorice in cases of high blood pressure.

1. Using juicer, process the orange, lime, and lemon. Whisk together and pour into a glass. Whisk in licorice.

Mint Julep

Serves 2 or 3

Sweet and only a little minty, this juice is best served in clear glasses so you can see the grape juice separate to the bottom. Use sprigs of mint for swizzle sticks.

If planning to use pulp in a frozen drink, remove and discard as many herb pieces as possible.

4	oranges, peeled and quartered	4
1	handful mint leaves, washed	1
6	sprigs lemon balm, washed	6
3 cups	washed red grapes	750 mL
1	lemon, peeled and halved	1

1. Using juicer, process oranges, mint, lemon balm, grapes and lemon. Whisk together and pour into glasses.

Orange Crush

Serves 1 or 2

3	oranges, peeled and quartered	3
1	carrot, scrubbed	1
1/2 cup	washed cranberries, fresh or frozen	125 mL
1 tsp	ground cinnamon	5 mL

1. Using juicer, process oranges, carrot and cranberries. Whisk together and pour into 1 or 2 glasses. Whisk in cinnamon.

Orange Zinger

Serves 1

1	orange, peeled and quartered	1
3	carrots, scrubbed	3
1	1/2-inch (1 cm) ginger root	1
1	apple, washed and cut into pieces	1

1. Using juicer, process orange, carrots, ginger and apple. Whisk together and pour into a glass.

Pear-Fennel

Serves 1

2	pears, washed and cut into pieces	2
Quarter	head fennel, washed and cut into pieces	Quarter
2	apples, washed and cut into pieces	2
1/2 tsp	powdered licorice (see note at left)	2 mL

Do not use licorice in cases of high blood pressure.

1. Using juicer, process pears, fennel and apples. Whisk together and pour into a glass. Whisk in licorice.

Pear Pineapple

Serves 1

2	pears, washed and cut into pieces	2
2	spears pineapple	2
1 cup	washed red or green grapes	250 mL
1	lemon, peeled and halved	1

1. Using juicer, process pears, pineapple, grapes and lemon. Whisk together and pour into a glass.

Pineapple-Citrus

Serves 1

Use pulp in Pineapple Sage Frappé (see recipe, page 171). Be sure to remove white pith and seeds from oranges and lime before juicing.

Half	pineapple, cut into spears	Half
2	oranges, peeled and quartered	2
1	lime, peeled and halved	1

1. Using juicer, process pineapple, oranges and lime. Whisk together and pour into a glass.

Pine-Berry

Serves 1

2	spears pineapple	2
1 cup	washed blueberries	250 mL
1 cup	washed pitted cherries	250 mL
1/2 cup	washed blackcurrants	125 mL

1. Using juicer, process pineapple, blueberries, cherries and blackcurrants. Whisk together and pour into a glass.

Raspberry Juice

Serves 1

1 cup	washed raspberries	250 mL
1	apple, washed and cut into pieces	1
2	oranges, peeled and halved	2

1. Using juicer, process raspberries, apple and oranges. Whisk together and pour into a glass.

Rhubarb

Serves 1

2	stalks fresh rhubarb, washed, trimmed	2
1 cup	washed fresh strawberries	250 mL
1	orange, peeled, quartered	1
1	1/2-inch (1 cm) piece ginger root	1

1. Using juicer, process rhubarb, strawberries, orange and ginger. Whisk together and pour into a glass.

Strawberry-Orange Lemonade

Serves 3

1 cup	washed strawberries	250 mL
1	lemon, peeled and halved	1
2	oranges, peeled and quartered	2
1 cup	sparkling mineral water	250 mL

1. Using juicer, process strawberries, lemon and oranges. Whisk together and pour into a pitcher. Whisk in mineral water.

Summer Nectar

Serves 2

3	nectarines, washed, pitted and halved	3
2	apricots, washed, pitted and halved	2
1 cup	washed blueberries	250 mL
2	peaches, washed, pitted and halved	2
2	plums, washed, pitted and halved	2

1. Using juicer, process nectarines, apricots, blueberries, peaches and plums. Whisk together and pour into glasses.

Summer Swizzle

Serves 2

4	apricots, washed, pitted and halved	4
1 cup	washed grapes	250 mL
4	peaches, washed, pitted and halved	4
1	2-inch slice watermelon, cut into chunks	1

1. Using juicer, process the apricots, grapes, peaches and watermelon. Whisk together and pour into glasses.

Sunrise Supreme

Serves 1

1 cup	washed strawberries	250 mL
1 cup	washed red grapes	250 mL
1	orange, peeled and halved	1

1. Using juicer, process strawberries, grapes and orange. Whisk together and pour into a glass.

Watermelon Cooler

Serves 1

1	2-inch slice (5 cm) watermelon, cut into chunks	1
1/2 cup	washed strawberries	125 mL
Quarter	head fennel, washed and cut into pieces	Quarter
1	lemon, peeled and halved	1

1. Using juicer, process watermelon, strawberries, fennel and lemon. Whisk together and pour into a glass.

Watermelon Strawberry

Serves 1

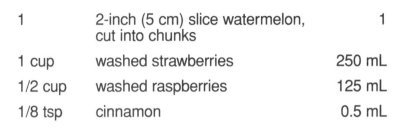

1	2-inch (5 cm) slice watermelon, cut into chunks	1
1 cup	washed strawberries	250 mL
1/2 cup	washed raspberries	125 mL
1/8 tsp	cinnamon	0.5 mL

1. Using juicer, process watermelon, strawberries and raspberries. Whisk together and pour into a glass. Whisk in cinnamon.

3PO

Serves 1

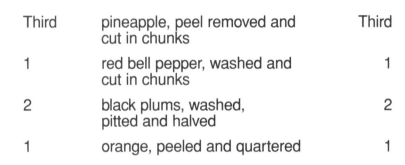

Third	pineapple, peel removed and cut in chunks	Third
1	red bell pepper, washed and cut in chunks	1
2	black plums, washed, pitted and halved	2
1	orange, peeled and quartered	1

1. Using juicer, process the pineapple, pepper, plums and orange. Whisk together and pour into a glass.

Vegetable Juices

ABC Juice

It's as easy as... well, A-B-C!

10	spears asparagus, washed	10
1	apple, washed and cut into pieces	1
1	stalk broccoli, washed and cut into pieces	1
2	carrots, scrubbed	2

1. Using juicer, process asparagus, apple, broccoli and carrots. Whisk together and pour into a glass.

Allium Antioxidant

Beware — this drink is very strong. Just preparing it will make your eyes water. But, for antioxidant and anti-bacterial power, it can't be beat.

3	stalks celery, washed	3
Half	onion, quartered	Half
1	clove garlic	1
1	stalk broccoli, washed and cut into pieces	1
1	apple, washed and cut into pieces	1

1. Using juicer, process celery, onion, garlic, broccoli and apple. Whisk together and pour into a glass.

THE POWER OF GARLIC

Garlic provides strong antioxidant action to protect cell membranes against free-radical formation. Some studies show that even in low doses, garlic stimulates the immune system, increasing the activity of natural "killer cells" to ward off pathogens.

Garlic also has strong antibiotic properties. It kills intestinal parasites and worms, as well as gram-negative bacteria. In recent studies, researchers using fresh and powdered garlic solutions discovered that garlic inhibited many bacteria, including staphylococcus auras, E. coli, proteus vulgaris, salmonella enteritidis, Klebsiella pneumonia and many others.

And when compared to antibiotics such as penicillin, tetracycline, erythromycin and others commonly prescribed, garlic proved to be as effective. One medium-sized garlic clove delivers the anti-bacterial equivalent of about 100,000 units of penicillin (typical oral penicillin doses range from 600,000 units to 900,000 units). Therefore a dose of 6 to 9 garlic cloves has roughly the same effect as a shot of penicillin.

Artichoke-Carrot

Serves 1

In this immune-boosting combination, you can reduce or increase the amount of thyme according to taste.

1 cup	scrubbed chopped Jerusalem artichoke	250 mL
3	carrots, scrubbed	3
1	apple, washed and cut into pieces	1
1 tbsp	chopped washed thyme leaves, (or 1 tsp [5 mL] dried)	15 mL

1. Using juicer, process artichokes, carrots and apple. Whisk together and pour into a glass. Whisk in thyme.

Artichoke Eight

Serves 1 or 2

1 cup	scrubbed Jerusalem artichokes	250 mL
2	stalks celery, washed	2
2	carrots, scrubbed	2
1	parsnip, washed and split	1
Quarter	head cabbage, washed and cut into chunks	Quarter
1 cup	washed spinach leaves	250 mL
1	apple, washed and cut into pieces	1
Half	leek, washed	Half

1. Using juicer, process artichokes, celery, carrots, parsnip, cabbage, spinach, apple and leek. Whisk together and pour into 1 large or 2 smaller glasses.

Beet

Serves 1 or 2

This combination nourishes the immune system, is an excellent lymphatic cleanser and is believed to reduce tumors. Make it fresh each day. Take one serving daily for at least 5 days in one week.

2	beets (with tops), scrubbed and cut into pieces	2
2	carrots, scrubbed	2
2	apples, washed and cut into pieces	2

1. Using juicer, process beets, beet tops, carrots and apples. Whisk together and pour into glasses.

Blazing Beets

Serves 1

3	beets (with tops), scrubbed and cut into pieces	3
1	1/2-inch (1 cm) piece ginger root	1
1	chile pepper, washed	1
2	apples, washed and cut into pieces	2
1	clove garlic	1
2	stalks celery, washed and cut into pieces	2

1. Using juicer, process beets, beet tops, ginger, chile, apples, garlic and celery. Whisk together and pour into a glass.

Bone Builder

Serves 1 or 2

The calcium, boron and magnesium delivered by the ingredients in this drink make it good for bones.

Parsley should be avoided during pregnancy.

1/2 cup	kelp or other sea herb	125 mL
1 cup	hot water	250 mL
2	stalks broccoli, washed and cut into pieces	2
2	kale leaves, washed	2
2	stalks celery, washed	2
Half	green pepper, washed and cut into pieces	Half
4	sprigs parsley (see note at left)	4
1	apple, washed and cut into pieces	1

1. In a medium bowl, pour water over kelp. Soak for 15 to 20 minutes or until kelp is reconstituted. Drain soaking water, reserving for another use.

2. Using juicer, process kelp, broccoli, kale, celery, green pepper, parsley and apple. Whisk together and pour into glasses.

Brocco-Artichoke

Serves 1

1	stalk broccoli, washed and cut into pieces	1
2	Jerusalem artichokes, scrubbed and cut into pieces	2
Quarter	head fennel, washed and cut into pieces	Quarter
3	sprigs parsley, washed	3

1. Using juicer, process broccoli, artichokes, fennel and parsley. Whisk together and pour into a glass.

CHILES: THE CULINARY FIREBRANDS

Chiles (capsicum spp.), the pods that bite back, are a unique and diverse group of perennial shrubs (annual in northern climates) native to South and Central America and Mexico. The term "pepper" when appended to chile, is misleading because the capsicum genus is not at all related to black pepper (piper nigrum) but was mistakenly given the pepper moniker by early European spice seekers who confused their hot spiciness with the coveted and elusive pepper berries of India and the Spice Islands (Malaysia and Indonesia).

Ranging from fiery hot to sweet and mild, chiles are a study in contradiction. Well known by chefs for its ability to cause severe burns to the skin and eyes, the powerful element in all chiles — capsaicin — is the main ingredient in skin creams used to soothe the excruciating pain of arthritis and shingles. Chiles are often shunned by those who believe that they cause or irritate ulcers. Yet in Mexico, a long-standing remedy for stomach problems has been to consume a whole serrano or jalapeño chile.

And the confusion doesn't stop with their folk remedies. Chiles are a hot-bed of conflicting species, varieties and pod types. The names change from region to region; just attempting to sort out the American/ Mexican nomenclature is a huge challenge. Typically the fresh and dried version of the same chile bear different names, which are different again when the chile is smoked, or green or ripe. Botanically, they are classified as berries. Horticulturally they are fruits. We use them fresh as vegetables but when dried, they're a spice.

But that confusion aside, why is it that we love the palate-searing experience of eating chiles? Capsaicin irritates the pain receptors on the tongue that ignite the pain center in the brain, triggering a release of morphine-like natural pain killers — endorphins. They try to douse the fire by setting the body awash in a sense of well-being and we ride the wave of euphoria throughout the rest of the meal.

But that's not the only reason people are all fired up over chiles. In addition to their distinctive aroma and delicious taste, 1/4 cup (50 mL) of the fresh, diced scorching orbs yields 4,031 IU of vitamin A, which becomes even more concentrated as the pod turns red and dries. Simply eating 1 tsp (5 mL) of red chili sauce supplies the body with the Recommended Dietary Allowance for vitamin A. The same 1/4 cup (50 mL) of chopped fresh chile pepper delivers 91 mg of vitamin C — as compared to 66 mg in 1 orange. And while the vitamin C diminishes by more than half in the dried red pods, the effect is still more than a flash in the pan. See page 49 for more on the health actions of chiles.

Brocco-Carrot

Serves 1

1	stalk broccoli, washed and cut into pieces	1
2	carrots, scrubbed	2
1	apple, washed and cut into pieces	1

1. Using juicer, process broccoli, carrots and apple. Whisk together and pour into a glass.

Cabbage Rose

Serves 1

Use the pulp from this juice as a salad. Be sure to peel, core and seed apple before juicing.

Eighth	cabbage, washed and cut into chunks	Eighth
4	spinach leaves, washed	4
2	sprigs rosemary, washed (or 1/2 tsp [2 mL] dried)	2
2	carrots, washed	2
1	apple, washed and cut into pieces	1

1. Using juicer, process cabbage, spinach, rosemary sprigs, carrots and apple. If using dried rosemary, whisk into juice. Whisk together and pour into a glass.

Carrot-Allium

Serves 1

3	carrots, scrubbed	3
6	spinach leaves, washed	6
1	clove garlic	1
Half	lemon, peeled, cut in half	Half
Pinch	cayenne	Pinch

1. Using juicer, process carrots, spinach, garlic and lemon, whisk together. Whisk together and pour into a glass. Whisk in cayenne.

Carrot-Apple

Serves 1

Use the pulp from this juice in quick breads or muffins. Be sure to peel, core and seed apple before juicing.

Parsley should be avoided during pregnancy.

4	carrots, scrubbed	4
2	stalks celery, washed	2
1	apple, washed and cut into pieces	1
4	sprigs parsley, washed (see note, left)	4

1. Using juicer, process carrots, celery, apple and parsley. Whisk together and pour into a glass.

Cauli-Slaw

Serves 1

Use the pulp from this juice as a salad. Be sure to peel, core and seed apple before juicing.

Half	head cauliflower, washed and cut into pieces	Half
Eighth	head cabbage, washed and cut into chunks	Eighth
2	carrots, scrubbed	2
2	stalks celery, washed	2
Quarter	onion	Quarter
1	apple, washed and cut into pieces	1

1. Using juicer, process cauliflower, cabbage, carrots, celery, onion and apple. Whisk together and pour into glasses.

Celery

Serves 1

For more antioxidant power, add one clove garlic.

4	stalks celery, washed	4
2	carrots, scrubbed	2
Quarter	head fennel, washed, cut in pieces	Quarter
1/2 tsp	ground cumin	2 mL

1. Using juicer, process the celery, carrots and fennel. Whisk together and pour into glass. Whisk in cumin.

C-Green

Serves 1 or 2

Parsley should be avoided during pregnancy.

3	sprigs parsley, washed (see note, left)	3
1	handful spinach leaves, washed	1
1	handful watercress, washed	1
1	apple, washed and cut into pieces	1

1. Using juicer, process parsley, spinach, watercress and apple. Whisk together and pour into a glass.

Cucumber Cooler

Serves 1 or 2

1	cucumber, scrubbed and cut into pieces	1
2 cups	washed green grapes	500 mL
1	handful borage leaves, washed	1
1	handful mint, washed	1
2	apples, washed and cut into pieces	2
Half	lemon, peeled and halved	Half

1. Using juicer, process cucumber, grapes, borage, mint, apples and lemon. Whisk together and pour into 1 large or 2 smaller glasses.

Cruciferous

Serves 1 or 2

The term *cruciferous* refers to the small cross formed when the flowers of particular plants are growing. Cruciferous vegetables include cabbage, broccoli, brussels sprouts and cauliflower.

1	stalk broccoli, washed and cut into pieces	1
Quarter	head cabbage, washed and cut into chunks	Quarter
Quarter	head cauliflower, washed and cut into pieces	Quarter
2	kale leaves, washed	2
Half	lemon, peeled and halved	Half
2	apples, washed and cut into pieces	2

1. Using juicer, process the broccoli, cabbage, cauliflower, kale, lemon and apples. Whisk together and pour into 1 large or 2 smaller glasses.

Dandelion Bitters

Serves 1

3	fresh young dandelions (roots and leaves), scrubbed	3
2	radishes, scrubbed	2
1	handful watercress, washed	1
1	apple, washed and cut into pieces	1
Half	lemon, peeled	Half
1	1/2-inch (1 cm) piece ginger root	1

1. Using juicer, process dandelion roots and leaves, radishes, watercress, apple, lemon and ginger. Whisk together and pour into a glass.

Flaming Antibiotic

Serves 1

If you're unaccustomed to the heat of chiles, start with a small piece and add more once you become accustomed to the fire.

See pages 49 and 136 for how to handle and use chiles for juices.

2	carrots, scrubbed	2
1	clove garlic	1
1	handful thyme, washed	1
1	chile, washed	1
Half	cucumber, washed and cut into chunks	Half
1	apple, washed and cut into pieces	1

1. Using juicer, process carrots, garlic, thyme, chile, cucumber and apple. Whisk together and pour into a glass.

Folic Plus

Serves 1

This juice is packed with folic acid, an essential nutrient for childbearing women.

2	oranges, peeled and quartered	2
3	kale leaves, washed	3
1/2 cup	washed spinach leaves	125 mL
5	stalks asparagus, washed	5
1 tbsp	soy protein powder	15 mL

1. Using juicer, process oranges, kale, spinach and asparagus. Whisk together and pour into a glass. Whisk in protein powder.

Gallstone Solvent

Serves 2

As the name implies, this drink is used as a bitter tonic for treating gallstones.

3	tomatoes, washed and quartered	3
2	carrots, scrubbed	2
2	stalks celery, washed	2
1	handful watercress, washed	1
4	radishes, washed	4
2	sprigs fresh parsley, washed	2
Half	lemon, peeled and halved	Half

1. Using juicer, process tomatoes, carrots, celery, watercress, radishes, parsley and lemon. Whisk together and pour into 2 glasses.

Gingered Broccoli

Serves 1

2	stalks broccoli, washed and cut into pieces	2
1	clove garlic	1
Eighth	head cabbage, washed, cut into cubes	Eighth
1	1/2-inch (1 cm) piece ginger root	1

1. Using juicer, process broccoli, garlic, cabbage and ginger. Whisk together and pour into a glass.

TRIAL BY FIRE: COMMON CHILE PEPPERS

There are five cultivated species of the capsicum genus — c. annuum, c. frutescens, c. chinense, c. baccatum and c. pubescens — and over 20 wild varieties.

For juicing, use fresh chiles. Wash, remove stems and juice whole (or cut larger varieties in half). The hot, irritating component, capsaicin, is concentrated in the ribs of the flesh, not the seeds (as is commonly thought), so leave the seeds intact. When first using chile peppers for juicing, juice after all other ingredients have been put through the machine and keep the juice separate. Add it to vegetable juice blends by the teaspoon (5 mL) in order to gage the amount with which you are comfortable.

As an alternative to fresh chiles, whisk in a drop of hot or jerk sauce or 1/4 tsp (1 mL) of powdered cayenne to juices and blended drinks. Adding yogurt to blended drinks helps to extinguish the fire. Dried or smoked chiles may be added to smoothies in small quantities. Remember to handle all chiles with care, washing hands thoroughly after touching.

Listed from mildest to hottest, the following are just a few of the hundreds of varieties enjoyed today.

New Mexican. Formerly called "Anaheim", the long green, mild chiles are available fresh, canned, roasted or left on the bush to turn red in the fall. Their taste is similar to mild

Gout Buster

Serves 1

Parsley should be avoided during pregnancy.

4	stalks celery, washed	4
3	sprigs parsley, washed (see note at left)	3
1	carrot, washed	1
1	clove garlic	1
1 cup	washed kale leaves	250 mL
1	1/2-inch (1 cm) piece ginger root	1

1. Using juicer, process celery, parsley, carrot, garlic, spinach and ginger. Whisk together and pour into a glass.

Green Beet

Serves 1

1/2 cup	kelp or other sea herb	125 mL
1 cup	hot water	250 mL
1	beet (with top) washed and cut into pieces	1
1 cup	washed spinach leaves	250 mL
1	apple, washed and cut into pieces	1

1. In a medium bowl, pour water over kelp. Soak for 15 to 20 minutes or until kelp is reconstituted. Drain soaking water, reserving for another use.

2. Using juicer, process kelp, beet, beet top, spinach and apple. Whisk together and pour into a glass.

bell peppers. They are used in most classic Tex-Mex dishes and are a good choice for novice chile users.

Poblano/Ancho. Poblano is the name of the fresh version of this big flat pepper, the widest of the hot peppers. Called ancho when dried, it acquires a nutty taste and raisin-like appearance and is the most commonly used variety in Mexico.

Jalapeño. Widely known, and at the halfway point on the Scoville Heat Unit Scale, they lend a meaty tex-

ture and rich flavor to dishes. Their thick flesh makes jalapeños an excellent juicing chile. When smoked and dried, jalapeños are called chipotles.

Serrano. More flavorful than jalapeño, the name serrano means "from the mountains." They are the most popular choice for fresh salsas, stews and moles.

Cayenne. Grown commercially in New Mexico, Africa, India, Japan and Mexico, the most common form is dried. A favorite in African and

Cajun dishes, cayenne is a major ingredient in barbecue rubs and powders. See page 49 for health actions.

Habanero. Also known also as Scotch Bonnet and rated a blazing 10+ on the Scoville Heat Unit Scale, this small, round chile really packs a punch in hot pepper and Caribbean jerk sauces, where it imparts a unique fruity, apricot-like aroma.

Visit www.chileheads.netimages for more information and links on chiles.

Green Goddess

Parsley should be avoided during pregnancy.

1	stalk broccoli, washed and cut into pieces	1
Half	cucumber, washed, cut into chunks	Half
Half	red bell pepper, washed	Half
2	sprigs parsley, washed (see note, left)	2

1. Using juicer, process broccoli, cucumber, pepper and parsley. Whisk together and pour into a glass.

Green Magic

2	stalks celery, washed	2
Eighth	cabbage, washed and cut into chunks	Eighth
6	spinach leaves, washed	6
1/4 cup	cubed pumpkin	50 mL
1 tsp	powdered ginkgo (optional)	5 mL

1. Using juicer, process celery, cabbage, spinach and pumpkin. Whisk together and pour into a glass. Whisk in ginkgo if using.

Immunity

2	stalks celery, washed	2
2	carrots, scrubbed	2
1	clove garlic	1
1	apple, washed and cut into pieces	1
1	1/2-inch (1 cm) piece ginger root	1
Half	lemon, peeled and cut in half	Half

1. Using juicer, process celery, carrots, garlic, apple, ginger and lemon. Whisk together and pour into a glass.

Kelp

Serves 1

6	kale leaves, washed	6
Quarter	head fennel, washed and cut into pieces	Quarter
2	carrots, scrubbed	2
1 tsp	crumbled dried kelp	5 mL
Pinch	nutmeg	Pinch

1. Using juicer, process kale, fennel and carrots. Whisk together and pour into a glass. Whisk in kelp and nutmeg.

Leafy Greens

Serves 1

Substitute lettuce or cabbage leaves for any of the leaves in this recipe. Use the celery and carrots to tap the leaves through the feed tube.

4	spinach leaves, washed	4
2	kale leaves, washed	2
1	beet (with top) or turnip, scrubbed and cut into pieces	1
2	stalks celery, washed	2
1	apple, washed and cut into pieces	1

1. Using juicer, process spinach, kale, beet, beet top, celery and apple. Whisk together and pour into a glass.

Liquid Lunch

Serves 1

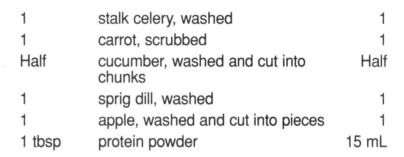

1	stalk celery, washed	1
1	carrot, scrubbed	1
Half	cucumber, washed and cut into chunks	Half
1	sprig dill, washed	1
1	apple, washed and cut into pieces	1
1 tbsp	protein powder	15 mL

1. Using juicer, process celery, carrot, cucumber, dill and apple. Whisk together and pour into a glass. Whisk in protein powder.

Liquid Salsa

Serves 1

2	tomatoes, washed and quartered	2
1	jalapeño pepper, washed	1
Quarter	onion	Quarter
6	sprigs cilantro, washed	6
Half	lime, peeled	Half

1. Using juicer, process tomatoes, pepper, onion, cilantro and lime. Whisk together and pour into a glass.

Moist & Juicy

Serves 1

1	leek, split and washed	1
2	kale leaves, washed	2
2	carrots, scrubbed	2
2	apples, washed and cut into pieces	2
1 tsp	powdered ginkgo	5 mL

1. Using juicer, process leek, kale, carrots and apples. Whisk together and pour into a glass. Whisk in ginkgo.

Nip of Goodness

Serves 1

1	turnip, scrubbed and cut into pieces	1
3	parsnips, scrubbed and halved	3
1	apple, washed and cut into pieces	1
Quarter	head fennel, washed and cut into pieces	Quarter

1. Using juicer, process turnip, parsnips, apple and fennel. Whisk together and pour into a glass.

Peas and Carrots

Serves 1

1 cup	washed peas	250 mL
2	carrots, scrubbed	2
1	parsnip, scrubbed and halved	1
Quarter	onion	Quarter
Quarter	head fennel, washed and cut into pieces	Quarter

1. Using juicer, process peas, carrots, parsnip, onion and fennel. Whisk together and pour into a glass.

Peas Please

Serves 1

1 cup	washed peas	250 mL
2	carrots, scrubbed	2
6	sprigs parsley, washed	6

1. Using juicer, process peas, carrots and parsley. Whisk together and pour into a glass.

Peppers Please

Serves 1

1	red bell pepper, washed and cut in pieces	1
1	green pepper, washed and cut in pieces	1
Half	cucumber, washed, cut in pieces	Half
1	carrot, washed	1

1. Using juicer, process peppers, cucumber and carrot, whisk together. Pour into a glass.

Popeye's Power

Serves 1

2	kale leaves, washed	2
6	spinach leaves, washed	6
1	beet (with top), scrubbed and cut into pieces	1
1	dandelion root, scrubbed	1
2 tsp	blackstrap molasses	10 mL

1. Using juicer, process kale, spinach, beet, beet leaves and dandelion root. Whisk together and pour into a glass. Whisk in molasses.

Red Devil

Serves 1

4	tomatoes, washed and quartered	4
5	radishes, scrubbed	5
Half	red bell pepper, washed and cut into chunks	Half
1	beet, scrubbed and cut into pieces	1
Pinch	cayenne pepper	Pinch

1. Using juicer, process tomatoes, radishes, pepper and beet. Pour into a glass and whisk in cayenne pepper.

Root Combo

Serves 1

Try 1/2 tsp (5 mL) curry powder or turmeric whisked into this drink.

1	parsnip, scrubbed and halved	1
2	carrots, scrubbed	2
1	beet, scrubbed and cut into pieces	1
1	apple, washed and cut into pieces	1

1. Using juicer, process parsnip, carrots, beet and apple. Whisk together and pour into a glass.

Rust Proofer #1

Serves 1

1	apple, washed and cut into pieces	1
3	sprigs parsley, washed (see note, left)	3
1	carrot, scrubbed	1
2	tomatoes, washed and quartered	2

1. Using juicer, process apple, parsley, carrot and tomatoes. Whisk together and pour into a glass.

Rust Proofer #2

Serves 1

In simple terms, aging is the process whereby our cells are damaged by oxidation. In truth, we are rusting from the inside out.

Antioxidant herbs and vitamins help prevent the damage to cells by oxidizing agents, which makes them a kind of rust proofer!

Half	sweet potato, scrubbed and cut into pieces	Half
3	carrots, scrubbed	3
1	stalk broccoli, washed and cut into pieces	1
4	sprigs peppermint, washed	4

1. Using juicer, process sweet potato. Set aside. Using another container, process the carrots, broccoli and peppermint.

2. When white starch has settled on the bottom of the container, pour sweet potato juice carefully into carrot juice mixture, being sure to leave starch behind. Discard starch, whisk juices together and pour into a glass.

Sea Herb Surprise

Serves 2

Wakame, hijiki, nori or kelp can be substituted for the dulse.

3	stalks celery, washed	3
2	carrots, scrubbed	2
1 cup	cubed squash	250 mL
1 tsp	extra virgin olive oil *or* hemp oil	5 mL
1 tsp	crumbled dried dulse	5 mL

1. Using juicer, process celery, carrots and squash. Whisk together and pour into a glass. Whisk in oil and dulse.

Slippery Beet

Serves 1

2	beets, scrubbed and cut into pieces	2
1	clove garlic	1
1	apple, washed and cut into pieces	1
1 tbsp	powdered slippery elm (optional)	15 mL

1. Using juicer, process beets, garlic and apple. Whisk together and pour into a glass. Whisk in slippery elm, if using.

Soft Salad

Serves 1

Half	head bok choy, washed and cut in wedges	Half
1	carrot, scrubbed	1
2	stalks celery, washed	2
1/4 cup	washed bean sprouts	50 mL
1	spear pineapple	1

1. Using juicer, process bok choy, carrot, celery, bean sprouts and pineapple. Whisk together and pour into a glass.

Spiced Carrot

Serves 1

3	carrots, washed	3
1	stalk broccoli, washed and cut into pieces	1
1/2 cup	spinach leaves, washed	125 mL
1	1/2-inch (1 cm) piece ginger root	1
1/2 tsp	ground cinnamon	2 mL
1/8 tsp	cayenne pepper, or to taste	0.5 mL

1. Using juicer, process carrots, broccoli, spinach and ginger. Whisk together and pour into a glass. Whisk in cinnamon and cayenne.

Spring Celebration

Serves 1

10	spears asparagus, washed	10
2	beets (with tops), scrubbed and cut into pieces	2
6	spinach leaves, washed	6
1	handful watercress or dandelion leaves, washed	1
1	apple, washed and cut into pieces	1
2 tbsp	maple sap (optional)	25 mL

1. Using juicer, process asparagus, beets, beet tops, spinach, watercress and apple. Whisk together and pour into a glass. Whisk in maple sap, if using.

Squash Special

Serves 1

1	sweet potato, scrubbed and cut into pieces	1
1 cup	cubed squash	250 mL
1/2 tsp	cayenne pepper	2 mL
1/2 tsp	dried dill	2 mL
1/2 tsp	ground cumin	2 mL

1. Using juicer, process sweet potato; set aside. Using another container, process squash. Whisk in cayenne, dill and cumin.

2. When starch from sweet potato has settled on the bottom of the container, pour juice carefully into squash juice, being sure to leave starch behind. Discard starch. Whisk juices together and pour into a glass.

The Chiller

Serves 1 or 2

1	carrot, scrubbed	1
2	stalks celery, washed	2
1	apple, washed and cut into pieces	1
Half	cucumber, washed and cut into spears	Half
Half	zucchini, washed and cut into spears	Half
Half	red bell pepper, washed	Half

1. Using juicer, process carrot, celery, apple, cucumber, zucchini and red pepper. Whisk together and pour into a glass.

Tomato Tang

Serves 1

2	large tomatoes, washed and quartered	2
2	carrots, scrubbed	2
1	beet, scrubbed and cut into pieces	1
1/4 cup	washed whole cranberries	50 mL

1. Using juicer, process tomatoes, carrots, beet and cranberries. Whisk together and pour into a glass.

Watercress

Serves 1

3	handfuls fresh watercress, washed	3
2	stalks celery, washed	2
2	sprigs basil, washed	2
1	parsnip, washed and halved lengthwise	1
Half	green pepper, washed and cut into pieces	Half

1. Using juicer, process watercress, celery, basil, parsnip and green pepper. Whisk together and pour into a glass.

Zippy Tomato

Serves 1

Parsley should be avoided during pregnancy.

1	Large tomato, washed and quartered	1
1	1/2-inch (1 cm) piece ginger root	1
4	sprigs parsley, washed (see note at left)	4
Half	lemon, peeled, cut into pieces	Half

1. Using juicer, process tomatoes, ginger, parsley and lemon. Whisk together and pour into a glass.

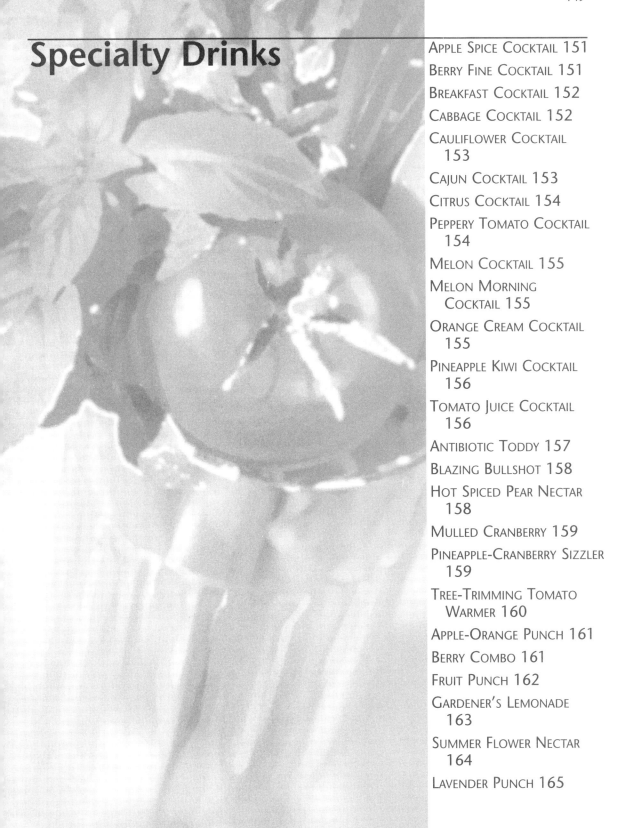

Specialty Drinks

COCKTAIL JUICES

Cocktails are relatively new inventions, arising early in the eighteenth century as brandy-sugar-champagne mixtures. Today, any short, cold drink based on alcohol or liqueur, stirred or shaken, served neat, on the rocks or blended with ice, is called a *cocktail*.

The following drinks have all the pizzazz of traditional cocktails with one exception: the fruit and vegetables *are* the drink, not just the decoration. They are the new-age cocktails, still using the term because of their complex blend of ingredients, spices and herbs. With these drinks, cocktail hour starts at breakfast and continues all day!

Apple Spice Cocktail

Serves 2

4	apples, washed and cut into pieces	4
1	carrot, scrubbed	1
1	stalk celery, washed	1
1	1-inch (2.5 cm) piece ginger root	1
1/4 tsp	ground cardamom	1 mL
1/4 tsp	ground nutmeg	1 mL

1. Using juicer, process apples, carrot, celery and ginger. Pour into a carafe or pitcher and whisk in cardamom and nutmeg. Pour into glasses.

Berry Fine Cocktail

Serves 2

2 cups	washed raspberries	500 mL
2	oranges, peeled and quartered	2
1/2 cup	washed cranberries, fresh or frozen	125 mL
1/2 cup	washed strawberries	125 mL

1. Using juicer, process raspberries, oranges, cranberries and strawberries. Whisk together and pour into glasses.

Breakfast Cocktail

Serves 1 or 2

A sweet blend of goodness — even the pastel orange color lends a cheerful note. Save pulp for use in Curry Sauce (see recipe, page 185). Peel, core and seed squash and apples if planning to use pulp later.

Quarter	acorn or butternut squash, scrubbed and cut into chunks	Quarter
2	medium apples, washed and cut into pieces	2
1	carrot, scrubbed	1
1	1-inch (2.5 cm) piece ginger root	1
1/4 cup	natural yogurt	50 mL

1. Using a juicer, process squash, apples, carrot and ginger. Whisk in yogurt. Pour into a carafe or large glasses.

Cabbage Cocktail

Serves 2 or 3

Quarter	head cabbage, washed and cut into chunks	Quarter
2	carrots, scrubbed	2
2	stalks celery, washed	2
1	clove garlic	1
3	sprigs parsley, washed	3
2	parsnips, scrubbed and cut into pieces	2
2	sprigs dill, washed	2
1	beet, scrubbed and cut into pieces	1
1	apple, washed and cut into pieces	1
1/2 tsp	dried fennel seeds (optional)	2 mL

1. Using juicer, process cabbage, carrots, celery, garlic, parsley, parsnips, dill, beet and apple. Whisk together and pour into a carafe or large glasses. Whisk in fennel seeds, if using.

Cauliflower Cocktail

Serves 2 or 3

Use any sea herbs in place of the kelp.

Half	head cauliflower, washed and cut into pieces	Half
1	stalk broccoli, washed and cut into pieces	1
3	tomatoes, washed and cut into wedges	3
2	carrots, scrubbed	2
2	stalks celery, washed	2
1	apple, washed and cut into pieces	1
1 tsp	crumbled dried kelp	5 mL

1. Using juicer, process cauliflower, broccoli, tomatoes, carrots, celery and apple. Whisk together and pour into glasses. Sprinkle with kelp.

Cajun Cocktail

Serves 2 or 3

If fresh chile pepper if not available, substitute 1 or 2 drops hot sauce or Jamaican jerk sauce. See page 49 for directions on juicing chile peppers. Plan to use pulp for Cajun Salsa (see recipe, page 184).

Parsley should be avoided during pregnancy.

3	large tomatoes, washed and cut into wedges	3
3	sprigs parsley, washed (see note, left)	3
2	stalks celery (with leaves), washed	2
1	clove garlic	1
Half	cucumber, washed and cut into cubes	Half
Half	lime, peeled	Half
Dash	Worcestershire sauce	Dash
1/2 tsp	prepared horseradish	2 mL
1	chile pepper, washed and halved	1

1. Using juicer, process tomatoes, parsley, celery, garlic, cucumber and lime. Pour into a carafe or pitcher. Whisk in Worcestershire sauce and horseradish.

2. In a separate container, juice chile pepper (see note at left). Whisk chile juice into cocktail 1/2 tsp (2 mL) at a time, tasting before adding more. Pour into glasses.

Citrus Cocktail

Serves 2

Use any melon or cantaloupe for this recipe.

Half	melon, peeled and cut into pieces	Half
1 cup	washed strawberries	250 mL
1	1-inch (2.5 cm) piece ginger root	1
1	orange, peeled and quartered	1
1	grapefruit, peeled and quartered	1
1/4 cup	natural yogurt	50 mL
1 tbsp	wheat germ *or* finely ground almonds	15 mL

1. Using juicer, process melon, strawberries, ginger, orange and grapefruit. Pour into a carafe. Whisk in yogurt and wheat germ. Pour into glasses.

Peppery Tomato Cocktail

Serves 1 or 2

3	large tomatoes, washed and cut into wedges	3
1	handful watercress, washed	1
1	green pepper, washed and cut into chunks	1
1	clove garlic	1
3	sprigs parsley, washed	3
2	carrots, scrubbed	2
Quarter	head fennel, washed	Quarter
1/2 tsp	cayenne pepper	2 mL

1. Using juicer, process tomatoes, watercress, green pepper, garlic, parsley, carrots and fennel. Pour into a carafe or pitcher. Whisk in cayenne pepper.

Melon Cocktail

Serves 2

Half	melon, peeled and cut into pieces	Half
4	oranges, peeled and quartered	4
1	carrot, scrubbed	1
1	2-inch (5 cm) slice watermelon, cut into pieces	1

1. Using juicer, process melon, oranges, carrot and watermelon. Whisk together and pour into glasses.

Melon Morning Cocktail

Serves 2

1	2-inch (5 cm) slice watermelon, cut into pieces	1
Quarter	cantaloupe, peeled and cut into pieces	Quarter
2	oranges, peeled and quartered	2
2	spears pineapple	2

1. Using juicer, process watermelon, cantaloupe, oranges and pineapple. Whisk together and pour into glasses.

Orange Cream Cocktail

Serves 2

3	oranges, peeled and quartered	3
2	spears pineapple	2
1	lime, peeled and halved	1
1	lemon, peeled and halved	1
1/4 cup	orange sherbet	50 mL
2	sprigs mint, washed	2

1. Using juicer, process oranges, pineapple, lime and lemon. Whisk together and pour into glasses. Scoop half sherbet into each glass. Garnish with mint sprig.

Pineapple Kiwi Cocktail

Serves 4

This is a very sweet drink, so you may wish to balance it by adding a lemon and up to 2 cups (500 mL) mineral water.

Half	pineapple, cut into spears	Half
3	kiwi, peeled and halved	3
2	oranges, peeled and quartered	2

1. Using juicer, process pineapple, kiwi and oranges. Whisk together and pour into glasses.

Tomato Juice Cocktail

Serves 4

The sodium in the celery lends its natural salt to this refreshing late-summer cooler.

3	large tomatoes, washed and cut into wedges	3
1	handful basil leaves, washed	1
1	small zucchini, scrubbed and cut into chunks	1
1	clove garlic	1
3	sprigs parsley, washed	3
1	stalk celery, washed and cut into pieces	1
1	beet, scrubbed and cut into pieces	1
1/8 tsp	cayenne pepper (optional)	0.5 mL

1. Using juicer, process tomatoes, basil, zucchini, garlic, parsley, celery and beet. Pour into a carafe or pitcher. Whisk in cayenne pepper.

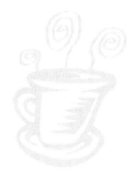

MULLED JUICES

Heating juices gives them a warming quality that's ideal when you have a cold or simply when it's cold outside. Keep in mind that heat-sensitive nutrients are lost when juices are heated. Our use of the term "mulled" is taking liberty with the term, since it usually applies only to red wine.

Use preheated mugs or glasses to keep the mulled juice warm longer. To preheat, pour boiling water into mugs and let stand; drain, then fill with hot mulled juice.

Serves 2

Antibiotic Toddy

For a heartier drink, which retains the goodness of the roots, do not strain mixture after it has simmered. Use a Vita-Mix® to liquefy and blend all ingredients before pouring into mugs and topping with orange or lemon slices. If the blended mixture is too thick, dilute it with boiled water.

2 cups	apple cider	500 mL
2 cups	orange juice	500 mL
1/2 cup	dried elderberries	125 mL
1	3-inch (7.5 cm) piece dried echinacea root	1
1	3-inch (7.5 cm) piece dried ginseng root	1
1	3-inch (7.5 cm) piece cinnamon stick	1
2 tbsp	finely chopped ginger root	25 mL
3	whole cloves	3
3	allspice berries	3
1 tbsp	dried stevia leaves	15 mL
1 tbsp	honey	15 mL
1 tbsp	apple cider vinegar	15 mL
1	lemon, juiced	1
	Orange or lemon slices for garnish	

1. In a saucepan over medium heat, combine apple cider, orange juice, elderberries, echinacea root, ginseng root, cinnamon stick, ginger, cloves, allspice berries and stevia leaves; heat until just under a boil. Cover, reduce heat and simmer for 10 minutes.

2. Strain mixture through a sieve, pressing on solids to extract all liquid. Stir in honey, vinegar and lemon juice. Pour into glasses and serve hot with orange or lemon slices.

Blazing Bullshot

Serves 4

Use any combination of vegetables for the vegetable juice.

3 cups	beef bouillon *or* vegetable stock	750 mL
1	chile pepper	1
1 cup	tomato or mixed vegetable juice	250 mL
1	lemon, juiced	1
Splash	Worcestershire sauce	Splash
1 tsp	garam masala (optional)	5 mL
4	stalks celery (with leaves) for garnish (optional)	4

1. In a saucepan over medium heat, combine bouillon
    and chile pepper; heat until just simmering. Cover,
    reduce heat and simmer for 10 minutes.

2. Remove from heat and whisk in tomato juice, lemon
    juice, Worcestershire sauce and, if using, garam masala.
    Remove chile pepper and pour hot mixture into
    glasses. Cut pepper lengthwise into quarters; use as
    garnish with celery stalks, if desired.

Hot Spiced Pear Nectar

Serves 2 or 3

If New Mexican chiles are not
available, substitute a poblano
chile.

6	pears, washed and cut into pieces	6
2	apples, washed and cut into pieces	2
1	lemon, peeled and cut in half	1
Half	New Mexican chile	Half
2 tbsp	maple syrup *or* molasses	25 mL
3	allspice berries	3
1	2-inch (5 cm) cinnamon stick	1

1. Using juicer, process pears, apples, lemon and chile.
    Transfer juice to a saucepan. Over medium heat, stir
    in maple syrup, allspice berries and cinnamon. Bring
    to just under a boil; cover, reduce heat and simmer
    for 5 minutes. Strain into heated mugs.

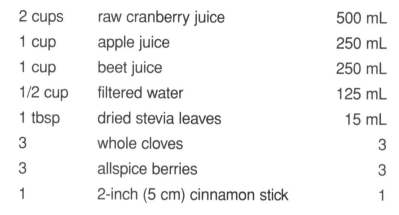

Mulled Cranberry

Serves 2

2 cups	raw cranberry juice	500 mL
1 cup	apple juice	250 mL
1 cup	beet juice	250 mL
1/2 cup	filtered water	125 mL
1 tbsp	dried stevia leaves	15 mL
3	whole cloves	3
3	allspice berries	3
1	2-inch (5 cm) cinnamon stick	1

1. In a saucepan over medium heat, combine cranberry juice, apple juice, beet juice, water, stevia leaves, cloves, allspice berries and cinnamon. Bring to just under a boil; cover, reduce heat and simmer for 5 minutes. Strain into hot mugs.

Pineapple-Cranberry Sizzler

Serves 6

For a deeper pineapple taste, add 2 or 3 bruised pineapple sage leaves *(salvia elegans)*, if available, to the pot while it is simmering.

2 cups	pineapple juice	500 mL
1 cup	raw cranberry juice	250 mL
1/2 cup	apple cider or apple juice	125 mL
1	2-inch (5 cm) piece licorice root	1
5	whole coriander seeds	5
1 tsp	fenugreek seeds	5 mL
2 tbsp	honey	25 mL

1. In a saucepan over medium heat, combine pineapple juice, cranberry juice, apple cider, licorice, coriander, fenugreek and honey. Bring to just under a boil; cover, reduce heat and simmer for 5 minutes. Strain into hot mugs.

Tree-Trimming Tomato Warmer

Serves 4

4	apples, washed and cut into pieces	4
1	lemon, peeled and halved	1
1 tbsp	curry powder	15 mL
1 tsp	ground cinnamon	5 mL
1 tsp	ground cumin	5 mL
4 cups	tomato juice	1 L
4	stalks celery (for garnish)	4

1. Using juicer, process apples and lemon.

2. In a saucepan over low heat, combine curry, cinnamon and cumin. Cook, stirring, for 2 minutes or until spices are aromatic. (Be careful not to let the spices burn.) Add apple-lemon juice and tomato juice. Bring to a light boil, stirring.

3. Remove from heat, pour into heated mugs and garnish with celery stalks.

JUICE PUNCHES

The *Dictionary of Gastronomy* suggests that the word "punch" comes from the Hindi word *panch*, meaning five, because five ingredients — arrack, lime, sugar, spices and water — were used. In its "Glossary of Culinary Terms", *Mrs. Beeton's Household Management* gives the following definition: "Punch á la Romaine (Fr). A kind of soft white ice, made from lemon-juice, white of egg, sugar, and rum. It is served in goblets and acts as a digestive." And the *New Larousse Gastronomique* explains it thus: "Punch: A drink said to have originated among English sailors, and which, about 1552, consisted of a simple mixture of cane spirit and sugar, heated."

Whatever its origins, punch has come to be known as a mixture of fruit juices served over ice with or without alcohol. Some punches require a simple syrup (a mixture of sugar and water, boiled to thicken it) especially if lemons are a major ingredient. Most of the recipes here rely on the natural sugars in the fruit.

Apple-Orange Punch

Serves 6

Make this punch in the fall, when apple cider is fresh and widely available. Use some of the orange and lime peel as garnish.

4	beets, scrubbed and cut into pieces	4
6	apples, washed and cut into pieces	6
3	oranges, peeled and quartered	3
1	lime, peeled and halved	1
1	1-inch (2.5 cm) piece ginger root	1
4 cups	fresh apple cider	1 L
6	scoops frozen Orange-Melon Sherbet (see recipe page 177)	6

1. Using juicer, process beets, apples, oranges, lime and ginger. Whisk together with cider and chill. To serve: Pour into a punch bowl and float sherbet on top.

Berry Combo

Serves 6

Perfect for spring gatherings, this punch has a vibrant pink color that brightens the buffet table. If available, float sweet cicely flowers or rose petals on top.

Native Cranberries

Chief Pakimintzen of the Delaware Indians offered cranberries as a gesture of peace. Over time, "pakimintzen" came to be the Delawares' word for "cranberry eater."

The Pequot Indians of Cape Cod and the Leni-Lenape tribes of New Jersey called the cranberry *ibimi*, meaning "bitter berry."

1 1/2 cups	sliced washed rhubarb	375 mL
1 cup	washed cranberries, chopped, fresh or frozen	250 mL
2 cups	washed blackberries or raspberries, fresh or frozen	500 mL
4 cups	water	1 L
2 tbsp	granulated sugar (or to taste)	25 mL
1 tsp	powdered stevia	5 mL
Half	pineapple, cut into wedges	Half
4	beets, scrubbed and cut into pieces	4
1	lemon, peeled and halved	1
1/4 cup	chopped sweet cicely leaves	50 mL
2 tbsp	finely grated ginger root	25 mL

1. In a saucepan over medium–high heat, bring rhubarb, cranberries, blackberries, water, sugar and stevia to a boil. Reduce heat and simmer, stirring occasionally, for 15 minutes. Strain through a sieve, pressing on solids to extract all liquid; discard solids. Chill.

2. To serve: Using a juicer, process pineapple, beets and lemon. Whisk together and add to punch bowl, with chilled rhubarb-berry juice. Whisk in sweet cicely and ginger.

Fruit Punch

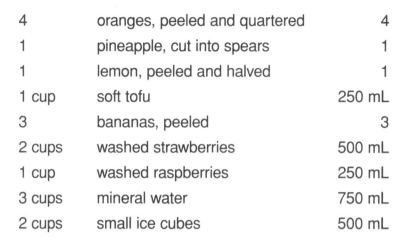

Serves 6

4	oranges, peeled and quartered	4
1	pineapple, cut into spears	1
1	lemon, peeled and halved	1
1 cup	soft tofu	250 mL
3	bananas, peeled	3
2 cups	washed strawberries	500 mL
1 cup	washed raspberries	250 mL
3 cups	mineral water	750 mL
2 cups	small ice cubes	500 mL

1. Using juicer, process oranges, pineapple and lemon. Whisk together and pour into a large glass jar with a lid. Chill until ready to serve.

2. Just before serving, divide each of tofu, bananas, strawberries and raspberries into 2 equal portions. Measure 2 cups (500 mL) of chilled orange-pineapple juice and set aside. Pour remaining juice into punch bowl.

3. Using a blender, process 1 cup (250 mL) of reserved orange-pineapple juice with one portion of tofu, bananas, strawberries and raspberries; add to punch bowl. Process remaining 1 cup (250 mL) juice, tofu and fruit. Add to punch bowl. Whisk until combined. Stir in mineral water, add ice and serve immediately.

Gardener's Lemonade

Serves 6

TEA HERBS
The following herbs make excellent herbal teas. Use them alone or in combination.

Mint (*Mentha*, see pages 35 and 39) Many varieties available including Ginger, Lime, Apple.

Chamomile (*Matricaria*, see page 27) Lends a flowery, apple-like taste.

Bergamot (*Mondara*) The whole plant smells pleasantly of orange and the taste is slightly citrus.

Anise Hyssop (*Agastache foeniclum*, see Hyssop, page 30) Scented of anise and mint. Best if blended with other tea herbs.

Roses (*Rosa*, see page 37) Use petals and hip.

Lemon Balm (*Melissa officianalis*, see page 31) The sweet, strong lemon smell and taste makes it a popular tea herb, alone or in blends.

Lemon Verbena (*Aloysia triphylla*, see page 31) Rich lemon taste.

Scented Geraniums (*Pelagonium*) Use the highly aromatic leaves from over 150 different Pelagoniums.

Sweet Cicely (*Myrrhis odoratat*) A very sweet, anise-flavored leaf that is commonly used in tea blends.

Thyme (*Thymus*, see page 41) Many different flavors including nutmeg, orange and lemon.

Lavender (*Lavendula*, see page 30) A flowery, distinct flavor. Best blended with other tea herbs.

Linden Flower (*Tilia cordata*, see page 32) A mild-flavored, gently calming herb.

1/3 cup	granulated sugar	75 mL
1 cup	water	250 mL
6	lemons, washed	6
3 cups	hot water	750 mL
1 tbsp	chopped lemon balm	15 mL
1 tbsp	chopped mint	15 mL
1 tbsp	washed bergamot leaves	15 mL
3	linden flowers, washed	3
	Extra tea herbs for garnish	

1. In a small saucepan over medium heat, combine sugar and 1 cup (250 mL) water. Heat, stirring constantly, until the sugar has completely dissolved. Bring to a boil and cook, without stirring, for 1 minute or until the syrup is clear. Set aside to cool.

2. Peel the rind of 2 lemons in one continuous strip; set strips aside. Cut all 6 lemons in half.

3. Using electric or cone hand juicer, juice lemons; strain into a large pitcher. Stir in cooled syrup, hot water, lemon balm, mint, bergamot, linden flowers and reserved lemon rind strips. Set in sun or leave on kitchen counter to steep for 1 hour or more. Remove herbs and lemon peel and chill or serve over ice. Garnish with fresh leaves of lemon balm, bergamot or linden flowers and mint sprigs.

Summer Flower Nectar

Serves 6

1/4 cup	washed calendula petals	50 mL
1/4 cup	washed chopped lemon balm	50 mL
3 tbsp	washed rose petals	45 mL
1 tbsp	washed lavender flowers	15 mL
1 tbsp	grated orange zest	15 mL
1 tsp	chopped ginger root	5 mL
4 cups	boiling water	1 L
5 tbsp	honey	75 mL
3	peaches, peeled, pitted and quartered	3
3	apricots, peeled, pitted and quartered	3
3	nectarines, peeled, pitted and quartered	3
2	oranges, peeled and quartered	2
2	2-inch (5 cm) slices watermelon, cut into pieces	2
3 cups	mineral water	750 mL
3	whole roses, washed (for garnish, optional)	3
3	whole calendula flowers, washed (for garnish, optional)	3

1. Place calendula, lemon balm, rose petals, lavender, orange peel, and ginger in a teapot. Pour in boiling water and steep for 5 minutes. Strain tea into a pitcher or container; discard solids. Add honey and stir until dissolved. Chill until ready to serve.

2. To serve: Using juicer, process peaches, apricots, nectarines, oranges and watermelon. Whisk together and pour into a punch bowl. Stir in mineral water and chilled tea. Garnish with whole flowers, if desired, and serve over ice.

Lavender Punch

Serves 6

2 cups	water	500 mL
1	2-inch (5 cm) cinnamon	1
2	star anise pods and seeds	2
3	allspice berries	3
2	whole cloves	2
1	stick astragalus root (optional)	1
3 tbsp	washed fresh lavender flower buds (or 1 tbsp [15 mL] dried)	45 mL
4	oranges, peeled and quartered	4
3	lemons, peeled and halved	3
3 cups	washed red grapes	750 mL
3 cups	mineral water	750 mL

1. In a medium saucepan over medium heat, combine water, cinnamon, star anise, allspice, cloves and, if using, astragalus. Bring to a light boil; cover, reduce heat and simmer gently for 5 minutes. Remove from heat and stir in lavender flowers; cover and let stand for 10 minutes. Strain into a covered jar or container; discard solids. Chill until ready to serve.

2. To serve: Using juicer, process oranges, lemons and grapes. Whisk together and add to punch bowl. Stir in chilled lavender water and mineral water. Serve over ice, and sweeten to taste with honey if desired.

Roman Punch No. 1

Serves 8

"Grate the yellow rind of four lemons and two oranges upon two pounds of sugar. Squeeze the juice of the lemons and oranges; cover it and let it stand until next day. Strain it through a sieve, mix with the sugar; add a bottle of champagne and the whites of eight eggs beaten to a stiff froth. It may be frozen or not, as desired. For winter use snow instead of ice."

From the *White House Cookbook* by Hugo Zieman and Mrs. F.L. Gilette, Toronto: The Copp Clark Co. Limited, 1887.

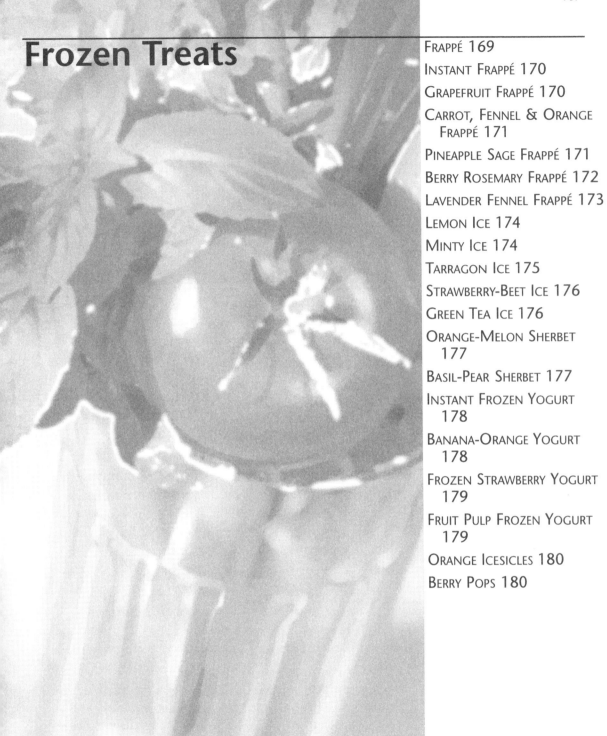

Frozen Treats

Frozen Treats

Holistic health practitioners all agree that sugar is a major contributor to diabetes, hypoglycemia and tooth decay — and, for this reason, should be avoided. Similarly, honey and other natural, non-herb sweeteners should be used only in very small amounts or not at all. Stevia (see page 40) is a good substitute in cases where the specific chemistry of sugar is not essential. Unfortunately, sugar (or honey) is necessary in frozen desserts — without it, the dessert crystallizes and freezes the liquids into one solid block. To ensure a soft, spoonable texture, frozen desserts must contain enough sugar to lower their freezing point; the more sugar, the softer the consistency.

The recipes in this section represent something of a compromise: They do not contain enough sugar to keep them from freezing completely, but they do have enough to give them a pleasant texture. We have included only as much sugar (or honey) as is absolutely necessary, so don't try to reduce the amounts any further or the recipes won't work.

Still, given that sugar is so undesirable, why provide these recipes at all? Simply because they enable you to use some of the pulp that is produced from juicing. Besides, these frozen treats are certainly preferable to commercial ice cream and sherbet. They contain far less sugar and only fresh, natural ingredients that contain no other chemicals or additives. And the popsicles in this section are a better bet for kids than the colored, sugared water they get from the store.

Of course, boiling and freezing juice, no matter how fresh it is, will destroy vitamin C, enzymes and other heat-sensitive phytonutrients. The best alternative is to make "instant" frappé or frozen yogurt using the Vita-Mix® (see page 170). This uses the whole fruit with pulp and does not require any sweeteners, except a small amount according to individual taste.

To use pulp from juice recipes: Pulp from any of the fruit juice or fruit juice cocktails may be used to make sherbets, ices or frappés, frozen yogurt or popsicles. Pulp from some of the sweeter vegetable juices such as carrot, beet, parsnip or fennel may also be used if blended with fruit pulp. To use pulp for frozen desserts, cut out the core and seeds and peel the fruit or vegetable before juicing. For best results, blend pulp using blender or food processor before using in frozen treats. Measure 2 cups (500 mL) of the blended pulp and chill if the frozen dessert will be made within a day, or label and freeze until ready to use.

Frappé

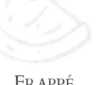

9- BY 5-INCH (22.5 BY 12.5 CM) METAL LOAF PAN

2 cups	chilled or frozen pulp	500 mL
2 cups	orange juice *or* apple juice *or* any other fruit juice	500 mL
1	lemon, juiced	1
3/4 cup	granulated sugar *or* honey	175 mL

FRAPPÉ

The term frappé comes from the French, meaning "chilled" or "iced." Simple mixtures made from water, sugar and chopped fruit, frappés are frozen to a mushy consistency. Frappés are coarser (with a texture resembling that of coarse rock salt) than any of the other iced desserts.

To make frappé from chilled or frozen pulp, the pulp need only be thawed enough to blend with other ingredients.

1. In a blender combine pulp, orange juice, lemon juice and sugar. Blend for 10 seconds on High. Pour into loaf pan. Freeze for 2 hours or until a mushy consistency is reached.

2. Stir mixture and return to freezer for 1 hour or just until firm enough to scoop. If it freezes solid, ripen in the refrigerator (see below) to soften.

Freezing ices, frappés, sherbets and yogurt. Freezing times given in recipe are approximate. Actual results will depend on the freezer and the pan. Deep-sided metal loaf pans are best because with each stirring, air is incorporated and the mixture tends to expand. The recipes in this section give directions for freezing the mixture in a 9- x 5-inch (22.5 by 12.5 cm) metal loaf pan in a chest freezer. However, if your freezer has a "fast freeze" compartment or if a square, shallow metal pan is used, freezing times will be shorter. All of the frozen treats can be made with an ice cream machine. Follow manufacturer's directions.

To "ripen" frozen ices. Unless timed perfectly, most ices will be too hard to serve directly from the freezer. In order to spoon and serve and to bring out their best flavor, iced desserts require "ripening" or softening. To ripen, set the iced dessert in the refrigerator for 45 minutes to 2 hours before serving, depending on the pan (wide, shallow pans thaw more quickly) and the degree to which the ice is frozen.

Instant Frappé

To make instant frappé: you will need a Vita-Mix® machine. The benefits of this method are that you can use the peel, core and seeds of most fruit, and sugar is not required. To sweeten, just add 1/2 tsp (2 mL) powdered or liquid stevia to taste.

1/2 cup	fruit juice	125 mL
2 cups	fruit or fruit-vegetable pulp	500 mL
1 to 2 tbsp	liquid honey *or* maple syrup *or* corn syrup (optional)	15 to 25 mL
3 cups	ice cubes	750 mL

1. Add juice, pulp, honey (if using) and ice cubes to Vita-Mix®. Secure lid. Process at variable speed #1, increasing speed to #10, then to High. Process for 30 to 60 seconds or until ice is chopped (but no longer). Serve immediately.

Grapefruit Frappé

Serves 4 to 6

Be sure to trim off the white pith and remove seeds before juicing the citrus fruits used in this recipe.

9- BY 5-INCH (22.5 BY 12.5 CM) METAL LOAF PAN

2 cups	water	500 mL
3/4 cup	granulated sugar	175 mL
1 cup	pulp from Grapefruit Juice (see recipe, page 119)	250 mL

1. In a saucepan over medium-high heat, combine water and sugar. Bring to a boil and cook 3 minutes without stirring. Remove from heat and set aside to cool.

2. In loaf pan, combine sugar syrup and grapefruit pulp. Freeze for 2 hours or until a mushy consistency is reached. Stir with a fork and return to freezer for 1 hour or until firm. If consistency is too hard, ripen in the refrigerator to soften.

Carrot, Fennel & Orange Frappé

Serves 4 to 6

9- BY 5-INCH (22.5 BY 12.5 CM) METAL LOAF PAN

2 cups	water	500 mL
1/2 cup	granulated sugar	125 mL
2 cups	pulp from Carrot Fennel Orange juice (see recipe, page 115)	500 mL

1. In a saucepan over medium-high heat, combine water and sugar. Bring to a boil and cook for 3 minutes without stirring. Remove from heat and set aside to cool.

2. In loaf pan, combine sugar syrup and pulp. Freeze for 2 hours or until a mushy consistency is reached. Stir with a fork and return to freezer for 1 hour or until firm. If consistency is too hard, ripen in the refrigerator to soften.

Pineapple Sage Frappé

Serves 4 to 6

Pineapple sage is a tender perennial with sweet, fragrantly pineapple flavor. If you can find any, use it in this or any of the fruit juice recipes.

9- BY 5-INCH (22.5 BY 12.5 CM) METAL LOAF PAN

2 cups	water	500 mL
2 cups	pulp from Pineapple-Citrus juice (see recipe, page 123)	500 mL
1/2 cup	honey	125 mL
2 tbsp	chopped sage leaves (optional)	25 mL

1. Using a blender, process water, pulp, honey and sage leaves until blended. Pour mixture into loaf pan. Freeze for 2 hours or until a mushy consistency is reached. Stir with a fork and return to freezer for 1 hour or until firm. If consistency is too hard, ripen in the refrigerator to soften.

Berry Rosemary Frappé

Serves 4 to 6

The rosemary is optional here, but it adds a fragrant bite that compliments the sweetness of the berries.

9- BY 5-INCH (22.5 BY 12.5 CM) METAL LOAF PAN

2 cups	water	500 mL
2 cups	pulp from any berry juice (such as Berry Best, page 113)	500 mL
1 tbsp	rosemary leaves (optional)	15 mL
1/2 cup	honey	125 mL

1. Using a blender, process water, pulp, rosemary leaves (if using) and honey until blended.

2. Pour mixture into loaf pan. Freeze for 2 hours or until a mushy consistency is reached. Stir with a fork and return to freezer for 1 hour or until firm. If consistency is too hard, ripen in the refrigerator to soften.

HONEY

Referred to as "the white man's fly" by Native Americans, the honeybee was introduced to North America in the seventeenth century by English colonists. It quickly became important for pollinating food crops and providing a sweet alternative to sugar from cane, beets and molasses.

To produce 1 tsp (5 mL) of honey, worker bees, which collect the nectar and flower pollen, will fly a distance equivalent to once around the world. A colony of workers must visit and extract nectar from about 2 million flowers to produce only 1 lb (500 g). In early human history, when honey was taken from hives, they were often destroyed in the process. Thankfully, in the mid-1800s, a wooden hive structure was invented that permitted the harvesting of honey without harming the bees. Variations on that box are still used by modern beekeepers.

The color and flavor of honey differs from region to region and country to country, depending on the types of flowers from which the nectar is gathered. Some common North American bee plants are listed below.

Alfalfa. An important honey plant in most of western North America, alfalfa honey is white or extra light amber in color and mild in taste.

Buckwheat. Plants grow in cool, moist climates and produce a dark brown, and distinct strongly flavored honey early in the season.

Clover. The most important (and popular) honey plant in North America, clover produces a honey that varies in color from water-white to extra light amber and has a mild, delicate flavor.

Eucalyptus. With over 500 distinct species and hybrids of eucalyptus, the honey from this plant varies greatly in color and taste but is generally a bold-flavored honey with a slightly medicinal aftertaste.

Orange blossom. Often derived from a combination of citrus blossom sources, the honey is white to extra light amber with the distinctive fragrance of oranges. This honey is abundant in the southern United States.

Sage. Found mostly along the California coast and Sierra Nevada mountain range, sage shrubs produce a mild, delicately flavored honey that is usually white in color.

Sunflower. A gold colored honey with a unique but delicate flavor from sunflowers that grow in abundance in Manitoba and the central United States.

For more information about honey and honey production, visit www.honey.com or www.agr.ca/cb/factsheets/honey.html

Lavender Fennel Frappé

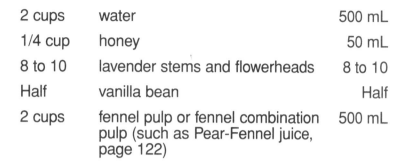

9- BY 5-INCH (22.5 BY 12.5 CM) METAL LOAF PAN

2 cups	water	500 mL
1/4 cup	honey	50 mL
8 to 10	lavender stems and flowerheads	8 to 10
Half	vanilla bean	Half
2 cups	fennel pulp or fennel combination pulp (such as Pear-Fennel juice, page 122)	500 mL

1. In a saucepan over medium-high heat, combine water and honey. Bring to a boil and cook for 2 to 3 minutes without stirring. Remove from heat and stir in lavender and vanilla bean. Set aside to cool.

2. When cooled, strain lavender mixture into loaf pan, discarding solids. Stir in pulp and freeze for 2 hours or until a mushy consistency is reached. Stir with a fork and return to freezer for 1 hour or until firm. If consistency is too hard, ripen in the refrigerator to soften.

SUGAR, SUGAR EVERYWHERE

The human predilection (or weakness) for sugar is such that it is now added (in significant quantities) to many commercially prepared food products, ranging from baby foods and vegetables to sauces, juices — even salt! We can't get away from it. Sugar comes from sugarcane, sorghum, corn syrup, sugar beets,

and sugar maple. Its component parts — dextrose (corn sugar), sucrose (cane sugar), fructose (fruit sugar), glucose or lactose (milk sugar) — are what we find in most commercially prepared foods.

And the result of eating all that sugar? Apart from supplying excess

calories, sugar depletes the immune system, causes tooth decay, and contributes to diabetes and hypoglycemia. Worse for children, high-sugar foods can replace nutritious foods and deprive young bodies of the nutrients necessary for growth and good health.

Lemon Ice

Serves 4 to 6

A wonderfully tart, lip-smuckering frozen dessert.

9- BY 5-INCH (22.5 BY 12.5 CM) METAL LOAF PAN

4	lemons	4
1/2 cup	lightly packed lemon balm leaves	125 mL
2 cups	boiled water	500 mL
1/3 cup	honey	75 mL

1. Grate the zest from one lemon; set aside. Using a hand or electric juicer, juice lemons. Chop the lemon balm.

2. In loaf pan, combine water, lemon juice, lemon zest, chopped lemon balm and honey. Freeze for 2 hours or until a mushy consistency is reached. Stir with a fork and return to freezer for 1 hour or until firm. If consistency is too hard, ripen in the refrigerator to soften.

Minty Ice

Serves 4 to 6

ICES

Made only from water, flavored water, fruit juices and syrup (no pulp is used in true ices), the texture of ices falls between the coarse frappé and the finer sherbet.

9- BY 5-INCH (22.5 BY 12.5 CM) METAL LOAF PAN

2 cups	water	500 mL
1/4 cup	chopped mint leaves	50 mL
1/2 cup	granulated sugar	125 mL
1	lime, juiced	1

1. In a saucepan over medium-high heat, combine water, mint and sugar. Bring to a boil and cook for 3 minutes without stirring. Remove from heat and set aside to cool.

2. Stir lime juice into cooled mint mixture; pour into loaf pan. Freeze for 2 hours or until a mushy consistency is reached. Stir with a fork and return to freezer for 1 hour or until firm. If consistency is too hard, ripen in the refrigerator to soften.

Tarragon Ice

Serves 4 to 6

9- BY 5-INCH (22.5 BY 12.5 CM) METAL LOAF PAN

2 cups	water	500 mL
3 tbsp	chopped tarragon leaves	45 mL
1/2 cup	granulated sugar	125 mL
2	lemons, juiced	2

1. In a saucepan over medium-high heat, combine water, tarragon and sugar. Bring to a boil and cook for 3 minutes without stirring. Remove from heat and set aside to cool.

2. Stir lemon juice into cooled tarragon mixture; pour into loaf pan. Freeze for 2 hours or until a mushy consistency is reached. Stir with a fork and return to freezer for 1 hour or until firm. If consistency is too hard, ripen in the refrigerator to soften.

Strawberry-Beet Ice

Serves 4 to 6

9- BY 5-INCH (22.5 BY 12.5 CM) METAL LOAF PAN

2 cups	strawberry and beet pulp	500 mL
2 cups	water	500 mL
1/3 cup	liquid honey	75 mL

1. In loaf pan combine pulp, water and honey. Freeze for 2 hours or until a mushy consistency is reached. Stir with a fork and return to freezer for 1 hour or until firm. If consistency is too hard, ripen in the refrigerator to soften.

Green Tea Ice

Serves 4 to 6

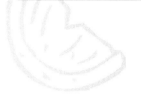

9- BY 5-INCH (22.5 BY 12.5 CM) METAL LOAF PAN

1	bag green tea (or 1 tsp [5 mL] loose green tea leaves)	1
2 tsp	Digestive Seed Tea (see recipe, page 204) *or* fennel seeds	10 mL
1	star anise pod (with seeds)	1
Half	vanilla bean	Half
3 cups	boiling water	750 mL
1/2 cup	granulated sugar	125 mL
2 tbsp	lemon juice	25 mL

1. In a large, non-reactive teapot, combine green tea, Digestive Seed Tea, anise and vanilla bean. Pour in boiling water, cover and steep for 5 minutes.

2. In a loaf pan, strain hot tea over sugar, stirring to dissolve. Set aside to cool.

3. When cooled, stir in lemon juice. Freeze for 2 hours or until a mushy consistency is reached. Stir with a fork and return to freezer for 1 hour or until firm. If frozen solid when ready to serve, ripen in the refrigerator to soften.

Sweet Alternatives

Aztec sweet herb (Phyla scaberrima, formerly Lippia dulcis). A perennial herb used by the Aztecs. The compound hernandulcin, found in the leaves, stems and roots, is about three times as sweet as sucrose but has a somewhat bitter aftertaste.

Date sugar. A coarse, dark mealy substance from ground-up dehydrated dates. High in fiber, vitamins and minerals, it is fine in baked products but does not dissolve in drinks or liquids.

Honey. See page 172.

Katemfe (Thaumatococcus daniellii). A perennial herb of the arrowroot family found in the East and West African rain forests. The sweet protein thaumatin, found in fruit of the plant, is up to 1600 times as sweet as sucrose but loses its sweetness if heated.

Licorice (Glycyrrhiza glabra, see page 31). Its wrinkled, thick brown roots contain glycyrrhizin, a compound that is 50 to 150 times as sweet as cane sugar. The elderly or people with high blood pressure or heart, kidney, or liver disease should avoid licorice.

Molasses (see page 52). The stronger tasting, crude blackstrap molasses is preferred nutritionally to the other lighter types. Molasses is a concentrated syrupy by-product of sugar cane refining and is rich in B vitamins, vitamin E, iron, calcium, magnesium, potassium, chromium, manganese and zinc.

Stevia (Stevia rebaudiana, see page 40). Known as the "sweet herb" and used in Paraguay and Central America since pre-Columbian times, stevia is 200 to 300 times as sweet as sucrose with none of the side effects or calories. A mild aftertaste is detectable in juices or fruit desserts where stevia is used. Widely available in alternative/health stores, stevia is the easiest of the sweet herbs to find and use even though it is still prevented from being used as a sugar substitute in the Unites States.

Other fruits and berries offering sweet alternatives to sugar include serendipity berries (Dioscoreophyllum cumminsii) and miracle fruit (Synsepalum dulcificum).

Orange-Melon Sherbet

Serves 4 to 6

SHERBET

Also called sorbet, sherbet is a smooth, frozen sugar-fruit-water mixture. Because of their high liquid content, sherbets require stabilizers to keep the texture solid and smooth but without freezing too hard. Dissolved gelatin, softened marshmallows and beaten egg whites are used for this purpose.

Sherbets are usually served in chilled sherbet glasses but individual servings can be molded in the shape of an egg and served on a chilled dessert plate with fruit or herb garnishes. Unlike mousses or cream molded frozen desserts, sherbets are not usually served with sauces.

9- BY 5-INCH (22.5 BY 12.5 CM) METAL LOAF PAN

2 cups	melon pulp (from any juice recipe containing melon)	500 mL
2 1/2 cups	orange juice	625 mL
2 tbsp	grated orange zest	25 mL
1	lemon, juiced	1
1/2 cup	granulated sugar	125 mL
1 cup	water	250 mL
2	egg whites	2

1. In loaf pan combine pulp, orange juice, orange zest, lemon juice, sugar and water. Freeze for 1 to 2 hours or until a mushy consistency is reached.

2. Beat egg whites in a bowl until stiff but not dry. Remove sherbet from freezer and beat with a fork for 20 seconds. Whisk in beaten egg whites. Return to freezer for 1 hour or until firm. If consistency is too hard, ripen in the refrigerator to soften.

Basil-Pear Sherbet

Serves 4 to 6

9- BY 5-INCH (22.5 BY 12.5 CM) METAL LOAF PAN

2 cups	pulp from Autumn Refresher juice (see recipe, page 113)	500 mL
1/2 cup	granulated sugar	125 mL
2 cups	water	500 mL
2 tbsp	chopped fresh basil	25 mL
2	egg whites	2

1. In loaf pan combine pulp, sugar, water and basil. Freeze for 1 to 2 hours or until a mushy consistency is reached.

2. Beat egg whites in a bowl until stiff but not dry. Remove sherbet from freezer and beat with a fork for 20 seconds. Whisk in beaten egg whites. Return to freezer for 1 hour or until firm. If consistency is too hard, ripen in the refrigerator to soften.

Instant Frozen Yogurt

Serves 4 to 6

To make instant frozen yogurt you will need a Vita-Mix® machine. Pineapple Citrus juice and pulp (see recipe, page 123) works well for this recipe and requires no sweetening.

1/2 cup	fruit juice	125 mL
2 cups	chilled or frozen fruit pulp (see note at left)	500 mL
1 cup	natural yogurt	250 mL
2 tbsp	honey (optional)	25 mL
3 cups	ice cubes	750 mL

1. Add juice, pulp, yogurt, honey (if using) and ice cubes to Vita-Mix®; secure lid. Process starting at variable speed #1, increasing speed to #10, then to High. Use the tamper while machine is processing. The process takes only 30 to 60 seconds. Serve immediately.

Banana-Orange Yogurt

Serves 4 to 6

Frozen yogurt
In these desserts, natural yogurt replaces the heavy cream of ice creams, mousses and parfaits. Substitute soft tofu for yogurt. Homemade frozen yogurt is truly healthier than the sweeter ices and fat-laden desserts made with 18% to 36% butterfat creams. It is superior to some commercial frozen yogurts which can contain much more sugar and chemical additives.

9- BY 5-INCH (22.5 BY 12.5 CM) METAL LOAF PAN

1 cup	natural yogurt	250 mL
1	ripe banana, mashed	1
2 cups	pulp from C-Blend juice (see recipe, page 116)	500 mL
2 tbsp	liquid honey	25 mL

1. In loaf pan combine yogurt, banana, pulp and honey. Freeze for 1 to 2 hours or until firm. If consistency is too hard, ripen in the refrigerator to soften.

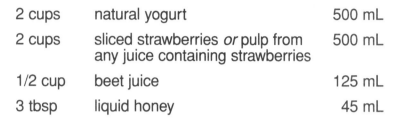

Frozen Strawberry Yogurt

Serves 4 to 6

9- BY 5-INCH (22.5 BY 12.5 CM) METAL LOAF PAN

2 cups	natural yogurt	500 mL
2 cups	sliced strawberries *or* pulp from any juice containing strawberries	500 mL
1/2 cup	beet juice	125 mL
3 tbsp	liquid honey	45 mL

1. In loaf pan combine yogurt, strawberries, beet juice and honey. Freeze for 1 to 2 hours or until firm. If consistency is too hard, ripen in the refrigerator to soften.

Fruit Pulp Frozen Yogurt

Serves 4 to 6

If desired, add up to 2 tbsp (25 mL) chopped fresh sage, thyme, basil, tarragon, mint, lemon balm or hyssop.

9- BY 5-INCH (22.5 BY 12.5 CM) METAL LOAF PAN

1 cup	natural yogurt	250 mL
2 cups	fruit pulp *or* sweet vegetable pulp	500 mL
1 tbsp	lemon juice	15 mL
3 tbsp	liquid honey (optional)	45 mL

1. In loaf pan combine yogurt, pulp, lemon juice and honey. Freeze for 1 to 2 hours or until firm. If consistency is too hard, ripen in the refrigerator to soften.

Berry Pops

Makes 12

POPSICLES

Kids love popsicles. If started young enough, they will also love frozen fruit juices or a mixture of pulp and juice with no sweetener at all. To wean older children off commercial popsicles, make this recipe with 2 to 3 tbsp (25 to 45 mL) liquid honey, then gradually reduce it.

Use juice or a 1:2 ratio of pulp to juice. Always process pulp in the blender before using in popsicles. Carrot, fennel and beet juice can be mixed with sweeter fruit juices. If herbs are recommended for a particular condition, a tea may be made, strained and blended with fruit juice, then frozen to make it easier for a child to take.

12 WAXED PAPER CUPS AND 12 WOODEN STICKS

2 cups	raspberry, strawberry or cherry juice	500 mL
1/2 cup	orange juice	125 mL
1/2 cup	beet juice	125 mL
2 tbsp	liquid honey (optional)	25 mL

1. In a medium bowl, combine raspberry juice, orange juice, beet juice and, if using, honey. Pour 1/4 cup (50 mL) juice into each waxed paper cup. Freeze for 1 hour or until firm enough to hold a stick. Insert wooden stick in middle and return to freezer for 1 hour or until hard.

Makes 12

Orange Icesicles

To freeze popsicles:
Pour 1/4 cup (50 mL) juice into waxed paper cups, freeze for 1 hour or until firm enough to hold stick. Insert wooden stick in middle and return to freezer for 1 hour or until hard. Reuseable plastic containers are available for making these refreshing treats at home.

12 WAXED PAPER CUPS AND 12 WOODEN STICKS

2 cups	orange juice	500 mL
1 cup	carrot juice	250 mL
2 tbsp	liquid honey (optional)	25 mL
2 tbsp	grated orange zest	25 mL

1. In a medium bowl, combine orange juice, carrot juice, honey and zest. Pour 1/4 cup (50 mL) juice into each waxed paper cup. Freeze for 1 hour or until firm enough to hold a stick. Insert wooden stick in middle and return to freezer for 1 hour or until hard.

Roughies and Smoothies

Roughies

Our definition of "roughies" is any food that has been made with the pulp from juicing. When fruits, vegetables or herbs are processed in a juice machine, two products are the result — pure raw juice and pulp. While juices contain a concentrated amount of nutrients, the pulp retains the fiber and a substantial amount of nutrients as well. Plan to use pulp from juicing in as many favorite recipes as possible — soup stocks, stews, dips, baked products, sauces and any recipe that calls for a purée of fruit or vegetable.

Versatile fruits or vegetables such as apples, carrots and tomatoes can be juiced first, the pulp collected and kept separate from other juice ingredients to keep their flavors pure for apple sauce, muffins, cakes or tomato sauces and salsas. See the Frozen Treats chapter (pages 167 to 180) for cooling recipes that use pulp.

To use pulp in recipes: Cut out the core and seeds and peel the fruit or vegetable before juicing. For best results, blend pulp using blender or food processor before using or freezing. Measure 2 cups (500 mL) of the blended pulp and transfer to a freezer bag or covered container. Store in the refrigerator if the pulp will be used within a day, or label and freeze until needed.

Apple-Rice Pudding

Serves 4

Dairy-free and low in fat, this alternative dessert is delicious. Substitute nut or fruit milk (see pages 214 and 215) for soy milk. Strain the yogurt through a cheesecloth-lined sieve.

2 cups	soy milk	500 mL
3/4 cup	rice	175 mL
1 cup	apple pulp	250 mL
1/2 cup	apple juice	125 mL
3 tbsp	honey	45 mL
1/2 cup	strained yogurt	125 mL
1 tbsp	finely chopped candied ginger	15 mL
1/2 tsp	ground cinnamon	2 mL
1/4 tsp	ground nutmeg	1 mL

1. In a saucepan over medium–high heat, combine soy milk and rice; bring to a light boil. Reduce heat and simmer gently, covered, for 20 minutes or until rice is cooked but still firm.

2. Increase heat slightly and stir in apple pulp, apple juice and honey. Simmer gently for 10 minutes or until liquid is slightly reduced, rice is tender and mixture is thick. Remove from heat and stir in yogurt, ginger, cinnamon and nutmeg.

Applesauce

Add 1/2 tsp (2 mL) powdered licorice for treating constipation or 1/2 tsp (2 mL) cayenne pepper or other herbs recommended for specific conditions. Try carrot and beet juices and more or less water to vary the thickness of the sauce.

2 cups	apple pulp	500 mL
2 cups	filtered water	500 mL
2 cups	apple juice	500 mL
3 tbsp	honey	45 mL
1/2 tsp	ground cinnamon	2 mL
1/4 tsp	ground nutmeg	1 mL

1. In a nonreactive saucepan over medium-high heat, combine pulp, water and juice; bring to a boil. Reduce heat and simmer for 20 to 30 minutes or until sauce is thick. Stir in honey, cinnamon and nutmeg. Serve warm or at room temperature. Store in covered container in refrigerator.

Avocado Gazpacho

Serves 4

Use any vegetable pulp for this great summer soup.

2 cups	vegetable or chicken stock	500 mL
1	lemon, juiced	1
1 tbsp	vinegar	15 mL
2 cups	vegetable pulp	500 mL
2	celery stalks, washed and cut into chunks	2
Half	cucumber, washed, seeded and cut into chunks	Half
2	cloves garlic	2
4	sprigs basil, washed	4
1	ripe avocado, peeled, pitted and cut into chunks	1
1 tbsp	dried chopped dulse	15 mL
4	basil or parsley sprigs, washed	4

1. In a Vita-Mix®, food processor or blender, combine stock, lemon juice, vinegar, pulp, celery, cucumber, garlic, basil and avocado; process until smooth (if necessary, process in two batches). Chill and serve garnished with dulse and fresh basil.

Cabbage Salad

Serves 4 to 6

2 cups	cabbage pulp	500 mL
1 cup	carrot-apple pulp	250 mL
3 tbsp	sunflower seeds	45 mL
2 tbsp	raisins	25 mL
2 tbsp	flax seeds	25 mL
1 tbsp	chopped apricot	15 mL
1/4 cup	hemp oil *or* olive oil	50 mL
2 tbsp	lemon juice	25 mL
2 tbsp	soy sauce	25 mL
2	cloves garlic, minced	2
1/4 cup	crumbled feta cheese (optional)	50 mL

1. In a large salad bowl, combine cabbage pulp, carrot-apple pulp, sunflower seeds, raisins, flax seeds and apricots. Toss to combine.

2. In a small jar with a tight-fitting lid or in a bowl, combine oil, lemon juice, soy sauce and garlic. Shake or whisk to mix thoroughly. Drizzle dressing over salad and toss to coat well. Sprinkle with feta cheese if using.

Cajun Salsa

Makes 1 cup (250 mL)

Use as a dip for nachos, a spread with bread, or a hot relish for chicken or fish. If you like your salsa hot, add a few drops of hot sauce or freshly chopped hot pepper to taste.

1 cup	Cajun Cocktail pulp (see recipe, page 153)	250 mL
2	medium tomatoes, washed, seeded and coarsely chopped	2
1	clove garlic, finely chopped	1
3 tbsp	olive oil	45 mL

1. In a medium bowl, combine pulp, tomatoes, garlic and olive oil. Toss to combine.

Curry Sauce

Try using the pulp from Breakfast Cocktail Juice (see recipe, page 152). Serve with cooked rice and steamed or stir-fried vegetables.

2 tbsp	butter	25 mL
1 tbsp	curry powder	15 mL
1 tbsp	garam masala	15 mL
2 cups	nut milk (see pages 214–215) *or* soy milk	500 mL
1 cup	onion-celery-apple pulp (see note at left)	250 mL
	Salt and black pepper	

1. In a small nonreactive saucepan, melt butter over medium heat. Stir in curry and garam masala; cook, stirring, for 1 minute.

2. Whisk in milk and stir in pulp, adjusting heat to keep the mixture at a slight boil. Cook, stirring constantly, for 5 minutes or until sauce is thick. Season to taste with salt and pepper.

Lemon Sauce

Lemon Rice Pudding: In a bowl combine Lemon Sauce with 2 cups (500 mL) cooked rice, 1 cup (250 mL) almond milk and 1/2 tsp (2 mL) ground cinnamon.

1 cup	pulp from Lemon Aid juice (see recipe, page 120)	250 mL
1/3 cup	lemon juice	75 mL
3 tbsp	honey	45 mL

1. In a small nonreactive saucepan over medium heat, combine pulp, lemon juice and honey; bring to a boil. Reduce heat slightly and boil gently, stirring, for 5 minutes or until sauce is thick. Serve warm or at room temperature. Store in covered container in refrigerator.

Papaya Marinade

**Makes 1 1/4 cups
(300 mL)**

This marinade is delicious with fish and poultry. Use kiwi, orange or pineapple pulp if papaya not available.

1 cup	papaya pulp (see note at left)	250 mL
2/3 cup	orange juice	150 mL
1/3 cup	soya sauce	75 mL
1	clove garlic, minced	1

1. In a shallow baking dish, combine pulp, orange juice, soya sauce and garlic. Arrange items to be marinated in dish, spooning marinade over top to coat both sides. Allow to stand, covered, in refrigerator for 1 hour, turning once or twice.

Tomato Sauce

Makes 4 cups (1 L)

Pulp from most tomato juices (such as Cajun Cocktail [see recipe, page 153], Peppery Tomato Cocktail [see recipe, page 154] or Tomato Juice Cocktail [see recipe, page 156]) will work in this recipe.

2 tbsp	olive oil	25 mL
3	cloves garlic, minced	3
1	large onion, chopped	1
2 cups	tomato pulp (see note at left)	500 mL
1 cup	filtered water	250 mL
3 tbsp	soya sauce	45 mL
1 tbsp	balsamic vinegar	15 mL
3 tbsp	chopped washed basil (or 1 tbsp [15 mL] dried)	45 mL
2 tbsp	chopped washed oregano (or 1 tbsp [15 mL] dried)	25 mL
2 tbsp	chopped washed thyme (or 1 tbsp [15 mL] dried)	25 mL
	Salt and black pepper	

1. In a nonreactive saucepan, heat oil over medium heat. Add garlic and onion; sauté for 5 minutes or until soft. Add tomato pulp, water, soya sauce, vinegar, basil, oregano and thyme; bring to a boil. Reduce heat and simmer, stirring occasionally, for 45 minutes to 1 hour or until reduced slightly. Season to taste with salt and pepper.

Makes 1 loaf

Thyme-Pumpkin Bread

PREHEAT OVEN TO 350° F (180° C)
8- BY 4-INCH (1.5 L) LOAF PAN, GREASED

2	eggs	2
2 tbsp	granulated sugar	25 mL
2 tbsp	honey	25 mL
1/2 cup	olive oil	125 mL
1 cup	pumpkin pulp or squash pulp	250 mL
1/2 cup	apple pulp	125 mL
Half	medium onion, peeled and chopped	Half
1 tbsp	Dijon mustard	15 mL
1 cup	all-purpose flour	250 mL
1/2 cup	whole-wheat flour	125 mL
3/4 tsp	baking powder	4 mL
1/2 tsp	baking soda	2 mL
1 tbsp	chopped washed thyme (or 1 tsp [5 mL] dried)	15 mL
1 tbsp	chopped washed oregano (or 1 tsp [5 mL] dried)	15 mL

1. In a large bowl, beat eggs. Beat in sugar, honey and oil. Stir in squash and apple pulp, onion and mustard.

2. In a medium bowl, stir together all-purpose flour, whole-wheat flour, baking powder, baking soda, thyme and oregano.

3. Stir flour mixture into pumpkin mixture. Pour into prepared loaf pan. Bake in preheated oven for 50 to 60 minutes or until a tester comes out clean.

Smoothies

Smoothies are thick, creamy fruit dishes that are delicious anytime. They are simple combinations of 1/2 to 1 cup (125 to 250 mL) fresh fruit juice and 1 cup (250 mL) fresh fruit. Bananas are usually included because they thicken the drink. Small amounts of other ingredients such as nuts, seeds, spices and herbs are optional. Nut milks may be used in place of soy milk or some fruit juices. Fruit milks, especially apricot milk, can be substituted for any of the fruit juices in smoothies. See page 214 for information on how to make nut and fruit milks.

To make smoothies: Using a blender or Vita-Mix®, place juice or liquid in container, then add other ingredients in the order given. Blend for 30 seconds to 1 minute or until smooth. Garnish if desired.

TEXTURE

The thick, creamy texture of smoothies makes them as satisfying as a traditional milkshake, but without the use of dairy products (milk, cream or ice cream) or any sweetener. While banana is the most popular thickener in smoothies, other ingredients can be used to produce a similar texture. Nut milks (see page 214), oatmeal or spelt flakes, flax or sesame seeds and nuts serve this purpose as well. Check the texture of the drink while it is still in the container. If too thin, add 1 tbsp (15 mL) oatmeal, nuts or seeds and process again. Make a note to substitute a nut milk the next time. If too thick, add any fruit juice in increments of 1/4 cup (50 mL) until the right texture is attained.

Almond-Banana Milk

Serves 1

Almonds work best, but any nut milk is good in this creamy drink. See page 217 for directions on freezing bananas.

1 cup	almond milk or soy milk	250 mL
2	bananas, fresh or frozen	2
Pinch	ground nutmeg	Pinch

1. Using a blender, process milk and bananas until smooth. Pour into a glass and sprinkle with nutmeg.

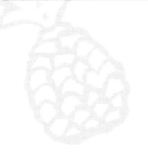

Avocado Pineapple

Serves 1

3/4 cup	raspberry juice	175 mL
1 cup	pineapple chunks,fresh or frozen	250 mL
1	avocado, peeled and pitted	1

1. Using a blender, process raspberry juice, pineapple and avocado until smooth. Pour into a glass.

B-Vitamin

Serves 1

Wheat germ is rich in B vitamins. Fish oil, evening primrose oil, flax seed oil, and hemp oil are all rich in the essential fatty acids important to health. Use any of them in this recipe.

1/4 cup	almond milk *or* soy milk	50 mL
1/2 cup	pineapple juice	125 mL
1 cup	pineapple chunks, fresh or frozen	250 mL
1	banana, peeled	1
2 tsp	flax seeds	10 mL
1 tbsp	wheat germ	15 mL
1 tsp	hemp oil	5 mL

1. Using a blender, process milk, pineapple juice, pineapple chunks, banana, flax seeds, wheat germ and oil until smooth. Pour into a glass.

Best Berries

Serves 1

Use any berry — raspberry, strawberry, blueberry or blackberry — for this sweet summer drink.

3/4 cup	pineapple juice	175 mL
3 tbsp	natural yogurt	45 mL
1 cup	fresh or frozen berries	250 mL
1	banana, peeled	1

1. Using a blender, process pineapple juice, yogurt, berries and banana until smooth. Pour into a glass.

Beta Blast

Serves 1

When available, substitute 2
fresh pitted apricots for dried.

1/2 cup	orange juice	125 mL
1/4 cup	carrot juice	50 mL
Half	cantaloupe, peeled (with seeds)	Half
1/4 cup	dried apricots	50 mL
1/4 cup	soft tofu	50 mL

1. Using a blender, process orange juice, carrot juice, cantaloupe, apricots and tofu until smooth. Pour into a glass.

Blue Cherry

Serves 1

1/2 cup	soy milk *or* nut milk	125 mL
1/4 cup	cranberry juice	50 mL
1/2 cup	fresh or frozen blueberries	125 mL
1/2 cup	fresh or frozen pitted cherries	125 mL
1	banana, peeled	1

1. Using a blender, process soy milk, cranberry juice, blueberries, cherries and banana until smooth. Pour into a glass.

Calming Chamomile

Serves 1

Add 1 tbsp (15 mL) sesame
seeds to thicken this drink.

1/2 cup	soy milk *or* nut milk	125 mL
1	apple, peeled, cored and cut into pieces	1
Quarter	cantaloupe, peeled (with seeds)	Quarter
1 tbsp	washed German chamomile flowers	15 mL
2 tbsp	natural yogurt	25 mL

1. Using a blender, process soy milk, apple, cantaloupe, chamomile and yogurt until smooth. Pour into a glass.

Cherries Jubilee

Serves 1

1/2 cup	soy milk	125 mL
2 cups	pitted washed cherries	500 mL
2	pineapple spears	2
1	banana, peeled	1
1 tbsp	flax seeds	15 mL
1/8 tsp	almond extract (optional)	0.5 mL

1. Using a blender, process soy milk, cherries, pineapple, banana, flax seeds and almond extract (if using) until smooth. Pour into a glass.

Cran-Orange

Serves 1

Dried cranberries are available
at health/alternative and bulk
food stores.

1/4 cup	orange juice	50 mL
1/4 cup	soft tofu	50 mL
1/2 cup	dried cranberries	125 mL
1	orange, peeled and seeded	1
1 tbsp	grated ginger root	15 mL
1 tbsp	honey	15 mL

1. Using a blender, process orange juice, tofu, cranberries, orange, ginger and honey until smooth. Pour into a glass.

Figgy Duff

Serves 1

If fig milk is available, use it instead of pineapple juice, then use 2 pineapple spears in place of the figs and omit the flax seeds.

1/2 cup	pineapple juice	125 mL
5	figs (fresh or dried), washed	5
2 tbsp	flax seeds	25 mL
2 tsp	oats	10 mL
1 tsp	extra virgin olive oil *or* hemp oil	5 mL

1. Using a blender, process pineapple juice, figs, flax seeds, oats and oil until smooth. Pour into a glass.

Frozen Fruit Slurry

Serves 2

Freeze whole fresh berries when in season and freeze fruit pulp from the juicing process in 2-oz (50 g) paper cups and pop into the Vita-Mix® to use in this easy slushy drink you eat with a spoon. See page 217 for how to freeze bananas.

If using a blender, allow fruit and juice to thaw until soft enough to process.

1/2 cup	orange juice	125 mL
1	banana, frozen and cut into chunks	1
4	strawberries, frozen	4
1/4 cup	frozen fruit juice	50 mL
1 cup	ice cubes	250 mL

1. In a Vita-Mix® or blender, combine orange juice, banana, strawberries, frozen juice and ice cubes; secure lid. Process starting at variable speed #1, increasing speed to #10 (or Medium), then to High. Process for 30 to 60 seconds or until ice is chopped (but no longer). Use the tamper while machine is processing. Serve immediately.

Green Energy

Serves 1

A "green" taste, not unpleasant but a definite departure from the traditional smoothie flavors.

Reduce amount of soy milk to 1/4 cup (50 mL) if using frozen spinach.

1/2 cup	soy milk	125 mL
1/4 cup	apricot milk	50 mL
2 cups	washed spinach fresh or frozen	500 mL
3 tbsp	chopped wheat or barley grass	45 mL
1 tbsp	pumpkin seeds	15 mL
1 tsp	ginkgo (optional)	5 mL

1. Using a blender, process soy milk, apricot milk, spinach, grass, pumpkin seeds and ginkgo (if using) until smooth. Pour into a glass.

Liquid Gold

For a change, use half orange juice and half apricot milk (see page 216) and eliminate the dried apricots.

1 cup	orange juice	250 mL
3 tbsp	lemon juice	45 mL
2	peaches, peeled and pitted	2
1	mango, peeled and pitted	1
4	dried apricots	4
1	banana, peeled	1
1	pineapple spear	1

1. Using a blender, process orange juice, lemon juice, peaches, mango, apricots, banana and pineapple until smooth. Pour into glasses.

Mango Madness

If using a blender, omit the grapes because the skins are difficult to blend.

1/2 cup	orange juice	125 mL
1	mango, peeled and pitted	1
1	banana, peeled	1
1 cup	washed red or green seedless grapes	250 mL
1	1/4-inch (5 mm) piece ginger root, peeled	1
1/2 tsp	ground cinnamon (optional)	2 mL

1. Using a Vita-Mix®, process orange juice, mango, banana, grapes, ginger and cinnamon (if using) until smooth. Pour into a glass.

Pineapple-C

Serves 1

1/2 cup	orange juice	125 mL
2 tbsp	lemon juice	25 mL
1	lime, juiced	1
1 cup	pineapple chunks	250 mL
1/4 cup	washed, strawberries fresh or frozen	50 mL

1. Using a blender, process orange juice, lemon juice, lime juice, pineapple and strawberries until smooth. Pour into a glass.

Prune Smoothie

Serves 1 or 2

A good morning starter.

1 cup	soy milk	250 mL
1/4 cup	pitted prunes	50 mL
1	banana, peeled	1

1. Using a blender, process soy milk, prunes and banana until smooth. Pour into a glass.

Plum Lico

Serves 1

Overconsumption of licorice (more than 1 tsp [5 mL] per 1 cup [250 mL]) leads to low potassium levels and water-retention. If potassium is a concern, add a banana to this or any smoothie recipe.

1/4 cup	pineapple juice	50 mL
1/4 cup	yogurt	50 mL
2	plums, washed, pitted and quartered	2
1 cup	washed pitted cherries	250 mL
1	grapefruit, peeled and quartered	1
1 tsp	powdered licorice (optional)	5 mL

1. Using a blender, process pineapple juice, yogurt, plums, cherries, grapefruit and licorice (if using) until smooth. Pour into a glass.

Pump It Up

With its natural sugar carbohydrates, and with potassium from the banana, this drink helps to prepare the body for intensive activity. Drink it before exercising, walking or any strenuous work. If using nut milk, omit the almonds.

1 cup	soy milk *or* nut milk	250 mL
1	banana, peeled	1
1/2 cup	washed pitted cherries	125 mL
1/4 cup	washed blueberries fresh or frozen	50 mL
1 tbsp	protein powder	15 mL
2 tbsp	ground almonds	25 mL

1. Using a blender, process soy milk, banana, cherries, blueberries and protein powder until smooth. Pour into glasses and garnish with ground almonds.

Sea-Straw Smoothie

Use kelp or any other sea herb in this high-calcium drink.

1/2 cup	grapefruit juice	125 mL
6	large strawberries, washed, fresh or frozen	6
3 tbsp	chopped dried dates	45 mL
1 tsp	crushed dried dulse	5 mL

1. Using a blender, process grapefruit juice, strawberries, dates and kelp until smooth. Pour into a glass.

Spa Special

1/4 cup	grapefruit juice	50 mL
1/4 cup	soft tofu	50 mL
1/4 cup	blueberries	50 mL
3	large strawberries, washed fresh or frozen	3
1 tsp	milk thistle	5 mL

1. Using a blender, process grapefruit juice, tofu, blueberries, strawberries and milk thistle until smooth. Pour into a glass.

Smart Smoothie

Serves 2

1/2 cup	orange juice	125 mL
1/4 cup	washed blueberries, fresh or frozen	50 mL
1/4 cup	washed seedless grapes	50 mL
1 cup	washed spinach, fresh or frozen	250 mL
1 tsp	ginkgo leaves (optional)	5 mL
1 tbsp	flax seeds	15 mL
1 tsp	skullcap	5 mL
1 tsp	lecithin	5 mL

1. Using a blender, process orange juice, blueberries, grapes, spinach, ginkgo, (if using) flax seeds, skullcap and lecithin until smooth. Pour into glasses.

The Cool Down

Serves 1

The natural calming effect of lemon balm and the potassium-rich banana refresh the body after any type of activity.

1/2 cup	carrot juice	125 mL
2	pineapple spears	2
1	banana, peeled	1
1	sprig lemon balm, washed	1

1. Using a blender, process carrot juice, pineapple, banana and lemon balm until smooth. Pour into a glass.

The Regular

Serves 1

Orange juice, strawberries and banana is the usual combination for a smoothie.

For extra punch, add 1 tsp (5 mL) [or the contents of 1 gel capsule] evening primrose oil or ginkgo to this smoothie.

1/2 cup	orange juice	125 mL
4	large strawberries, washed fresh or frozen	4
1	banana, peeled	1
2 tbsp	wheat germ	25 mL
1 tbsp	chopped almonds	15 mL

1. Using a blender, process orange juice, strawberries, banana, wheat germ and almonds until smooth. Pour into a glass.

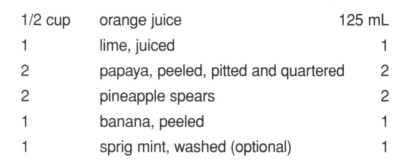

Taste of the Tropics

Serves 1

1/2 cup	orange juice	125 mL
1	lime, juiced	1
2	papaya, peeled, pitted and quartered	2
2	pineapple spears	2
1	banana, peeled	1
1	sprig mint, washed (optional)	1

1. Using a blender, process orange juice, lime juice, papaya, pineapple, banana and mint (if using) until smooth. Pour into a glass.

Tropics

Serves 2

For extra relief from heart-burn, add 1 tbsp (15 mL) slippery elm powder.

1/2 cup	coconut milk	125 mL
1	fresh papaya, peeled and seeded (or 1/4 cup [50 mL] dried)	1
1	banana, peeled	1
1	kiwi, peeled and cut into chunks	1
1/2 cup	pineapple chunks	125 mL

1. Using a blender, process coconut milk, papaya, banana, kiwi and pineapple until smooth. Pour into glasses.

Tropi-Cocktail

Serves 2

1/4 cup	apricot milk	50 mL
1/2 cup	natural yogurt	125 mL
1	fresh papaya, peeled and seeded (or 1/4 cup [50 mL] dried)	1
1	banana, peeled	1
1	mango, peeled and seeded	1
Quarter	cantaloupe, peeled	Quarter

1. Using a blender, process apricot milk, yogurt, papaya, banana, mango and cantaloupe until smooth. Pour into glasses.

Watermelon Smoothie

Serves 1

1/3 cup	natural yogurt	75 mL
1 cup	watermelon chunks	250 mL
1 cup	washed blueberries	250 mL
2 tbsp	pumpkin seeds (optional)	25 mL

1. Using a blender, process yogurt, watermelon, blueberries and, pumpkin seeds (if using) until smooth. Pour into glass.

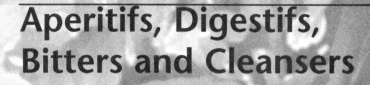

Aperitifs, Digestifs, Bitters and Cleansers

Aperitifs

The old pharmacopoeia recognized major bitters (roots of parsley, fennel, asparagus and butcher's broom) and minor bitters (roots of maidenhair fern, couchgrass, thistle, rest-harrow and strawberry-plant). The term as used today only applies to stimulants of appetite.

Aperitifs served in cafés are drinks of a greater or lesser degree of bitterness, variously flavored, which are drunk neat or diluted with water. They generally have a strong alcoholic content, because the essences of which they are composed are not soluble except in strong alcohol (which is why they go cloudy when mixed with water) and this alcohol content to a great extent nullifies the beneficial action of the bitters.

But through sheer force of habit (or perhaps through imagination), some people think that they have no appetite unless they have their daily aperitif (or aperitifs). It is this fact which has led to the coining of the phrase that if an aperitif can open the appetite, it does so with a skeleton key. Be this as it may, the aperitif was, and still is, a traditional rite in certain circles.

The New Larousse Gastronomique, P. Montagné. Crown Publishers, Inc., New York: 1977.

NATURAL AIDS TO DIGESTION

Acidophilus (see Yogurt, page 54). *Lactobacillus acidophilus* is a "friendly" type of bacteria used to ferment milk into yogurt. It replaces the intestinal bacteria necessary for digestion which are destroyed by antibiotics.

Calendula (*Calendula officinalis*, see page 21). Stimulates bile production and in this way, aids digestion. Calendula may be included in aperitifs and makes an attractive garnish for drinks.

Cinnamon (*Cinnamomum zeylan-icum,* see page 22). A warming carminative used to promote digestion, cinnamon adds a pleasant taste to aperitif and digestif drinks.

Dandelion root (*Taraxacum officinalis,* see page 24). Easily obtained, fairly mild but bitter laxative that stimulates the liver and gall bladder and increases the flow of bile to aid digestion. Dandelion leaves act as a diuretic.

Fennel (*Foeniculum vulgare,* see page 25). Juice the bulb or make tea from the seeds to aid digestion and soothe discomfort from heartburn and indigestion.

Fiber (see page 262). Insoluble fiber in fruits, vegetables and whole grains helps prevent constipation and digestive diseases such as diverticulosis and colon cancer.

German Chamomile (*Matricaria recutita,* see page 27). As Peter Rabbit's mother knew, chamomile soothes upset tummies and inflammations and reduces flatulence and pain caused by gas.

Digestifs

Digestive problems, or *indigestion*, is the inability to digest food and absorb the nutrients from it. Gas and bloating are often the result. These problems may mask more serious medical conditions that should always be attended to by a medical practitioner. Age often plays a major role in the decline of the body's digestive abilities; indigestion can be alleviated with foods or herbs. In many cases, eating foods in a specific order or following guidelines for food combining (see page 256) reduces gas, bloating, flatulence and burping.

The recipes in this section are meant to be made fresh, just before or after dinner. They are particularly useful in overcoming a feeling of fullness, and are sophisticated enough to accompany even the most elegant meal.

Ginger (*Zingeber officinalis*, see page 27). Ginger is used to stimulate blood flow to the digestive system and to increase absorption of nutrients. It increases the action of the gall bladder while protecting the liver against toxins.

Kiwi (*Actinidia chinensis*, see page 45). Enzymes in kiwi fruit help digestion.

Licorice (*Glycyrrhiza glabra*, see page 31). Soothes gastric mucus membranes and eases spasms of the large intestine. Should be avoided in cases of high blood pressure.

Papaya (*Carica papaya*, see page 46). Papaya is a traditional remedy for indigestion. It contains an enzyme called papain, which is similar to pepsin, an enzyme that helps digestion of protein.

Peppermint (*Mentha piperita*, see page 35). Peppermint contains flavonoids that stimulate the liver and gall bladder and increases the flow of bile. Its antispasmodic effect on the smooth muscles of the digestive tract make it a good choice in after-dinner drinks.

Pineapple (*Ananas comosus*, see page 46). Pineapple is rich in the anti-bacterial enzyme bromelain, which is anti-inflammatory and helps in the digestive process.

Turmeric (*Curcuma longa*, see page 41). Increases bile production and bile flow.

Before Dinner Mint

Serves 1

This aperitif is naturally sweet, with just a hint of mint. Take it before eating to help stimulate liver and gall bladder function by increasing bile flow to the liver and intestines. If fresh mint is not available, whisk 1 tbsp (15 mL) powdered dried peppermint into juice

3	kiwi, peeled and halved	3
1	apple, washed and cut into pieces	1
8	sprigs peppermint (leaves and stems)	8
	Ice (optional)	

1. Using juicer, process kiwi, apple and peppermint. Pour into a large glass. If desired, add ice.

After Dinner Cocktail Smoothie

Serves 4 to 6

Serve this feathery light drink (with its papain and bromelain enzymes) to aid in the digestive process.

2/3 cup	mineral water	150 mL
2	papaya, peeled, seeded and cut into pieces	2
1/2 cup	natural yogurt	125 mL
Half	pineapple, peeled and cut into pieces	Half
1	1/2-inch (1 cm) ginger root, peeled	1
	Ice (optional)	

1. Using a Vita-Mix® or a blender, process mineral water, papaya, yogurt, pineapple and ginger. Pour into cocktail glasses. If desired, add ice.

Digestive Cocktail Juice

Serves 2 or 3

This powerful drink will really get the digestive juices flowing. For a milder version, omit the garlic.

Serve before or after dinner in small glasses over ice and, for an extra kick, add a dash of cayenne.

2	tomatoes, washed and cut into wedges	2
2	carrots, scrubbed	2
Quarter	fennel bulb, cut into pieces	Quarter
1	clove garlic	1
4	basil leaves, washed	4
4	sprigs dill, washed	4
2	sprigs thyme, washed	2
2	stalks celery, washed	2
1	beet, scrubbed and cut into pieces	1
1/2 tsp	ground turmeric	2 mL
1/4 tsp	powdered mustard	1 mL
1/4 tsp	ground cumin	1 mL
Pinch	ground cloves (optional)	Pinch

1. Using juicer, process tomatoes, carrots, fennel, garlic, basil, dill, thyme, celery and beet. Pour into a pitcher and whisk in turmeric, mustard, cumin and cloves.

Digestive (Gripe) Water

Serves 1 adult

Fennel seeds are calming and antiflatulent and have been safely given to babies to treat colic for centuries. This water is also effective as a digestive for adults and especially recommended after eating oily fish or fried foods.

1 tsp	fennel seeds	5 mL
3	stevia leaves (optional)	3
1 1/4 cups	boiling water	300 mL

1. With a mortar and pestle, crush fennel and stevia. Transfer to a nonreactive teapot.

2. Pour boiling water over crushed herbs. Cover and steep for 20 minutes. Strain, discarding solids.

For adults: Sip 1 serving, warm or cold, after eating

For babies: Make sure all solids are strained out. Dilute 1/4 cup (50 mL) gripe water with 1/2 cup (125 mL) warm water or chamomile tea. Fill the baby's bottle with the warm mixture for drinking

To store: Pour into a clean (or sterile) jar, cover tightly and keep in refrigerator for up to 2 days.

Digestive Seed Tea

Anise seeds (Pimpinella anisum) or star anise (Illicium anisatum) can be used in this recipe. Both have digestive properties.

1 part	anise seed	1 part
1 part	dill seed	1 part
1 part	fennel seed	1 part

1. In a medium bowl, combine anise, dill and fennel. Transfer to a clean jar with lid and label. Store in a cool, dry dark place.

2. To make tea: Into a mortar or small electric grinder, measure 1 tsp (5 mL) blended seeds for every 1 cup (250 mL) to be made. Lightly crush seeds (with pestle or grinder.) Place crushed seeds in a nonreactive teapot and cover with boiling water; steep for 15 minutes. Strain and drink warm.

James Duke's Carminatea

The world's foremost authority on healing herbs and the healing traditions of different cultures, James Duke has written several books on the practical use of herbs for medicinal purposes. Here is a recipe for deflating flatus, based on his recipe for Carminatea from *The Green Pharmacy*.

2 tbsp	dried peppermint	25 mL
1 tbsp	dried German chamomile	15 mL
1 tbsp	dried lemon balm	15 mL
2 tsp	dill seeds	10 mL
1 tsp	fennel seeds	5 mL
1 tsp	powdered licorice	5 mL

1. In a medium bowl, mix together peppermint, chamomile, lemon balm, dill, fennel and licorice. Transfer to a clean jar with a lid and label. Store in a cool, dry dark place.

2. For each 1 cup (250 mL) tea, lightly crush 1 tsp (5 mL) blended seeds with a mortar and pestle or small food grinder. Add to a nonreactive warmed teapot and pour in boiling water; steep for 15 minutes. Strain and drink warm.

Rosy Peppermint Tea

Serves 1 or 2

Take this digestive tea after meals.

1 tbsp	washed peppermint leaves (or 1 tsp [5 mL] dried)	15 mL
1 tbsp	washed rose petals (or 1 tsp [5 mL] dried)	15 mL
2 cups	boiling water	500 mL
2	slices kiwi peeled (optional)	2

1. In a mortar lightly crush peppermint and rose petals. Place in a nonreactive teapot and pour in boiling water. Cover and steep for 10 minutes.

2. Strain the tea into mugs and, if desired, garnish with kiwi slices.

Spiced Papaya Tea

Serves 1 or 2

Sweet enough to enjoy on its own, this tea also brings a fine meal to a tasty conclusion.

2 tbsp	chopped, dried papaya	25 mL
1/2 tsp	slippery elm bark	2 mL
1/2 tsp	lightly crushed coriander seeds	2 mL
1/4 tsp	ground cinnamon	1 mL
1/4 tsp	ground cumin	1 mL
1/4 tsp	ground turmeric	1 mL
2 cups	boiling water	500 mL

1. In a nonreactive teapot, combine papaya, slippery elm bark, coriander, cinnamon, cumin and turmeric. Pour in boiling water, cover and steep for 15 minutes. Strain the tea into cups and drink warm.

BEANS AND THE DIGESTIVE SYSTEM

Dried beans are rich in oligosaccharides — complex sugars that can't be broken down by human digestive enzymes. When you eat legumes, the oligosaccharides enter the lower intestine where they are met by bacteria that eat the starches and, in the process, create gas. To combat this effect, some cultures combine savory (Satureja) with beans, peas and lentils. Drinking carminative herbs (cayenne, chamomile, cinnamon, clove, lavender, peppermint, parsley, rosemary) in teas is helpful as well.

Bitters

Bitter Herbs

Dandelion leaf (*Taraxacum officinale,* see page 23). Leaves may be dried for bitter tea blends.

Chicory (*Cichorium intybus*) Use fresh or dried root or leaves for bitter teas.

Endive (*Cichorium endivia*) Good for salads to start or end to a meal.

Radicchio (*Cichorium endivia*) A red version of Belgium endive.

Rapini (*Brassica rapa [Ruvo]*) Flowering stems and leaves have a mildly bitter flavor. Often found in European markets.

Sheep Sorrel (*Rumex acetoselia*) A close relative to French sorrel (*Rumex scutatus*). Use either in bitters. Traditionally used for fevers, inflammation, diarrhea, excessive menstruation and cancer (sheep sorrel is one of the four ingredients of the Essiac® anti-cancer remedy).

Watercress (*Nasturtium officinale,* see page 51). A sharp, peppery, but not unpleasant taste makes watercress a welcome addition to salads and sandwiches.

Yellow Dock (*Rumex crispus,* see page 43). Leaves have a distinctive, sour flavor that combines well with dandelion leaves, chickweed, chicory and the milder lettuces. Wash dock leaves before eating raw: the chrysophanic acid irritates the mouth and can cause a numbing sensation of the tongue and lips for several hours.

Herbalists agree that bitters support the heart, small intestines and liver, as well as reduce fever. The astringent taste of greens such as endive, chicory, sheep sorrel, radicchio, dandelion and yellow dock awakens the palate and makes it more receptive to appreciate other flavors. The digestive tonic action promotes the secretion of hydrochloric acid that aids digestion. A glass of bitter juice is an excellent tool for whetting the appetite, but may take some getting used to.

In Chinese medicine, bitters are cool and drying, and therefore used to reduce fevers and dry excess body fluids. In the Ayurvedic model, bitter foods have a similar function: to stimulate the digestion to absorb phlegm and to treat fevers or skin disease.

Scientists say we have about 10,000 taste buds, with each one living not much longer than a week before it is shed and regenerated. Taste buds are clusters of cells in the tongue and in the mouth that relay the four tastes — sweet, salty, bitter and sour — to the brain. Some herbalists and ancient traditions link the four tastes to effects on the mind. For example, a balanced intake of bitter flavors could be thought to encourage honesty, integrity, optimism and a loving heart.

To start enjoying the medicinal effects of bitters, it might be helpful to begin with a combination of bitter and slightly sweet juices, then gradually eliminate the sweeter juices until you are taking the bitters on their own. Keep in mind that the bitter taste must be present in order to realize the medicinal effects; to sweeten them is to cancel their effect.

Use any or all of the bitter herbs and vegetables listed here to blend your own bitters. Try to use them fresh in juices, teas and salads — all of them are easily grown, most are available fresh in supermarkets and some may be wildcrafted.

Dandelion Delight

Serves 1 or 2

1 tbsp	chopped dried dandelion root	15 mL
2 cups	water	500 mL
1 tbsp	fresh washed German chamomile (or 1 tsp [5 mL] dried)	15 mL
1 tsp	dried fennel seeds	5 mL

1. In a nonreactive saucepan over medium heat, bring dandelion root and water to a slow simmer. Cover pot, reduce heat and simmer for 20 minutes.

2. Place chamomile and fennel seeds in a teapot. Pour hot dandelion water over herbs, straining out dandelion and steep for 5 minutes. Drink hot or cool to room temperature.

Dandelion Bitters

Serves 1 or 2

As your taste for bitters increases, the apple can be gradually withdrawn from this drink.

Drink 1/4 cup (50 mL) at noon or just before dinner.

1	4-inch (10 cm) piece dandelion root, scrubbed	1
2	carrots, scrubbed	2
1	apple, washed and cut into pieces	1

1. Using juicer, process dandelion, carrots and apple. Pour into 1 large or 2 smaller glasses.

Spring Green Bitters

Serves 3 to 6

Use this drink sparingly. Make the recipe once in the spring and take daily for as long as it lasts (maximum 2 to 3 days). If desired repeat once again in the fall.

Sorrel leaves have a high oxalic acid content, so eat when young and tender in the spring, in small amounts.

6	yellow dock leaves with stems	6
4	endive leaves, washed	4
4	sprigs sheep sorrel, washed	4
4	stalks celery, washed	4
	Honey (optional)	

1. Using juicer, process yellow dock, endive, sheep sorrel and celery. Whisk in honey to taste. Take 1 or 2 tbsp (15 or 25 mL) before the main meal of the day.

CLEANSERS AND DETOXIFIERS

Astragalus root (*Astragalus membranacus,* see page 18). A tonic and immune-enhancing herb that can be used in vegetable soups and whisked into juices. Use dried astragalus in tea blends.

Burdock root (*Arctium lappa,* see page 20). A skin and blood cleanser, burdock stimulates urine flow and sweating while supporting the liver, lymphatic glands and digestive system. Use fresh root or leaves in juices or vegetable soups. Make teas from dried burdock.

Cayenne (*Capsicum,* see page 21). Stimulates blood circulation, purifies the blood, expels mucus and promotes fluid elimination and sweat. Juice fresh chile peppers with other cleansing fruits, vegetables and herbs or use dried in teas.

Dandelion root (*Taraxacum officinale,* see page 24). A common herb, dandelion cleans the liver and blood, filters toxins, acts as a mild laxative, and increases the flow of urine. Best blended with fruits or vegetables, juice the fresh root or leaves or use dried root in coffee substitutes and teas.

Echinacea root (*E. agustifolia* or *E. purpurea,* see page 24). Available in dried whole or cut form, and fresh from growers in the fall, echinacea helps stimulate the immune system while cleansing the lymph system.

People in central Europe began to juice cabbages, potatoes and beetroot to treat ulcers, cancer and leukemia in the late 1800's. But the practice of pressing the water from fruits and vegetables for health reasons is centuries old, being rooted in many religious faiths and indigenous cultures. Modern science is pointing to the fact that the future of health care in today's stressful and toxic environments will have as its core a whole food diet and regular, safe cleansing or detoxification of the body.

The goal of cleansing, detoxifying or fasting is to release and eliminate toxins stored in the colon and fat cells of the body. Those toxins re-enter the bloodstream where they re-circulate in the body. That is why at the beginning of a cleansing, fasting or detoxifying program, diarrhea, headaches, irritability and catarrh can occur. As toxins are released, they are able to unleash their damage again. So it is important to ensure that they are eliminated. After a 5- to 10-day cleanse, a 3- to 5-day fast, or a supervised detoxifying program, most people feel calmer with a sense of well being, more clear-headed and energetic.

A cleansing regime can consist of a restricted diet of vegetable soups, raw fresh salads, whole grains and other high-fiber foods, limited fruit juices, vegetable and herb juices, blended drinks and herbal teas. While cleansing, it is important to drink 8 to 10 glasses of pure water and eat only organic fruits, vegetables, herbs and grains while abstaining from fats (especially fried foods, red meats and milk products), alcohol, soft drinks, caffeine, refined foods and sugar or other sweeteners.

Fasting involves avoiding solid food for a prescribed period of time and should be undertaken with the help of a health practitioner. You should first define the purpose of the fast, whether it be to address a specific condition, to relieve and regenerate internal organs, or to simply lose weight. Then, with the help of a medical herbalist or other natural health practitioner, you can determine which of the five systems (digestion, circulation, elimination, respiration or nervous) or combinations of the five systems require support.

Fasting is always approached with a cleansing diet as described above for a minimum of 2 days preceding and following the actual fasting period. Fasts in the true sense call for water only, or water and clear juices only. However,

Elderberry (*Sambucus nigra,* see page 25). Supports detoxification by promoting bowel movements, urination, sweating, and secretion of mucus.

Ginger root (*Zingeber officinalis,* see page 27). Ginger helps elimination of toxins by stimulating circulation and sweating. Widely available, it is used in healing juices and grated into supportive teas and coffee substitutes.

Licorice root (*Glycyrrhiza glabra,* see page 31). With its gentle laxative effect, licorice is often included in cleansing supportive teas.

Milk thistle (*Silybum marianus,* see page 33). Containing some of the most potent liver cleansing and protecting compounds known, 1 tbsp (15 mL) milk thistle seed is an excellent addition to pulped drinks and cleansing supportive teas.

Yellow dock root (*Rumex crispus,* see page 43). A cleansing herb that supports the liver, lymphatic glands and digestive system, dock is a strong laxative. It can be blended with other herbs when used for detoxifying.

juice "fasts" have come into popular use, allowing all types of fruit or vegetable juices along with herbal teas. These fasts are simple and safe for everyone in general good health (except anyone with a chronic degenerative disease or those who suffer from hyperthyroidism or anemia and pregnant or lactating women).

To promote proper elimination of the released toxins, whether cleansing or fasting, the main organs of elimination — liver, kidney, respiratory and lymph systems and skin — must be supported. Fresh, raw juice is a natural choice for cleansing. The concentrated nutrients are assimilated quickly without putting stress on the organs of digestion or elimination. Also, many fruits, vegetables and herbs are high in antioxidants, which are necessary for the elimination of toxins and free radicals. Only fresh, organic fruit, vegetable and herb juices are used in cleanses or fasts. Some experts recommend using only vegetable juices; others claim that both fruit and vegetable juices may be used. If using both, take fruit juices in the morning and at lunch, then take only vegetable juices from mid-afternoon onward. Organ-supporting herbal teas and tonics, light to moderate exercise (sweating is one of the body's primary mechanisms for getting rid of toxic wastes) and saunas or baths, along with dry brushing, assist in the process of elimination. Psyllium seeds and a minimum of 10 glasses of pure, filtered water also help to remove toxins.

Short-term cleanses and juice fasts work best when part of a healthy lifestyle that includes a whole food diet (see Guidelines to Good Health, pages 10–11), regular exercise, and a strong commitment to inner growth and spiritual nurturing.

The herbs listed at left (on this and the facing page) provide support for cells, organs and the process of elimination and cleansing. Juice fresh herbs when available or whisk up to 1 tsp (5 mL) dried herbs into juices and blended drinks or add to supportive cleansing teas.

Cell Support Juice

Serves 1

While the cleansing effects of juicing are taking place, this drink supports and nourishes the cells.

3	apples, washed and cut into pieces	3
1	handful parsley, washed	1
1	handful alfalfa, washed (or 1 tbsp [15 mL] dried)	1

1. Using juicer, process apples, parsley and, if using fresh, the alfalfa. Whisk together and pour into a large glass. If using dried alfalfa, whisk into juice.

Crimson Cleanser Juice

Serves 1

The brilliant red color of beets signals a high beta carotene content. Coupled with the toxin-clearing ability of dandelion, it provides a pleasant internal wash.

1	apple, washed and cut into pieces	1
1	large handful dandelion leaves, washed	1
1	medium beet, scrubbed and cut into pieces	1
2 tsp	maple syrup (or to taste)	10 mL

1. Using a juicer, process apple, dandelion and beet. Whisk together and pour into a large glass. Whisk in maple syrup to taste.

Lemon Cleanser Juice

Serves 1

It is generally believed that lemon has "solvent properties", which makes this drink important when treating gallstones. Substitute 1/4 tsp (1 mL) powdered stevia for maple syrup, if desired.

2	lemons, peeled and halved	2
1	apple, washed and cut into pieces	1
2 tsp	maple syrup	10 mL
1/4 tsp	cayenne pepper	1 mL

1. Using juicer, process lemons and apple. Whisk together and pour into a large glass. Whisk in maple syrup and cayenne.

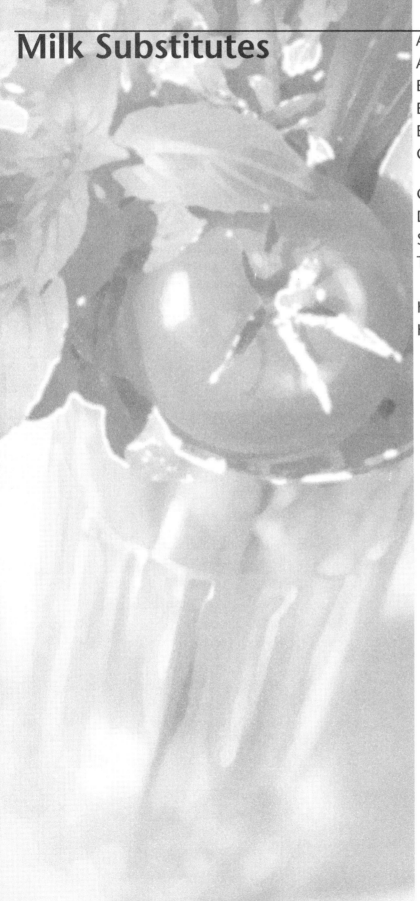

Milk Substitutes

Milk Substitutes

Milk allergies, or a separate condition called lactose intolerance (see page 263), cause a significant number of people to experience painful symptoms that make it necessary to eliminate milk and dairy products from their diet. In addition to milk, cream and butter, problematic foods can include processed products like cereals, baking mixes and baked goods that contain milk, milk solids, cheese (or cheese flavoring), whey, curds, and even margarine.

Fermented dairy foods, such as natural yogurt, contain live bacteria that help digest lactose and may not irritate allergies. Soy milk and nut milks are the best substitutes for dairy milk.

SOY MILK

Soy milk (and tofu) is widely available in supermarkets and health/alternative stores, but can easily be made at home (see *Rodale's* reference, Bibliography, page 266). Soy milk and tofu should be used with some caution, however, since there is growing concern over the use of genetically modified and chemically sprayed soybeans for most commercial soy products.

NUT MILKS

Nuts make a pleasant, thick liquid that can be used in some sauces and desserts. Use unsalted, organic almonds, pecans, cashews or walnuts (any nut or seed will work) with the skins still on. Nuts contribute protein, vitamin E and fiber to the diet, but should be taken in small amounts since they have a high fat content (although mostly unsaturated and with essential fatty acids). Nut milks make a thicker shake or smoothie than soy milk.

As you might expect, anyone with an allergy to nuts cannot use nut milks. However, for healthy teens with high energy demands, nut milks can be used regularly in any of the milk shake recipes in this section.

To make nut milk: Combine the nuts with other ingredients as listed below in a clean jar with a lid. Note that boiled water should not be boiling when added. Shake well, cool, blend using a blender or food processor, and use immediately. Or return to the jar and place in refrigerator for up to 2 or 3 days.

Almond: 1 cup (250 mL) finely chopped almonds, 1 tbsp (15 mL) finely chopped dates, 1 tbsp (15 mL) flax seed, 1-inch (2.5 cm) piece vanilla bean, 2 cups (500 mL) just-boiled water

Cashew: 1 cup (250 mL) finely chopped cashews, 1 tbsp (15 mL) finely chopped dried dulse, 1 tbsp (15 mL) finely chopped raisins, 1-inch (2.5 cm) piece vanilla bean, 2 cups (500 mL) just-boiled water

Pecan: 1 cup (250 mL) finely chopped pecans, 1 tbsp (15 mL) finely chopped raisins, 1 tbsp (15 mL) flax seed, 1-inch (2.5 cm) piece vanilla bean, 2 cups (500 mL) just-boiled water

Walnut: 1 cup (250 mL) finely chopped walnuts, 1 tbsp (15 mL) finely chopped dates, 1 tbsp (15 mL) flax seed, 1-inch (2.5 cm) piece vanilla bean, 2 cups (500 mL) just-boiled water

FRUIT MILKS

Coconut/Carob milk. Use fresh coconut and shred it, freezing the remainder if necessary. If fresh coconut is unavailable, use the unsweetened dried type available at some health/alternative stores. Coconut is naturally sweet and when blended with carob, it is even sweeter. Use coconut milk to replace dairy and sugar in shakes, puddings and other desserts.

To make coconut milk: In a blender or food processor, combine 1/2 cup (125 mL) shredded fresh coconut (or 1/3 cup [75 mL] shredded dried), 3 tbsp (45 mL) powdered carob (optional), 1-inch (2.5 cm) piece vanilla bean and 1/2 cup (125 mL) just-boiled water. Cool, then process until smooth. Add more water if a thinner product is desired. Use immediately or store in refrigerator up to a week.

Date milk. Date sugar is commonly used in commercial products as a sweetener. Using date milk is like using sugar (although it provides some fiber and a few nutrients), so use it sparingly. Make the milk with dried, pitted dates.

To make date milk: In a blender or food processor, combine 1/4 cup (50 mL) chopped dates, 1-inch (2.5 cm) piece vanilla bean and 1/2 cup (125 mL) just-boiled water. Cool, then process until smooth. Use immediately or store in refrigerator for up to 1 week.

Fig milk. Figs have anti-bacterial, cancer-fighting properties and make a sweet milk that can be used with yogurt or tofu in shakes and other recipes. Use fresh figs if available. Dried figs are tough and should be coarsely chopped by hand before processing in the blender or food processor.

To make fig milk: In a blender or food processor, combine 1/4 cup (50 mL) chopped figs, 1-inch (2.5 cm) piece vanilla bean and 1/2 cup (125 mL) just-boiled water. Cool, then process until smooth. Use immediately or store in refrigerator for up to 1 week.

Apricot milk. Sweet, yet slightly tart, this fruit milk has a unique taste. Use it in any of the fruit shakes or smoothies in this book. Look for organic apricots without sulphur added in the drying process.

To make apricot milk: In a blender or food processor, combine 1/4 cup (50 mL) chopped dried apricots, 1-inch (2.5 cm) piece vanilla bean and 1/2 cup (125 mL) just-boiled water. Cool, then process until smooth. Use immediately or store in refrigerator for up to 1 week.

Apple Pie

Serves 1

1 cup	soy milk *or* apricot milk	250 mL
2	apples, washed, peeled, cored and quartered	2
2 tbsp	spelt flakes	25 mL
1/4 tsp	ground cinnamon	1 mL
1/8 tsp	ground nutmeg	0.5 mL

1. In a blender process soy milk, apples, spelt, cinnamon and nutmeg until smooth. Pour into a glass.

Avocado Shake

Serves 1

1 cup	soy milk *or* nut milk	250 mL
1	avocado, peeled and pitted	1
1	grapefruit, peeled and quartered	1
Half	lemon, juiced	Half
1 tbsp	molasses	15 mL

1. In a blender process soy milk, avocado, grapefruit, lemon juice and molasses until smooth. Pour into a glass.

Banana Frappé

Serves 1 or 2

To freeze bananas: Peel several bananas, cut each into 4 chunks and spread on a baking sheet. Freeze in coldest part of the freezer for 30 minutes. Then place chunks in a freezer bag, seal and store in freezer until ready to use.

1 cup	almond milk *or* soy milk	250 mL
1/2 cup	soft tofu	125 mL
1	banana, frozen	1
1 tbsp	powdered carob	15 mL
1/4 tsp	almond extract (optional)	1 mL
	Pinch of nutmeg	

1. In a blender process almond milk, tofu, banana, carob and almond extract until smooth. Pour into glasses and garnish with nutmeg.

Berry Frappé

Any berries — blueberries, raspberries, strawberries, blackberries or even currants — work well in this shake.

1 cup	soy milk *or* nut milk	250 mL
1/2 cup	soft tofu	125 mL
1/2 cup	washed berries, fresh or frozen	125 mL
Half	lemon, juiced	Half

1. In a blender process soy milk, tofu, berries and lemon juice until smooth. Pour into 1 large or 2 smaller glasses.

Beta Whiz

This drink is thick with the distinctive taste of cantaloupe. For a thinner consistency, increase either the orange or carrot juice by 1/4 cup (50 mL) or to taste.

1/2 cup	apricot milk *or* fruit milk *or* soy milk	125 mL
1/4 cup	carrot juice	50 mL
Quarter	cantaloupe, peeled	Quarter
1 tbsp	chopped almonds	15 mL
1 tbsp	buckwheat flakes	15 mL

1. In a blender process apricot milk, carrot juice, cantaloupe, almonds and buckwheat until smooth. Pour into 1 large or 2 smaller glasses.

Carob-Orange Shake

Thicken with oats or banana if desired.

1 cup	orange juice	250 mL
1/2 cup	yogurt	125 mL
2 tbsp	powdered carob	25 mL
1 tsp	grated orange peel (optional)	5 mL

1. In a blender process orange juice, yogurt, carob and orange peel (if using) until smooth. Pour into a glass.

Chocolate Shake

Serves 1 or 2

1 cup	pecan milk *or* soy milk	250 mL
1/2 cup	soft tofu	125 mL
1	banana, frozen	1
2 tbsp	powdered carob	25 mL

1. In a blender process pecan milk, tofu, banana and carob until smooth. Pour into 1 large or 2 smaller glasses.

Date and Nut Shake

Serves 1 or 2

If not using date milk, add 1 tbsp (15 mL) chopped dates.

1 cup	date milk *or* soy milk	250 mL
1/2 cup	soft tofu	125 mL
2	pears, washed, peeled and cored	2
1 tbsp	chopped almonds	15 mL

1. In a blender process date milk, tofu, pears and almonds until smooth. Pour into 1 large or 2 smaller glasses.

Strawberry Shake

Serves 1

1/2 cup	orange juice	125 mL
1/2 cup	soft tofu	125 mL
1 1/2 cups	washed strawberries, fresh or frozen	375 mL
1/2 tsp	vanilla extract	2 mL

1. In a blender process orange juice, tofu, strawberries and vanilla until smooth. Pour into a glass.

Tropical Shake

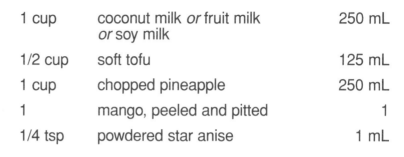

Serves 2

1 cup	coconut milk *or* fruit milk *or* soy milk	250 mL
1/2 cup	soft tofu	125 mL
1 cup	chopped pineapple	250 mL
1	mango, peeled and pitted	1
1/4 tsp	powdered star anise	1 mL

1. In a blender process coconut milk, tofu, pineapple, mango and star anise until smooth. Pour into glasses.

Hot Milk Drinks
Hot Carob

Serves 2

2 cups	date milk *or* fig milk *or* soy milk	500 mL
3 tbsp	powdered carob	45 mL
1/2 tsp	cinnamon	5 mL

1. In a saucepan over medium-low heat, scald milk (heat until little bubbles form around the edge of the pan). Whisk in carob and cinnamon and simmer gently until blended. Serve immediately in warmed mugs.

Hot Nut Chai

Serves 2

Use any nut milk for this recipe.

Add 1 tbsp (15 mL) powdered carob if desired.

2 cups	nut milk	500 mL
2 tsp	Indian Chai Blend (see recipe, page 227)	10 mL

1. In a saucepan over medium-low heat, scald milk (heat until little bubbles form around the edge of the pan). Whisk in Indian Chai Blend and simmer gently for about 10 minutes. Strain into hot mugs and serve immediately.

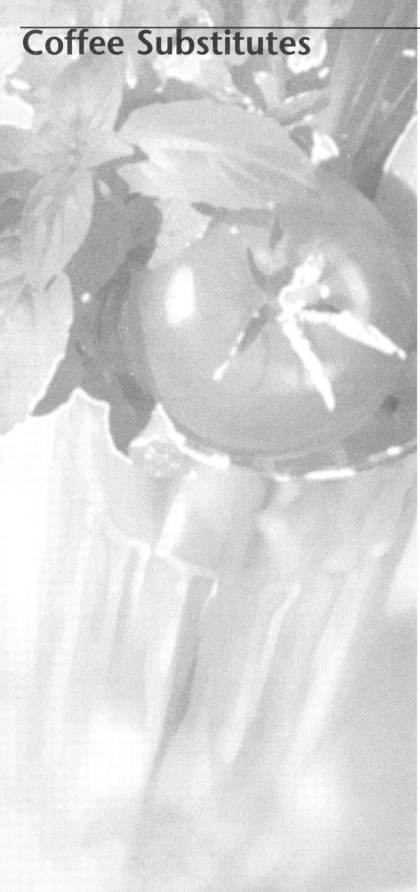

Coffee Substitutes

Coffee Substitutes

Astragalus root (*Astragalus membranacus,* see page 18). Either whole root or cut or powdered, astragalus can be used in coffee substitute blends.

Burdock root (*Arctium lappa,* see page 20). A healing root which lends a nutty taste to roasted herb root blends.

Chicory root (*Cichorium intybus*). The most common coffee substitute and closest in taste. However, unlike coffee, chicory does not have caffeine and is mildly liver-supportive. The large roots can be used alone but are best blended with other roasted herb roots, nuts, grains or seeds.

Dandelion root (*Taraxacum officinalis,* see page 24). A common root, fairly mild in taste, and best blended with other roasted herb roots.

Echinacea root (*Echinacea agustifolia or E. purpurea,* see page 24). Available in dried, whole or cut form (or fresh from growers in the fall). It is a good root to add to winter coffee blends, and helps stimulate the immune system.

Ginseng root (*Panax quinquefolius,* see page 28). An excellent coffee substitute that restores both physical and mental functions. If taken regularly, it improves resistance to disease and stress. And, unlike coffee, it is not addictive.

continued...

There is no herb that imitates the taste of coffee or that has the caffeine found in coffee. The recipes that follow have a fragrant taste quite unique and delicious on their own, and no milk is needed although you might try a drop or two of nut milk (see page 215) in them. When taken on a regular basis in place of coffee, they will act as tonics and provide significant healing benefits.

To harvest roots, you have grown or those gathered from the wild, wait until after the tops of the plants have died back in the fall (be sure to note the location of the plants first), but before the ground is frozen, to dig up the roots.

To roast fresh roots, preheat oven to 300° F (150° C). Scrub roots well and chop to a uniform medium size (about the size of dried peas). Spread on an ungreased baking sheet and bake in preheated oven, stirring after 20 minutes, for 45 minutes or until golden. Reduce oven temperature to 200° F (100° C); bake for 1 hour or until thoroughly dry, stirring every 20 minutes. Cool before blending or storing.

To roast dried roots: Most health/alternative stores sell the herb roots listed below in chopped, dried form. Roasting gives a richer taste to the blend but is strictly optional. Spread dried roots on an ungreased baking sheet and roast at 300° F (150° C), stirring once, for 20 minutes or until lightly browned.

To brew root coffee: Just before using, grind small amounts at a time with a mortar and pestle, coffee grinder or mini food processor. Use 1 tbsp (15 mL) ground roots for every 1 cup (250 mL) of water. Brew in a coffee maker as you would regular coffee. Use stevia or honey to sweeten if desired.

Use any or all of the roots listed in the sidebar to blend your own rich-tasting coffee substitute. All of the roots are available in dried form in alternative/health stores and most may be wildcrafted.

**Makes 3 cups (750 mL)
root blend**

Anxiety Antidote

This is a very mild-tasting blend. For a richer taste, add 1 tsp (5 mL) carob for each cup to be brewed.

A few drops of valerian tincture can be added to a cup of this soothing drink if taken before bedtime. Note, however, that some people experience adverse effects from valerian.

PREHEAT OVEN TO 300° F (150° C)
LARGE BAKING SHEET, UNGREASED

1 cup	chopped dried chicory roots	250 mL
1 cup	chopped dried marshmallow roots	250 mL
1/2 cup	finely chopped almonds	125 mL
1/2 cup	oat flakes	125 mL
1 tbsp	ground dried ginseng root	15 mL
1 tsp	ground cloves	5 mL
1/2 tsp	ground allspice (optional)	2 mL
1/4 tsp	ground nutmeg	1 mL

1. Spread chicory roots, marshmallow roots, almonds and oat flakes on baking sheet. Roast in preheated oven, stirring once, for 20 minutes or until lightly browned. Set aside to cool.

2. In a bowl combine roasted mixture with ginseng, cloves, allspice (if using) and nutmeg. Transfer to an airtight jar to store.

3. Grind a small amount and use 1 tbsp (15 mL) for every cup (250 mL) of water.

Licorice root (*Glycyrrhiza glabra,* see page 31). Adds a sweet, slightly anise taste to all root blends, and helps to activate healing properties in other herbs. Do not use in cases of high blood pressure.

Marshmallow root (*Althaea officinalis,* see page 32). A mild-tasting root that offers medicinal benefits.

Yellow dock root (*Rumex crispus,* see page 43). A cleansing herb with strong laxative properties, it can be blended with other roots and used for specific remedies, but is not a general coffee substitute.

Easy Root Coffee

Makes 1 1/4 cups (300 mL) root blend

Using the powdered form of roots makes them easy to blend — an "instant" coffee substitute. To make 1 cup (250 mL) Easy Root Coffee, measure 1 tbsp (15 mL) root blend into a mug and pour boiling water over. Stir and allow solids to settle on the bottom (or strain) before drinking.

1/2 cup	powdered chicory root	125 mL
1/4 cup	powdered dandelion root	50 mL
1/4 cup	powdered burdock root	50 mL
1/4 cup	powdered carob	50 mL
1 tbsp	ground dried ginseng root	15 mL

1. In a mixing bowl, combine chicory, dandelion, burdock, carob and ginseng root. Transfer to an airtight jar to store.

Immune Blend

Makes 1 3/4 cups (400 mL) root blend

A good all-round blend of herbs that will serve as a general tonic and keep the immune system healthy.

Use fresh roots if available.

PREHEAT OVEN TO 300° F (150° C)
LARGE BAKING SHEET, UNGREASED

1/2 cup	chopped dried burdock root	125 mL
1/2 cup	chopped dried ginseng root	125 mL
1/4 cup	chopped dried astragalus root	50 mL
1/4 cup	chopped dried licorice root	50 mL
1/4 cup	barley flakes	50 mL

1. Spread burdock, ginseng, astragalus, licorice and barley flakes on baking sheet. Bake in preheated oven, stirring once, for 20 minutes or until golden. Cool, mix well and transfer to an airtight jar to store.

2. Grind a small amount and use 1 tbsp (15 mL) for every cup (250 mL) of water.

COFFEE

When coffee (Coffea arabica) was introduced to Europeans in the 1600s, it was dispensed by physicians as a drug. But the stimulating beverage soon became popular and, in 1652, the first coffee shop had opened in London.

Now known to boost mental proficiency, act as a mild antidepressant, stimulate physical ability and stamina, mitigate asthma attacks, protect teeth from cavities and perhaps help deflect cancer, coffee taken in moderate amounts (no more than 2 cups [500 mL] per day) may actually be useful in specific circumstances.

But caffeine has many less desirable side effects: it directly stimulates the heart and raises blood pressure; it appears to promote heart disease in people at risk, as well as those who consume 5 cups (1.25 L) or more per day. Coffee may be a factor in fibrocystic breast disease. It depletes the body of B vitamins, magnesium, zinc and calcium. Excess coffee is associated with anxiety and depres-

Root Coffee Blend

Makes 2 1/2 cups (625 mL) root blend

See page 222 for tips on harvesting your own fresh roots.

PREHEAT OVEN TO 300° F (150° C)
LARGE BAKING SHEET, UNGREASED

6 to 8	dandelion roots	6 to 8
4 to 6	burdock roots	4 to 6
3 to 4	chicory roots	3 to 4
1	2-inch (5 cm) piece cinnamon stick	1
1/4 cup	chopped dried licorice root*	50 mL
1 tbsp	ground dried ginseng root	15 mL

*omit if prone to hypertension

1. Spread dandelion, burdock and chicory roots on baking sheet. Bake in preheated oven, stirring after 20 minutes, for 45 minutes or until golden. Reduce oven temperature to 200° F (100° C) and roast for 45 minutes to 1 hour or until thoroughly dry, stirring every 20 minutes. Set aside to cool.

2. Meanwhile, using a mortar and pestle, food processor or blender, crush cinnamon stick.

3. In a bowl combine roasted roots, crushed cinnamon, licorice and ginseng. Transfer to an airtight jar to store. Roots must be thoroughly dried before storing.

4. Grind a small amount and use 1 tbsp (15 mL) for every 1 cup (250 mL) water.

sion. Caffeine increases the effects of stress and aggravates symptoms of anxiety, tension, irritability and hypoglycemia. Coffee interferes with hormonal balance, disturbing the normal menstrual cycle. Coffee can trigger headaches in some people, even if taken moderately, and often when withdrawn. Coffee can serious-

ly impair the ability to get to sleep as well as the quality of sleep. Coffee is contraindicated in people prone to ulcers, chronic diarrhea, kidney stones and gout, anxiety, tension, depression, hypoglycaemia, menstrual disturbances, breast lumps, high blood pressure, arthritis, during pregnancy, and those who suffer

panic attacks.

All in all, herbalists believe that the benefits do not outweigh the negative effects of coffee consumption. They recommend juices and coffee substitutes as a healthier, more nutritious alternative .

Seed Power Coffee

PREHEAT OVEN TO 300° F (150° C)

LARGE BAKING SHEET, UNGREASED

Roasted or unroasted, this blend makes a delicate drink.

1 part	pumpkin seeds	1 part
1 part	sunflower seeds	1 part
1/2 part	sesame seeds	1/2 part
1 part	chopped dried chicory	1 part
1 part	ginkgo leaves	1 part
1/4 part	powdered carob	1/4 part

1. For an unroasted blend, proceed with step 2. Otherwise, spread pumpkin seeds, sunflower seeds, sesame seeds and chicory on baking sheet. Roast in preheated oven, stirring once, for 20 minutes or until lightly browned. Set aside to cool.

2. In a medium bowl, combine seeds, chicory, ginkgo leaves and carob. Stir well to mix. Transfer to a clean jar with lid.

3. Grind a small amount and use 1 tbsp (15 mL) for every cup (250 mL) of water.

Winter Coffee

Drying Citrus Peel

Herb tea and root coffee blends can be enriched with the use of dried citrus peel. Use organic fruit only — much of the chemicals from pesticides are concentrated in the peel. To dry, remove peel, coarsely chop and place on a drying rack or in a sieve so that air can circulate freely. Keep in a warm dark place for at least a week. When absolutely dry, transfer to a glass jar and store in a cool, dark, dry place.

1 part	chopped dried chicory root	1 part
1 part	chopped dried burdock root	1 part
3/4 part	powdered carob	3/4 part
1/2 part	chopped dried echinacea root	1/2 part
1/4 part	chopped dried astragalus root	1/4 part
1/4 part	chopped dried orange peel	1/4 part

1. In a medium bowl, combine chicory root, burdock root, carob, echinacea, astragalus and orange peel. Stir well to mix. Transfer to a clean jar with lid.

2. Grind a small amount and use 1 tbsp (15 mL) for every cup (250 mL) of water.

**Makes about 1/3 cup
(75 mL) blend**

Indian Chai Blend

For a sweet sip of the East, try this spice blend. If you need it sweeter than it already is, use any of the fruit milks when making the chai, or add powdered stevia (1/2 tsp [2 mL] to each 1/3 cup [75 mL] of the blend).

2 tbsp	fennel seeds	25 mL
1 tbsp	cardamom seeds	15 mL
1 tbsp	coriander seeds	15 mL
1 tbsp	fenugreek seeds	15 mL
2	whole cloves	2
2	star anise pods with seeds	2
1	2-inch (5 cm) cinnamon stick, crushed or broken into pieces	1

1. In a small saucepan over medium-high heat, combine fennel, cardamom, coriander, fenugreek, cloves, star anise and cinnamon pieces. Toast for 40 seconds or until seeds begin to sizzle and pop. Set aside to cool.

2. Using a mortar and pestle, coffee grinder or small food processor, grind toasted mixture. Transfer to a clean jar with a lid and store in a cool dry place. Use 1 tsp (5 mL) blend per 1 cup (250 mL) water.

INDIAN CHAI

Indian chai — tea boiled with spices and milk — is starting to bubble up in tony areas in cities and airport kiosks all over North America. Little has been written about this now trendy beverage, although one book describes as follows:
[In India...] generally the tea is boiled in an open pot together with a few green (unbleached) car-damom seeds, a pinch of fennel, and sugar. Milk is added to the boiling liquid — about one part milk to four parts water. This sweet, fragrant brew is served all over India, in cups and glasses in the cities and towns, and sometimes in crude earthenware "glasses" — which look like miniature flower pots — in remoter villages. Every station of the Indian railway has at least one tea stand, and at any hour of the day or night, as a train lumbers in, the air is filled with cries of the tea vendors — "chay-ya! chay-ya!"

The Book of Coffee and Tea: A Guide to the Appreciation of Fine Coffees, Teas, and Herbal Beverages. *Joel, David and Karl Schapira, New York: St. Martin's Press, 1975.*

Indian Chai Tea

Serves 1

A warming drink to take at bedtime, this tea can be prepared with any of the strained nut or fruit milks (see page 215). If using fruit milk, combine with an equal amount of regular or soy milk to make up 1 cup (250 mL). For more sweetness, increase the proportion of fruit milk.

2 tsp	Indian Chai Blend (see recipe, page 227)	10 mL
1/4 cup	water	50 mL
1 cup	skim milk *or* soy milk *or* almond milk	250 mL
1	bag green tea (or 1 tsp [5 mL] loose green tea)	1
Pinch	freshly grated nutmeg	Pinch

1. In a small saucepan over medium heat, combine Indian Chai Blend, water and milk. Bring to a boil, reduce heat and gently simmer for 10 minutes. Turn off heat and add green tea bag or stir in leaves. Cover and leave saucepan on burner. Steep for 3 to 5 minutes, then strain into a cup. Sprinkle with grated nutmeg and serve immediately.

Teas and Tonics

TEA BLENDS

Just as commercial tea producers blend several tea leaves for each kind of tea, so herbalists have learned that combining different herb leaves, flowers and seeds, adding spices and sometimes citrus peel, produces a richer tasting tea. Sweet cicely (see page 163) and stevia (see page 40) are often added to herbal tea blends because of their ability to add a sweetness to more bitter herbs. (See Tea Herbs, page 163.)

To make herb blends: Dry herbs for teas by hanging upside down in a dark, hot, dry place until they are crackling-dry. Strip leaves from the stems, but try to keep the leaves whole for storage. Blend the dried leaves according to your creative whim or use the following recipes for more specific effects. Store herb blends in a labeled airtight tin or dark-colored jar in a dark, cool, dry cupboard.

How to brew the perfect cup of tea: Bring fresh cold filtered water to the boil. Rinse a teapot with some of the boiling water, and pour off. (Do not use metal teapots and keep a teapot strictly for medicinal teas.) Measure 1 tsp (5 mL) crushed herbs per 1 cup (250 mL) water into the warmed pot. If making more than 2 cups of tea, add an extra 1 tsp (5 mL) dried herbs "for the pot." Pour boiling filtered water over; put a lid on the pot and a stopper in the spout. Steep 15 minutes before straining into cups. Herb teas should be consumed as soon as they are brewed. Otherwise, the volatile oils evaporate and the taste and medicinal benefit can be dispersed in the steam.

How to use tea as a gargle: Some herb teas — such Throat Saver (see recipe, page 247) — are excellent when used as a gargle for sore throats and to act as an antibiotic swab. Brew the tea following the directions given for the recipe. After steeping the tea, strain into a clean jar with a lid. Cool to room temperature with the lid on, store in the refrigerator. Gargle 1/4 to 1/2 cup (50 to 125 mL) at a time, every 1 to 2 hours or as needed.

Teas

Second only to water as the world's leading beverage, tea has been cultivated and harvested for at least 1700 years. During that time, green and black teas, along with herbs, have been used to aid digestion, lift the spirits, calm nerves and stomach upsets, induce sleep and stimulate the system. Herb teas are gaining in popularity now because of the health benefits of the active ingredients and the gentle, caffeine-free flavor.

Herb teas are effective as a therapeutic tool because when boiling water is poured over the herbs and then allowed to steep, the cell walls are broken, releasing soluble organic compounds and essences into the water.

While fresh herbs can be used to make nutritive teas, most medicinal tea recipes call for dried herbs because dried herbs are easiest to store, transport and use. In the following recipes, amounts given are for dried herbs unless otherwise stated. Fresh herbs cannot be substituted for dried in tea blends since they will mildew during storage.

Adrenal Support Tea

2 parts	borage leaves	2 parts
2 parts	stinging nettle leaves	2 parts
2 parts	oat straw	2 parts
1 part	basil leaves	1 part
1 part	gotu kola leaves	1 part
1/2 part	dried chopped ginger root (or 1/4 part ground ginger)	1/2 part
1/2 part	dried chopped licorice root (or 1/4 part powdered licorice)	1/2 part

1. In an airtight tin or dark-colored jar, blend together borage, stinging nettle, oat straw, basil, gotu kola, ginger and licorice. Store in a cool, dry, dark place.

2. To make tea: Crush a small amount of blend to a fine powder, then measure 1 tsp (5 mL) per 1 cup (250 mL). Place in a warmed ceramic teapot, add 1 tsp (5 mL) "for the pot" and pour boiling water over the herbs. Cover the pot and put a cork in the spout. Steep for about 15 minutes, then strain into cups.

Aller-free Tea

Helps to clear mucus and strengthen the immune system to resist allergies.

2 parts	stinging nettle leaves	2 parts
2 parts	elderflowers	2 parts
2 parts	rose hips	2 parts
2 parts	cinnamon bark, lightly crushed (or 1 part ground cinnamon)	2 parts
1 part	thyme leaves	1 part
1/2 part	dried chopped ginger root (or 1/4 part ground ginger)	1/2 part
1/2 part	peppermint leaves	1/2 part

1. In an airtight tin or dark-colored jar, blend together stinging nettle, elderflowers, rose hips, cinnamon, thyme, ginger and peppermint. Store in a cool, dry, dark place.

2. To make tea: Crush a small amount of blend to a fine powder, then measure 1 tsp (5 mL) per 1 cup (250 mL). Place in a warmed ceramic teapot, add 1 tsp (5 mL) "for the pot" and pour boiling water over the herbs. Cover the pot and put a cork in the spout. Steep for about 15 minutes, then strain into cups.

Antioxi-T

Scottish researchers have found that among the 75 chemicals found in thyme extract, 25% of them have antioxidant properties.

2 parts	thyme leaves	2 parts
1 part	peppermint leaves	1 part
1 part	rosemary leaves	1 part
1/2 part	sage leaves	1/2 part

1. In an airtight tin or dark-colored jar, blend together thyme, peppermint, rosemary and sage. Store in a cool, dry, dark place.

2. To make tea: Crush a small amount of blend to a fine powder, then measure 1 tsp (5 mL) per 1 cup (250 mL). Place in a warmed ceramic teapot, add 1 tsp (5 mL) "for the pot" and pour boiling water over the herbs. Cover the pot and put a cork in the spout. Steep for about 15 minutes, then strain into cups.

Bone Blend

Nourishes bone tissue and speeds repair. Horsetail (*Equisetum arvense*) is high in silica and, if used internally, should only be gathered from the wild early in the season (before June). Purchase from health/alternative stores.

2 parts	horsetail tops	2 parts
2 parts	stinging nettle leaves	2 parts
2 parts	oat straw	2 parts
1 part	red clover flowers	1 part
1 part	sage leaves	1 part
1/2 part	chopped dried licorice root (or 1/4 part powdered)	1/2 part

1. In an airtight tin or dark-colored jar, blend together horsetail, stinging nettle, oat straw, red clover, sage and licorice. Store in a cool, dark, dry place.

2. To make tea, crush a small amount of blend to a fine powder, then measure 1 tsp (5 mL) per 1 cup (250 mL). Place in a warmed ceramic teapot, add 1 tsp (5 mL) "for the pot" and pour boiling water over the herbs. Cover the pot and put a cork in the spout. Steep for about 15 minutes, then strain into cups.

Calming Cuppa Tea

Have a calming "cuppa" to ease stress any time of day, and to induce sleep at night.

2 parts	lemon balm leaves	2 parts
2 parts	skullcap leaves	2 parts
1 part	lemon verbena leaves	1 part
1 part	linden flowers	1 part
1 part	lavender flowers	1 part
1 part	passionflower	1 part

1. In an airtight tin or dark-colored jar, blend together lemon balm, skullcap, lemon verbena, linden flowers, lavender flowers and passionflower. Store in a cool, dark, dry place.

2. To make tea: Crush a small amount of blend to a fine powder, then measure 1 tsp (5 mL) per 1 cup (250 mL). Place in a warmed ceramic teapot, add 1 tsp (5 mL) "for the pot" and pour boiling water over the herbs. Cover the pot and put a cork in the spout. Steep for about 15 minutes, then strain into cups.

Chamomile-Licorice-Ginger

Serves 1 or 2

A calming, digestive and liver-supportive tea.

Do not use licorice in cases of high blood pressure.

1 tbsp	German chamomile flowers	15 mL
1 tsp	powdered licorice root (see note at left)	5 mL
1/2 tsp	ground ginger	2 mL
3 cups	boiling water	750 mL

1. In a nonreactive teapot, combine chamomile, licorice and ginger. Cover with boiling water and steep for 15 minutes. Strain into cups and serve.

Cleansing Tea

A mineral rich tea that stimulates the bowel, liver, kidneys and lymphatic glands to aid cleansing and hormone balancing.

1 part	chopped dried burdock root (or 1/2 part powdered burdock)	1 part
1 part	chopped dried dandelion root (or 1/2 part powdered dandelion)	1 part
1 part	chopped dried yellow dock root (or 1/2 part powdered yellow dock)	1 part
1 part	stinging nettle leaves	1 part
1 part	plantain leaves	1 part
1 part	red clover flowers	1 part
1/2 part	chopped dried ginger root (or 1/4 part ground ginger)	1/2 part
1/2 part	chopped dried licorice root (or 1/4 part powdered licorice)	1/2 part
1/2 part	fennel seeds	1/2 part

1. In an airtight tin or dark-colored jar, blend together burdock, dandelion, yellow dock, stinging nettle, plantain leaves, red clover, ginger, licorice and fennel seeds. Store in a cool, dark, dry place.

2. For each cup of tea, in a medium saucepan, combine 1 tsp (5 mL) of the lightly crushed herb mix with 1 cup (250 mL) water. Cover saucepan tightly and simmer for 15 minutes. Strain tea and serve. Drink 1/2 to 1 cup (125 to 250 mL) three times daily. To store, strain into a clean jar. Cover tightly and refrigerate for up to 2 days.

Circulation Tea

Stimulates blood circulation, enhancing the nourishment to all body cells. Make up 1 cup (250 mL) of this tea, strain and combine with the same amount of fresh carrot or beet juice for extra healing power.

3 parts	ginkgo leaves	3 parts
2 parts	stinging nettle leaves	2 parts
2 parts	rosemary leaves	2 parts
1 part	chopped dried ginger root (or 1/2 part ground ginger)	1 part
1 part	ground cinnamon	1 part
1 part	cardamom pods	1 part
1 part	yarrow aerial parts	1 part

1. In an airtight tin or dark-colored jar, blend together ginko, stinging nettle, rosemary, ginger, cinnamon, cardamom and yarrow. Store in a cool, dark, dry place.

2. To make tea: Crush a small amount of blend to a fine powder, then measure 1 tsp (5 mL) per 1 cup (250 mL). Place in a warmed ceramic teapot, add 1 tsp (5 mL) "for the pot" and pour boiling water over the herbs. Cover the pot and put a cork in the spout. Steep for about 15 minutes, then strain into cups.

Cold and Flu-T

Makes 4 cups (1 L) tea

Powerfully antibiotic and antiviral, this tea fights colds and flu. Garlic is one of the key ingredients in this blend and it must be taken fresh because the powdered form has little medicinal value. For this reason, make up in small quantities and use when cold and flu symptoms appear.

2 tsp	fresh thyme leaves (or 1 tsp [5 mL] dried thyme)	10 mL
1 tsp	fresh lemon balm leaves (or 1/2 tsp [2 mL] dried lemon balm)	5 mL
1	fresh clove garlic, finely chopped	1
1/2 tsp	finely grated ginger root (or 1/4 tsp [1 mL] ground ginger)	2 mL
1/2 tsp	chopped dried licorice root (or 1/4 tsp [1 mL] powdered licorice)	2 mL
4 cups	boiling water	1 L

1. In a nonreactive teapot, combine thyme, lemon balm, garlic, ginger and licorice. Cover with boiling water and steep for 15 minutes. Strain into a clean jar with a lid. Store in refrigerator for up to 2 days. Drink 1/2 to 1 cup (125 mL to 250 mL) four times per day.

Digestive Stress Soother

A tasty, mucilage-rich tea to soothe digestive tract inflammation. This tea can be taken after meals for indigestion and before bed to protect the digestive tract from acid damage at night. Make 1 cup (250 mL) of this tea, strain and combine with the same amount of fresh carrot or beet juice for extra healing power.

1 part	slippery elm bark powder	1 part
1 part	marshmallow leaf or dried chopped marshmallow root	1 part
1 part	German chamomile flowers	1 part
1/2 part	dried chopped licorice root (or 1/4 part powdered licorice)	1/2 part
1/2 part	fennel seeds	1/2 part

1. In an airtight tin or dark-colored jar, blend together elm bark, marshmallow, chamomile, licorice and fennel seeds. Store in a cool, dark, dry place.

2. To make tea: Crush a small amount of blend into a fine powder, then measure 1 tsp (5 mL) per 1 cup (250 mL). Place in a warmed ceramic teapot, add 1 tsp (5 mL) "for the pot" and pour boiling water over the herbs. Cover the pot and put a cork in the spout. Steep for about 15 minutes, then strain into cups.

Energizer

Basil leaves are difficult to dry at home. Use commercially dried basil found in health/ alternative stores.

1 part	sage leaves	1 part
1 part	rosemary leaves	1 part
1 part	thyme leaves	1 part
1 part	basil leaves	1 part
1/2 part	chopped dried ginger root (or 1/4 part ground ginger)	1/2 part
1/2 part	cinnamon bark, lightly crushed (or 1/4 part ground cinnamon)	1/2 part

1. In an airtight tin or dark-colored jar, blend together sage, rosemary, thyme, basil, ginger and cinnamon. Store in a cool, dark, dry place.

2. To make tea: Crush a small amount of blend to a fine powder, then measure 1 tsp (5 mL) per 1 cup (250 mL). Place in a warmed ceramic teapot, add 1 tsp (5 mL) "for the pot" and pour boiling water over the herbs. Cover the pot and put a cork in the spout. Steep for about 15 minutes, then strain into cups.

Flu Fighter

Promotes sweating to relieve symptoms of a cold or flu and helps speed recovery.	2 parts	chopped dried pineapple or papaya or mango	2 parts
	1 part	chopped dried ginger root (or 1/2 part ground ginger)	1 part
	1/2 part	finely cut dried echinacea root (or 1/4 part powdered)	1/2 part
	1/2 part	dried whole elderberries	1/2 part
	1/4 part	powdered boneset	1/4 part
	1/8 part	cayenne	1/8 part

1. In an airtight tin or dark-colored jar, blend together pineapple, ginger, echinacea, elderberries, boneset and cayenne. Store in a cool, dark, dry place.

2. To make tea, crush a small amount of blend to a fine powder, then measure 1 tsp (5 mL) per 1 cup (250 mL). Place in a warmed ceramic teapot, add 1 tsp (5 mL) "for the pot" and pour boiling water over the herbs. Cover the pot and put a cork in the spout. Steep for about 15 minutes, then strain into cups.

Free Flow Tea

Diuretic, anti-inflammatory, soothing and antiseptic to the urinary tract.	2 parts	marshmallow leaf	2 parts
	1 part	yarrow flower	1 part
	1 part	plantain leaves	1 part
	1 part	stinging nettle leaves	1 part
	1 part	goldenrod aerial parts	1 part
	1/2 part	ground cinnamon	1/2 part

1. In an airtight tin or dark-colored jar, blend together marshmallow, yarrow, plantain, stinging nettle, goldenrod and cinnamon. Store in a cool, dark, dry place.

2. To make tea: Crush a small amount of blend to a fine powder, then measure 1 tsp (5 mL) per 1 cup (250 mL). Place in a warmed ceramic teapot, add 1 tsp (5 mL) "for the pot" and pour boiling water over the herbs. Cover the pot and put a cork in the spout. Steep for about 15 minutes, then strain into cups.

Ginger Tea

Stimulates circulation and digestion.	1 part	chopped dried ginger root	1 part
	1/3 part	fennel seeds	1/3 part
	1/3 part	lemon balm leaves	1/3 part

1. In an airtight tin or dark-colored jar, blend together ginger, fennel and lemon balm. Store in a cool, dark, dry place.

2. To make tea: Crush a small amount of blend to a fine powder, then measure 1 tsp (5 mL) per 1 cup (250 mL). Place in a warmed ceramic teapot, add 1 tsp (5 mL) "for the pot" and pour boiling water over the herbs. Cover the pot and put a cork in the spout. Steep for about 15 minutes, then strain into cups.

Ginseng

Stimulates circulation, digestion and energy.	1 part	powdered ginseng root	1 part
	1 part	fennel seeds	1 part
	1 part	stinging nettle leaves	1 part
	1/2 part	ground ginger	1/2 part
	1/4 part	powdered stevia leaves	1/4 part

1. In an airtight tin or dark-colored jar, blend together ginseng, fennel, stinging nettle, ginger and stevia. Store in a cool, dark, dry place.

2. To make tea, crush a small amount of blend to a fine powder, then measure 1 tsp (5 mL) per 1 cup (250 mL). Place in a warmed ceramic teapot, add 1 tsp (5 mL) "for the pot" and pour boiling water over the herbs. Cover the pot and put a cork in the spout. Steep for about 15 minutes, then strain into cups.

Gout Buster

Stimulates elimination of wastes, including excess uric acid.	2 parts	stinging nettle leaves	2 parts
	1 part	burdock seed	1 part
	1 part	celery seed	1 part
Do not use licorice in cases of high blood pressure.	1/2 part	powdered licorice root (see note at left)	1/2 part

1. In an airtight tin or dark-colored jar, blend together stinging nettle, burdock, celery seed and licorice. Store in a cool, dark, dry place.

2. To make tea, crush a small amount of blend to a fine powder, then measure 1 tsp (5 mL) per 1 cup (250 mL). Place in a warmed ceramic teapot, add 1 tsp (5 mL) "for the pot" and pour boiling water over the herbs. Cover the pot and put a cork in the spout. Steep for about 15 minutes, then strain into cups.

Green Giant Tea Blend

An antioxidant tea that stimulates circulation and digestion.

2 parts	ginkgo leaves	2 parts
1 part	German chamomile flowers	1 part
1 part	green tea leaves	1 part
1/2 part	sweet cicely, aerial parts	1/2 part
1/4 part	sage leaves	1/4 part

1. In an airtight tin or dark-colored jar, blend together ginkgo, chamomile, green tea, sweet cicely and sage. Store in a cool, dark, dry place.

2. To make tea: Crush a small amount of blend to a fine powder, then measure 1 tsp (5 mL) per 1 cup (250 mL). Place in a warmed ceramic teapot, add 1 tsp (5 mL) "for the pot" and pour boiling water over the herbs. Cover the pot and put a cork in the spout. Steep for about 15 minutes, then strain into cups.

Hangover Rescue Tea

2 parts	German chamomile flowers	2 parts
1 part	meadowsweet leaves	1 part
1/2 part	ground ginger	1/2 part
1/4 part	lavender buds	1/4 part

1. In an airtight tin or dark-colored jar, blend together chamomile, meadowsweet, ginger and lavender. Store in a cool, dark, dry place.

2. To make tea, crush a small amount of blend to a fine powder, then measure 1 tsp (5 mL) per 1 cup (250 mL). Place in a warmed ceramic teapot, add 1 tsp (5 mL) "for the pot" and pour boiling water over the herbs. Cover the pot and put a cork in the spout. Steep for about 15 minutes, then strain into cups.

Herp-eze Tea

Nerve nourishing, immune
system supporting, and antiviral to the Herpes virus, these
herbs work to relieve, and
protect from infection.

2 parts	chopped dried echinacea root or leaf (or 1 part powdered)	2 parts
2 parts	lemon balm leaves	2 parts
1 part	St. John's wort flowers (see note)	1 part

Omit St. John's wort if taking prescription drugs

1 part	calendula flowers	1 part
1 part	red raspberry leaves	1 part
1 part	burdock leaf or chopped burdock root	1 part
1/2 part	peppermint leaves	1/2 part

1. In an airtight tin or dark-colored jar, blend together echinacea, lemon balm, St. John's wort, calendula, raspberry, burdock and peppermint. Store in a cool, dark, dry place.

2. To make tea: Crush a small amount of blend to a fine powder, then measure 1 tsp (5 mL) per 1 cup (250 mL). Place in a warmed ceramic teapot, add 1 tsp (5 mL) "for the pot" and pour boiling water over the herbs. Cover the pot and put a cork in the spout. Steep for about 15 minutes, then strain into cups.

Hormone Balancing Tea

Nourishes the reproductive area.

Caution: Not to be taken in pregnancy.

3 parts	red raspberry leaves	3 parts
2 parts	chaste berries	2 parts
2 parts	lemon balm leaves	2 parts
1 part	stinging nettle leaves	1 part
1 part	yarrow aerial parts	1 part
1 part	red clover flowers	1 part
1 part	chopped dried ginger root (or 1/2 part ground ginger)	1 part
1 part	German chamomile flowers	1 part
1 part	rosemary leaves	1 part

1. In an airtight tin or dark-colored jar, blend together raspberry, chaste berries, lemon balm, stinging nettle, yarrow, red clover, ginger, chamomile and rosemary. Store in a cool, dark, dry place.

2. To make tea: Crush a small amount of blend to a fine powder, then measure 1 tsp (5 mL) per 1 cup (250 mL). Place in a warmed ceramic teapot, add 1 tsp (5 mL) "for the pot" and pour boiling water over the herbs. Cover the pot and put a cork in the spout. Steep for about 15 minutes, then strain into cups.

Immune Regulator

These are excellent herbs for supporting the immune system.

2 parts	lemon balm leaves	2 parts
2 parts	rose hips	2 parts
1 part	German chamomile flowers	1 part
1 part	red clover flowers	1 part
1 part	thyme leaves	1 part
1/2 part	chopped dried licorice root	1/2 part
1/2 part	chopped dried ginger root	1/2 part

1. In an airtight tin or dark-colored jar, blend together lemon balm, rose hips, German chamomile, red clover, thyme, licorice and ginger. Store in a cool, dark, dry place.

2. To make tea: Crush a small amount of blend to a fine powder, then measure 1 tsp (5 mL) per 1 cup (250 mL). Place in a warmed ceramic teapot, add 1 tsp (5 mL) "for the pot" and pour boiling water over the herbs. Cover the pot and put a cork in the spout. Steep for about 15 minutes, then strain into cups.

Lavender Tea

Relaxing, digestive and liver supportive.

2 parts	lemon balm leaves	2 parts
1 part	lavender flowers	1 part
1 part	German chamomile flowers	1 part
1 part	passionflower	1 part

1. In an airtight tin or dark-colored jar, blend together lemon balm, lavender, chamomile and passionflower. Store in a cool, dark, dry place.

2. To make tea: Crush a small amount of blend to a fine powder, then measure 1 tsp (5 mL) per 1 cup (250 mL). Place in a warmed ceramic teapot, add 1 tsp (5 mL) "for the pot" and pour boiling water over the herbs. Cover the pot and put a cork in the spout. Steep for about 15 minutes, then strain into cups.

Lung Relief Tea

Expectorant, anti-bacterial
and soothing to the lungs.
Make up 1 cup (250 mL) of
this tea, strain and combine
with the same amount of
fresh carrot or beet juice for
extra healing power.

1 part	marshmallow leaves or root	1 part
1 part	hyssop leaves	1 part
1 part	thyme leaves	1 part
1/2 part	dried chopped licorice root (or 1/4 part powdered)	1/2 part

1. In an airtight tin or dark-colored jar, blend together marshmallow, hyssop, thyme and licorice. Store in a cool, dark, dry place.

2. To make tea: Crush a small amount of blend to a fine powder, then measure 1 tsp (5 mL) per 1 cup (250 mL). Place in a warmed ceramic teapot, add 1 tsp (5 mL) "for the pot" and pour boiling water over the herbs. Cover the pot and put a cork in the spout. Steep for about 15 minutes, then strain into cups.

Memory Booster Tea Blend

1 part	ginkgo leaves	1 part
1 part	dandelion leaves	1 part
1/4 part	rosemary leaves	1/4 part
1/4 part	sage leaves	1/4 part
1/4 part	dried chopped ginger (or 1/8 part powdered)	1/4 part
1/4 part	stevia leaves (or 1/8 part powdered)	1/4 part

1. In an airtight tin or dark-colored jar, blend together ginkgo, dandelion, rosemary, sage, ginger and stevia. Store in a cool, dark, dry place.

2. To make tea, crush a small amount of blend to a fine powder, then measure 1 tsp (5 mL) per 1 cup (250 mL). Place in a warmed ceramic teapot, add 1 tsp (5 mL) "for the pot" and pour boiling water over the herbs. Cover the pot and put a cork in the spout. Steep for about 15 minutes, then strain into cups.

Migraine Buster

According to James Duke, "In my own experience, and this is reflected in the medical literature, feverfew works [to prevent and even cure migraines and other headaches] for about two-thirds of those who use it consistently." Take 1 cup (250 mL) daily to avoid migraines.

1 part	feverfew leaves	1 part
1 part	ginkgo leaves	1 part
1/2 part	lemon balm leaves	1/2 part
1/2 part	German chamomile flowers	1/2 part

1. In an airtight tin or dark-colored jar, blend together feverfew, ginkgo, lemon balm and chamomile. Store in a cool, dark, dry place.

2. To make tea, crush a small amount of blend to a fine powder, then measure 1 tsp (5 mL) per 1 cup (250 mL). Place in a warmed ceramic teapot, add 1 tsp (5 mL) "for the pot" and pour boiling water over the herbs. Cover the pot and put a cork in the spout. Steep for about 15 minutes, then strain into cups.

Mother's Own

A nourishing tea that increases breast milk in nursing mothers.

2 parts	red raspberry leaves	2 parts
1 part	rose hips	1 part
1 part	stinging nettle leaves	1 part
1 part	lemon verbena leaves	1 part
1 part	fennel seeds	1 part
1/2 part	lemon balm leaves	1/2 part
1/2 part	alfalfa aerial parts	1/2 part

1. In an airtight tin or dark-colored jar, blend together raspberry, rose hips, stinging nettle, lemon verbena, fennel, lemon balm and alfalfa. Store in a cool, dark, dry place.

2. To make tea, crush a small amount of blend to a fine powder, then measure 1 tsp (5 mL) per 1 cup (250 mL). Place in a warmed ceramic teapot, add 1 tsp (5 mL) "for the pot" and pour boiling water over the herbs. Cover the pot and put a cork in the spout. Steep for about 15 minutes, then strain into cups.

Nerve Nourisher

Omit St. John's wort if taking prescription drugs

2 parts	oat straw	2 parts
2 parts	lemon balm leaves	2 parts
1 part	German chamomile flowers	1 part
1 part	chopped dried licorice root (or 1/2 part powdered)	1 part
1 part	rosemary leaves	1 part
1 part	vervain leaves	1 part
1 part	skullcap leaves	1 part
1 part	St. John's wort flowers (see note at left)	1 part

1. In an airtight tin or dark-colored jar, blend together oat straw, lemon balm, chamomile, licorice, rosemary, vervain, skullcap and St. John's wort. Store in a cool, dark, dry place.

2. To make tea, crush a small amount of blend to a fine powder, then measure 1 tsp (5 mL) per 1 cup (250 mL). Place in a warmed ceramic teapot, add 1 tsp (5 mL) "for the pot" and pour boiling water over the herbs. Cover the pot and put a cork in the spout. Steep for about 15 minutes, then strain into cups.

Nettle Tea

Water retention is gently reduced by this nourishing tea.

2 parts	stinging nettle leaves	2 parts
1 part	dandelion leaves	1 part
1 part	yarrow aerial parts	1 part

1. In an airtight tin or dark-colored jar, blend together stinging nettle, dandelion and yarrow. Store in a cool, dark, dry place.

2. To make tea, crush a small amount of blend to a fine powder, then measure 1 tsp (5 mL) per 1 cup (250 mL). Place in a warmed ceramic teapot, add 1 tsp (5 mL) "for the pot" and pour boiling water over the herbs. Cover the pot and put a cork in the spout. Steep for about 15 minutes, then strain into cups.

Raspberry Ginger

Serves 1 or 2

Slippery elm bark is, well, slippery. It tends to clump and float on the top of liquids. For this reason, whisk herbs with a wire whisk or fork while slowly pouring in hot water.

1 tbsp	raspberry leaves	15 mL
1 tsp	grated ginger root (or 1/2 tsp [2 mL] ground ginger)	5 mL
1 tsp	slippery elm bark	5 mL
1 1/2 cups	boiling water	375 mL

1. In a nonreactive teapot, combine raspberry, ginger and elm bark. Whisk while slowly adding boiling water; steep for 15 minutes. Strain into cups and drink warm.

Raspberry Tea

Serves 1 or 2

3 tbsp	washed raspberries, fresh or frozen	45 mL
1 tsp	dried raspberry leaves	5 mL
1 tsp	lemon balm leaves	5 mL
2 cups	boiling water	500 mL

1. In a nonreactive teapot, combine raspberries, raspberry leaves and lemon balm. Cover with boiling water and steep for 15 minutes. Strain into cups and drink warm.

Relax Tea

Calms the muscles and nerves.

2 parts	skullcap leaves	2 parts
2 parts	linden flower	2 parts
2 parts	lemon balm leaves	2 parts
1 part	cramp bark	1 part
1 part	lemon verbena leaves	1 part
1 part	passionflower	1 part
1 part	lavender flowers	1 part

1. In an airtight tin or dark-colored jar, blend together skullcap, linden flower, lemon balm, cramp bark, lemon verbena, passionflower and lavender. Store in a cool, dark, dry place.

2. To make tea: Crush a small amount of blend to a fine powder, then measure 1 tsp (5 mL) per 1 cup (250 mL). Place in a warmed ceramic teapot, add 1 tsp (5 mL) "for the pot" and pour boiling water over the herbs. Cover the pot and put a cork in the spout. Steep for about 15 minutes, then strain into cups.

Root Decoction

Serves 2 or 3

1 tbsp	chopped dried dandelion root	15 mL
1 tsp	chopped dried licorice root	5 mL
2 tsp	chopped dried ginseng root	10 mL
4 cups	water	1 L

1. In a saucepan over medium-high heat, combine dandelion, licorice, ginseng and water; bring to a light boil. Cover pan, reduce heat and lightly simmer for 15 minutes. Remove from heat and steep for 5 minutes. Strain into cups and serve.

Saw Palmetto

1 part	ground saw palmetto berries	1 part
1 part	green tea	1 part
1 part	chopped fresh nettle root (if available)	1 part
1/2 part	ground ginger	1/2 part

1. In an airtight tin or dark-colored jar, blend together palmetto berries, green tea, nettle root and ginger. Store in a cool, dark, dry place.

2. To make tea: Crush a small amount of blend to a fine powder, then measure 1 tsp (5 mL) per 1 cup (250 mL). Place in a warmed ceramic teapot, add 1 tsp (5 mL) "for the pot" and pour boiling water over the herbs. Cover the pot and put a cork in the spout. Steep for about 15 minutes, then strain into cups.

HIGH-BUSH CRANBERRY
(*VIBURNUM OPULUS*)

Also called cramp bark, high-bush cranberry is a completely different plant from the popular cranberry, but one that is highly regarded by the Catawba, Penobscot, Meskawaki and Menominee, who still use the bark to treat cramps, muscle tension, swollen glands, colic and diarrhea.

A simple tea to relieve menstrual cramps
1 cup (250 mL) boiling water poured over 1 tbsp (15 mL) dried cramp bark and allowed to steep for 15 minutes. Sip often throughout the day as long as the pains are present.

Spiced Papaya

3 parts	chopped dried papaya	3 parts
1/2 part	slippery elm bark	1/2 part
1/2 part	coriander seeds	1/2 part
1/4 part	crushed cinnamon bark (or 1/8 part ground cinnamon)	1/4 part
1/4 part	cumin seeds	1/4 part
1/4 part	ground turmeric root	1/4 part

1. In an airtight tin or dark-colored jar, blend together papaya, elm bark, coriander, cinnamon, cumin and turmeric. Store in a cool, dark, dry place.

2. To make tea: Crush a small amount of blend to a fine powder, then measure 1 tsp (5 mL) per 1 cup (250 mL). Place in a warmed ceramic teapot, add 1 tsp (5 mL) "for the pot" and pour boiling water over the herbs. Cover the pot and put a cork in the spout. Steep for about 15 minutes, then strain into cups.

Spirit Raising Tea

A pleasant tasting tea that can shift the blues.

Omit St. John's wort if taking prescription drugs

2 parts	linden flowers	2 parts
2 parts	lemon verbena leaves	2 parts
2 parts	St. John's wort flowers (see note)	2 parts
1 part	rosemary leaves	1 part
1 part	lavender flowers	1 part
1 part	vervain leaves	1 part
1 part	thyme leaves	1 part

1. In an airtight tin or dark-colored jar, blend together linden flowers, lemon verbena, St. John's wort, rosemary, lavender, vervain and thyme. Store in a cool, dark, dry place.

2. To make tea: Crush a small amount of blend to a fine powder, then measure 1 tsp (5 mL) per 1 cup (250 mL). Place in a warmed ceramic teapot, add 1 tsp (5 mL) "for the pot" and pour boiling water over the herbs. Cover the pot and put a cork in the spout. Steep for about 15 minutes, then strain into cups.

The Green Diablo

Serves 4

Garnished with slices of lime, this green devil is an excellent antioxidant tea.

Avoid parsley in pregnancy and kidney inflammation

2 tsp	green tea leaves	10 mL
1 tsp	dried parsley leaves (see note)	5 mL
1 tsp	dried citrus peel	5 mL
1 tsp	ground cayenne pepper	5 mL
1/2 tsp	stevia leaves	2 mL
5 cups	boiling water	1.25 L
4	slices lime (optional)	4

1. In a nonreactive teapot, combine green tea, parsley, citrus peel, cayenne pepper and stevia. Pour in boiling water and steep, covered, for 15 minutes. Strain the tea into cups and, if desired, garnish with lime slices.

Throat Saver Tea Blend

All elements in this soothing tea will help ease a sore throat.

1 part	thyme leaves	1 part
1 part	peppermint leaves	1 part
1 part	sage leaves	1 part
1/8 part	ground ginger	1/8 part
	Honey	

1. In an airtight tin or dark-colored jar, blend together thyme, peppermint, sage and ginger. Store in a cool, dark, dry place.

2. To make tea: Crush a small amount of blend to a fine powder, then measure 1 tsp (5 mL) per 1 cup (250 mL). Place in a warmed ceramic teapot, add 1 tsp (5 mL) "for the pot" and pour boiling water over the herbs. Cover the pot and put a cork in the spout. Steep for about 15 minutes, strain into cups and add honey to taste.

Varicosi Tea

Nourishes and tones the
veins.

1 part	dandelion leaves	1 part
1 part	yarrow aerial parts	1 part
1 part	hawthorn leaf and flower	1 part
1 part	linden flower	1 part
1/2 part	chopped dried ginger root (or 1/4 part ground ginger)	1/2 part

1. In an airtight tin or dark-colored jar, blend together dandelion, yarrow, hawthorn, linden flower and ginger. Store in a cool, dark, dry place.

2. To make tea: Crush a small amount of blend to a fine powder, then measure 1 tsp (5 mL) per 1 cup (250 mL). Place in a warmed ceramic teapot, add 1 tsp (5 mL) "for the pot" and pour boiling water over the herbs. Cover the pot and put a cork in the spout. Steep for about 15 minutes, then strain into cups.

Woman's Own

2 parts	motherwort aerial parts	2 parts
1 part	chaste berries	1 part
1 part	red clover flowers	1 part
1 part	powdered licorice root	1 part
1/2 part	fennel seeds	1/2 part
1/2 part	chopped dried ginseng root (or 1/4 part powdered)	1/2 part

1. In an airtight tin or dark-colored jar, blend together motherwort, chaste berries, red clover, licorice, fennel and ginseng. Store in a cool, dark, dry place.

2. To make tea: Crush a small amount of blend to a fine powder, then measure 1 tsp (5 mL) per 1 cup (250 mL). Place in a warmed ceramic teapot, add 1 tsp (5 mL) "for the pot" and pour boiling water over the herbs. Cover the pot and put a cork in the spout. Steep for about 15 minutes, then strain into cups.

Tonics

By definition, a tonic is an infusion of herbs that invigorates or strengthens the system. Often tonics act as stimulants and alteratives. Taken either hot or cold, tonics restore tone, purify the blood and act as nutritive builders. Tonic water is a vestige of earlier practices: in the 1500s, Europeans learned of chinchona bark (*Chinchona officinalis*), which contains quinine, (a tonic effective against maleria) and have used it ever since. Throughout history, and even as late as the twentieth century, spring tonics have been used in North America to cleanse the system after a long winter of preserved meats with no fresh fruit or vegetables. Spring tonics and fasts helped to prepare the body for the shock of astringent spring greens, and were even used as a kind of personal extension of the traditional household "spring cleaning."

Tonic herbs support the body's systems in maintaining health. Depending on what herbs are used, they can support the whole body or specific systems or organs. They are able to do this because they contain opposing groups of constituents that can lower (or raise), stimulate (or depress), increase (or decrease) individual biological processes. Tonics increase the tone of the body tissues, imparting strength and vitality by promoting the digestive process, improving blood circulation and increasing the supply of oxygen to the tissues.

Tonic herbs are safe to use daily except during pregnancy (see page 260). Following is a list of tonic herbs.

Alfalfa (*Medicago sativa*, see page 18). A nutritive tonic for the musculoskeletal system.

Astragalus (*Astragalus membranaceus*, see page 18). Promotes tissue regeneration, and is a heart tonic as well as a powerful immune system stimulator for virtually every phase of immune system activity.

Dandelion (*Taraxacum officinale*, see page 23). A liver and digestive tonic.

Devil's Claw (*Harpagophytum procumbens*). A liver tonic.

Echinacea (*Echinacea purpurea* or *E. angustifolia*, see page 24). An immune system tonic.

Ginseng (*Panex cinquefolium*, see page 28). An adaptogen used to relieve stress.

Licorice Root (*Glycyrrhiza glabra*, see page 31). Licorice root is considered to be one of the best tonic herbs because it provides nutrients to almost all body systems.

Parsley (*Petroselinum crispum*, see page 34). Acts as a general tonic.

For the Field or Workshop, Nourishing, as well as Allaying Thirst...

Make oatmeal into a thin gruel; then add a little salt and sugar to taste, with a little grated nutmeg and 1 well-beaten egg to each gallon, well stirred in while yet warm. This was first suggested by the Church of England leaflets, put out among the farmers and others, to discourage them from carrying whiskey into the field.

If the above plan is too much trouble, although it is, indeed, very nourishing and satisfactory, take the Scotch plan of stirring raw oatmeal into the bucket of cold water, and stir when dipped up to drink. I drank of this at the building of the New York and Brooklyn Bridge, which I visited with my son, while in New York, in the Centennial year of 1876, on our way from Philadelphia, and we were highly pleased with it. As near as I could judge, 1/2 to 1 pint was stirred into a common 12-quart pail. The workmen drank freely, preferring it to plain water very much."

from Dr. Chase's New Receipt Book or Information for Everybody. *Toronto: G.M. Rose & Sons Co. Limited. Date unknown.*

Makes 3 cups (750 mL)

Adaptogen

1 part	chopped dried or powdered ginseng root	1 part
1 part	chopped dried or powdered astragalus root	1 part
1/2 part	parsley leaves	1/2 part
1/2 part	alfalfa aerial parts	1/2 part
1/4 part	chopped dried or powdered licorice root	1/4 part

1. In an airtight tin or dark-colored jar, blend together ginseng, astragalus, parsley, alfalfa and licorice. Store in a cool, dark, dry place.

2. To make tonic: Crush a small amount of blend to a fine powder, then measure 1 tsp (5 mL) per 1 cup (250 mL). Place in a warmed ceramic teapot, add 1 tsp (5 mL) "for the pot" and pour boiling water over the herbs. Cover the pot and put a cork in the spout. Steep for about 5 minutes, then strain into cups.

Barley Water

1/4 cup	barley or spelt flakes	50 mL
1 cup	filtered water	250 mL
1 tbsp	lemon juice	15 mL
2 cups	mineral water	500 mL
Pinch	ground nutmeg	Pinch

1. In a saucepan over medium-high heat, combine barley and water; bring to a boil. Reduce heat and simmer gently, stirring often, for 10 minutes.

2. Turn off heat and allow mixture to cool sitting on the element. Stir in lemon juice, mineral water and nutmeg. Pour into a clean jar with a lid. Store in refrigerator for up to 3 days.

General Tonic

This tea feeds the cells of the body and boosts the immune system. It can be used every day with young and old. Make it up in larger quantity and store in a clean jar with a lid up to 2 days. Add 1 cup (250 mL) to soups and stocks and use in place of other liquids in cooking. This tonic may be used with cancer patients before, during and after treatment.

1 part	chopped dried astragalus root	1 part
1 part	parsley leaves	1 part
1 part	alfalfa aerial parts	1 part

1. In an airtight tin or dark-colored jar, blend together astragalus, parsley and alfalfa. Store in a cool, dark, dry place.

2. To make tonic: Crush a small amount of blend to a fine powder, then measure 1 tsp (5 mL) per 1 cup (250 mL). Place in a warmed ceramic teapot, add 1 tsp (5 mL) "for the pot" and pour boiling water over the herbs. Cover the pot and put a cork in the spout. Steep for about 5 minutes, then strain into cups.

Iron Builder

Serves 2 or 3

Young people experiencing puberty require extra iron to help them cope with the rapid changes within their bodies.

6	sprigs fresh peppermint	6
4	fresh stinging nettle tops (each 4 to 6 inches [10 to 15 cm])	4
1	fresh yellow dock root	1
1	small fresh burdock leaf, chopped	1
1/2 cup	chopped fresh sweet cicely	125 mL
3 cups	boiling water	750 mL

1. In a non-reactive teapot or heatproof jar, combine peppermint, stinging nettle, yellow dock, burdock and sweet cicely. Pour in boiling water and steep, covered, for at least 12 hours (the longer steeping time is necessary to extract the minerals from the herbs). Strain and drink 1/2 cup (125 mL) twice daily. Store tonic in a clean jar with a lid in the refrigerator for up to 3 days.

Nerve Support

*Omit St. John's wort if taking prescription drugs

1 part	German chamomile flowers	1 part
1 part	lemon balm leaves	1 part
1 part	linden flowers	1 part
1 part	St. John's wort* flowers	1 part

1. In an airtight tin or dark-colored jar, blend together chamomile, lemon balm, linden flowers and St. John's wort. Store in a cool, dark, dry place.

2. To make tonic: Crush a small amount of blend to a fine powder, then measure 1 tsp (5 mL) per 1 cup (250 mL). Place in a warmed ceramic teapot, add 1 tsp (5 mL) "for the pot" and pour boiling water over the herbs. Cover the pot and put a cork in the spout. Steep for about 5 minutes, then strain into cups.

Spring Tonic

Makes 3 cups (750 mL)

3 cups	filtered water	750 mL
1	2-inch (5 cm) piece fresh ginseng root, chopped	1
1	2-inch (5 cm) piece fresh dandelion root, chopped	1
1	2-inch (5 cm) piece fresh burdock root, chopped	1
2 tsp	chopped parsley leaves	10 mL
2 tsp	chopped stinging nettle tops	10 mL
1/4 cup	maple sap	50 mL

1. In a nonreactive saucepan over medium heat, pour water over ginseng, dandelion and burdock. Cover and bring to a boil. Turn off heat and steep, covered, for 5 minutes.

2. Stir in parsley and nettle. Steep, covered, for another 10 minutes. Strain into a clean jar. Stir in maple sap. Use immediately or cover tightly and keep in refrigerator for up to 2 days.

Appendices and References

APPENDIX A

FOOD ALLERGIES

Certain foods can trigger or aggravate conditions such as asthma, chronic fatigue syndrome, depression, chronic digestive problems, eczema, headaches, hives, irritable bowel syndrome, migraines, rheumatoid arthritis and ulcerative colitis in adults, and ear infections and epilepsy in children.

Symptoms of food allergies and intolerances can include chronic infections or inflammations, diarrhea, fatigue, anxiety, depression, joint pain, skin rashes, dark circles or puffiness under the eyes, itchy nose or throat, water retention, and swollen glands.

In the classic allergic reaction, a trigger (such as nuts) is mistakenly identified as an "enemy" by the immune system, which sets out to get rid of the offending toxin.

Food intolerances or sensitivities differ from "classic" allergies in that reactions do not happen immediately. As a result, allergy tests often cannot detect food intolerances. If you suspect that a food may be causing a chronic problem, the most effective method of identifying the culprit is to use an elimination diet.

Factors in food allergies include digestive system problems and lowered immune system functioning. While eliminating suspected foods from the diet, work to improve immunity (see Immune Deficiency page 82) and digestion (see Indigestion page 84). A key factor in digestion is liver functioning (see Liver Problems page 90). Regular daily exercise and stress-reduction activities, such as meditation and yoga, improve immunity.

The most common foods that provoke chronic conditions are dairy products, wheat, corn, caffeine, yeast and citrus fruits. Other common food problems occur with processed and refined foods, food additives and preservatives, eggs, strawberries, pork, tomatoes, peanuts and chocolate. In irritable bowel syndrome, potatoes and onions are also common triggers. Dairy products are the most common trigger for children's chronic ear infections.

Foods that are especially helpful in reducing allergic reactions are:

• plenty of antioxidant fruit and vegetables

• yogurt with live bacterial cultures to re-establish helpful digestive bacteria

• flavonoids in the skins of fruits and vegetables, especially citrus

• essential fatty acids in oily fish (herring, salmon, sardines, mackerel), fish oils, flax seeds and evening primrose oil are anti-inflammatory and reduce the severity of allergies

• vitamin C decreases allergic reactions. Broccoli, lemon juice and rosehip tea are sources that are unlikely to cause allergic reactions.

THE ELIMINATION DIET

Preparation
Before starting on an elimination diet, consult with your healthcare practitioner to eliminate the possibility of serious disease causing your symptoms. If disease is not evident, ask for (and follow) your healthcare practitioner's advice about trying the elimination diet.

Choosing foods to eliminate
Start with the Guidelines to Good Health (see pages 10–11). This will eliminate refined and processed food, which will improve immunity and digestion. Avoid food additives and preservatives, which are common food allergens. If you regularly drink coffee or alcohol and are eliminating them, you may experience headache. To avoid this side affect, cut down on these gradually.

You can choose to eliminate one food at a time, or multiple foods. It is important that you maintain a wide variety of different types of food in your diet. Choose to eliminate the most common food allergies from the list on page 254. Do not add foods to which you have known allergies.

Steps in the Elimination Diet
1. Start a daily "diet diary," noting all the foods you eat each day and the symptoms you experience.

2. Eliminate one food item from your diet for a period of 1 week. Start with a food that most commonly causes symptoms, especially one that you eat regularly. The food must be completely eliminated. If you are eliminating eggs, avoid cakes, salad dressings and any other food that may contain eggs. If eliminating dairy products, check the ingredients of all foods for lactose, lactic acid and whey. Margarine commonly contains these ingredients.

3. If you have fewer symptoms while eliminating the chosen food or foods, proceed to step 4 to check each food you have eliminated. If there is no improvement in your symptoms, go back to the Guidelines to Good Health diet while you choose another food to eliminate.

4. Add the food item back into your diet, by eating 2 servings a day for the next 3 days. If you experience any symptoms, stop eating the food immediately and avoid it for 6 months while you work on improving your immunity, digestion and liver functioning.

Reintroducing foods that cause adverse reactions
After eliminating the food from the diet for a period of 6 months, the food can often be slowly reintroduced to the diet without adverse effects.

APPENDIX B

FOOD COMBINING

Food combining is a disciplined method of eating foods in a specific order or *combination*. It is used as a short-term aid to digestive problems and, in simple terms, requires eating protein foods, carbohydrate foods and fruit at different times, thus allowing for complete and efficient digestion of these foods.

Protein foods — meat, poultry, fish, eggs, nuts, seeds, dairy products, soy products — require the most time and energy for the body to digest.

Carbohydrates are the starches and sugars found in foods that furnish most of the energy needed for the body's activities. Squash, legumes, grains (wheat, oats, rice, rye, etc.), pasta, beets, parsnips, carrots, sweet potato and pumpkin are starchy carbohydrate foods that break down faster than protein but not as quickly as fruit. Fruits are the high-sugar carbohydrate foods that are digested very quickly, and are thus considered separately in food combining

Fruit requires the least time and energy for digestion and should be eaten before a meal or at least 2 hours after a meal. When taken this way, fruit acts as a digestive cleanser, promoting digestive function. Fruit taken with a meal causes digestive problems. Melons and bananas should be eaten separately from other fruit.

The best food combination meals are given below.

• Fruit alone. This is best taken as a variety of fruits at breakfast.
• Proteins with non-starchy vegetables: leafy green vegetables, asparagus, broccoli, cabbage, celery, cucumber, onion, peppers, sea vegetables, tomatoes, zucchini.
• Grains with non-starchy vegetables.

Health conditions that may benefit from food combining are food allergies and intolerances, indigestion, inflammatory bowel, flatulence, fatigue and peptic ulcer.

Eating protein and carbohydrates in the same meal

Protein foods need to be in the stomach for 3 to 4 hours. Protein requires an acid medium in which to be digested. Pepsin, the enzyme that begins the digestion of protein, is active only in an acid medium.

Starches (elements that break down into sugars) and sugars (honey, sugar and sugar products) pass through the stomach within 20 to 45 minutes and are digested in the small intestine. Starch requires an alkaline medium in which to be digested. The enzyme ptyalin (salivary amylase), which initiates starch breakdown, is active in an alkaline medium only and is destroyed by the hydrochloric acids that the stomach secretes.

When starches and proteins are eaten together, acidic gastric juice destroys the ptyalin and the salivary digestion of starch. Starches cannot pass through to the small intestine and are left to rot and ferment, causing gas and abdominal pain. The undigested starch in the stomach interferes with the breakdown and absorption of protein, leading to undigested protein in the stool and protein deficiency in the body.

The hydrochloric acids normally produced by a healthy system can neutralize the putrefactive process if they are present in significant amounts. For many people, especially those over the age of 35, or those with weak secretions, hydrochloric acid is not produced in sufficient amounts.

APPENDIX C

HERBS TO AVOID IN PREGNANCY

Avoid medicinal doses of all herbs while pregnant unless you have full knowledge of the actions of the herb or recipe specific advice from a midwife. Following are some of the most common herbs to avoid during pregnancy.

Alder buckthorn *Rhamnus frangula*

Aloe *Aloe vera* (use externally only)

Angelica *Angelica archangelica*

Arbor vita *Thuja occidentalis*

Autumn crocus *Colchicum autumnale*

Barberry *Berberis vulgaris*

Bethroot *Trillium* (all species)

Black cohosh *Cimicifuga racemosa* (except as advised by midwife)

Blood root *Sanguinaria canadensis*

Blue cohosh *Caulophyllum thalacthroides* (except as advised by midwife)

Bogbean *Menyanthes trifoliata*

Broom *Sarothamnus scoparius*

Bryony *Bryonia dioica*

Buchu *Barosma betulina*

Calamus *Acorus calamus*

Cascara sagrada *Rhamnus purshiana*

Cayenne *Capsicum minimum* (use sparingly)

Celandine *Chelidonium majus*

Coffee *Coffea arabia*

Coltsfoot *Tussilago farfara*

Comfrey *Symphytum officinale*

Cotton root *Gossypium herbaceum*

Dong quai *Angelica sinensis*

Elecampane *Inula helenium*

Essential oils (except floral oils, use sparingly)

Fenugreek *Trigonella foenum-graecum*

Feverfew *Tanacetum parthenium*

Gentian *Gentiana lutea*

Ginger *Zingiber officinale* (use sparingly)

Ginkgo *Ginkgo biloba*

Ginseng *Panax ginseng, Panax quinquefolium, Eleutherococcus senticosus*

Goldenseal *Hydrastis canadensis*

Hops *Humulus lupulus*

Horehound *Marrubium vulgare*

Horseradish *Amoracia lapathifolia*

Hyssop *Hyssopus officinalis*

Jamaican dogwood *Piscidia erythrina*

Jimsonweed *Datura stramonium*

Juniper *Juniperus communis*

Licorice *Glycyrrhiza glabra*

Lobelia *Lobelia inflata*

Lomatium *Lomatium dissectum*

Ma huang (Ephedra) *Ephedra sinensis*

Male fern *Dryopteris felix-mas*

Mandrake *Podophyllum peltatum*

Mistletoe *Viscum album*

Mugwort *Artemesia vulgare*

Nutmeg *Myristica officinalis* (use sparingly)

Oregon/Mountain grape *Berberis aquafolia*

Osha root *Ligusticum porterii*

Parsley *Petroselinum crispum* (use sparingly)

Pennyroyal *Mentha pulegium*

Peruvian bark *Cinchona spp.*

Pleurisy root *Aesclepius tuberosa*

Poke root *Phytolacca decandra*

Poppy *Papiver somniferum*

Purging buckthorn *Rhamnus cathartica*

Rue *Ruta graveolens*

Sage *Salvia officinalis*

Saw palmetto *Serenoa serrulata*

Senna *Cassia senna*

Snake root *Polygala senega*

Southernwood *Artemesia arboratum*

Tansy *Tanacetum vulgare*

Thuja *Thuja occidentalis*

Thyme *Thymus vulgaris*

Turkey rhubarb root *Rheum palmatum*

Vervain *Verbena officinalis*

Wild indigo *Baptisia tinctoria*

Wormwood *Artemesia absinthum*

Yarrow *Achillea millefolium*

Yellow jasmine *Gelsemium sempervirens*

Yellow dock *Rumex crispus*

GLOSSARY

Adaptogen. A substance that builds resistance to stress by balancing the functions of the glands and immune response, thus strengthening the immune system, nervous system, and glandular system. Adaptogens promote overall vitality. *Examples: astragalus and ginseng.*

Alterative. A substance that gradually changes a condition by restoring health.

Analgesic. A substance that relieves pain by acting as a nervine, antiseptic or counterirritant. *Examples: German chamomile, meadowsweet, nutmeg and willow.*

Anodyne. Herbs that relieve pain. *Example: clove.*

Antibiotic. Meaning "against life", antibiotics are substances that work to destroy infectious agents, including bacteria and fungi, without endangering the patient's health. *Examples: garlic, green tea, lavender, sage and thyme.*

Anti-inflammatory. Controlling or reducing swelling, redness, pain and heat, which is a reaction of the body to injury or infection. *Examples: German chamomile and St. John's wort.*

Antioxidant. A compound that protects cells by preventing polyunsaturated fatty acids (PUFAs) in cell membranes from oxidizing, or breaking down. They do this by neutralizing free radicals. Vitamins C, E and beta carotene are antioxidant nutrients and foods high in them will have antioxidant properties. *Examples: alfalfa, beet tops, dandelion leaves, parsley, garlic, thyme and watercress.*

Antiseptic: Herbs used to prevent or counteract the growth of disease germs in order to prevent infection. *Examples: cabbage, calendula, German chamomile, clove, garlic, honey, nutmeg, onion, parsley, peppermint, rosemary, salt, thyme, turmeric and vinegar.*

Antispasmodic. Relieving muscle spasm or cramp, including colic. *Examples: German chamomile, ginger, licorice and peppermint.*

Astringent. Drying and contracting substances that aid in reducing secretions. *Examples: cinnamon, lemon, sage and thyme.*

Beta carotene. The natural coloring agent (carotenoids) that gives fruits and vegetables (such as carrots) their deep orange colour. It converts in the body to vitamin A. Benefits of eating foods high in beta carotene include cancer prevention, lowering the risk of heart disease, increased immunity, lower risk of cataracts and better mental functioning. *Examples: squash, carrots, yams, sweet potatoes, pumpkins and red peppers.*

Bitters. See pages 207–209.

Carbohydrates. An important group of plant foods that are composed of carbon, hydrogen and oxygen. A carbohydrate is a simple sugar or a substance formed by combination of simple sugars. The chief sources of carbohydrates in a whole foods diet are grains, vegetables and fruits. Other sources include sugars, natural sweeteners and syrups.

Carminative. Herbs that relax the stomach muscles and are taken to relieve gas and gripe. *Examples: allspice, cloves, caraway, dill, fennel, garlic, ginger, parsley, peppermint, sage and thyme.*

Cathartic. Herbs that have a laxative effort. *Examples: dandelion, licorice and parsley.*

Cholagogue. Promotes the secretion of bile, assisting digestion and bowel elimination. Examples: dandelion root, licorice, yellow dock

Decoction. A solution obtained by using the woody parts of plants (roots, seeds, bark) and boiling them in water for 10 to 20 minutes.

Demulcent. Soothing substances taken internally to protect damaged tissue. *Examples: barley, cucumber, honey, marshmallow and fenugreek.*

Depurative. Herbs taken to cleanse the blood. *Examples: burdock, dandelion root, garlic, onion stinging nettles and yellow dock.*

Diaphoretic. Herbs used to induce sweating. *Examples: cayenne, German chamomile, cinnamon, ginger and horseradish.*

Digestive. Substances that aid digestion. See Indigestion, page 84 and section on aperitifs and digestifs, pages 199 to 261.

Diuretic. Herbs that increase the flow of urine. Should be used for the short term only. *Examples: cucumber, burdock, dandelion leaf and root, fennel seed, lemon, linden, parsley and pumpkin seed.*

Dysmenorrhea. Condition of menstruation accompanied by cramping pains that may be incapacitating in their intensity.

Ellagic acid. A natural plant phenol thought to have powerful anti-cancer/anti-aging properties. Research indicates that it blocks cells' receptor sites from taking up chemically induced carcinogens.

Elixir. A tonic that invigorates or strengthens the body by stimulating or restoring health.

Emetic. A substance taken to provoke vomiting to expel poisons. *Examples: salt, nutmeg and mustard.*

Emmenagogue. Herbs that promote menstruation. *Examples: calendula and German chamomile.*

Enzymes. The elements found in food that act as the catalyst for chemical reactions within the body, allowing efficient digestion and absorption of food, and enabling the metabolic processes that support tissue growth, high levels of energy and promote good health. Enzymes are destroyed by heat but juicing leaves them intact and readily absorbed.

Essential fatty acids (EFA's). Fat is an essential part of a healthy diet — about 20 fatty acids are used by the human body to maintain normal function. Fats are necessary to maintain healthy skin and hair, transport the fat-soluble vitamins (A, D, E and K), and to signal the feeling of fullness after meals. The three fatty acids considered to be most important — essential — are omega-6 linoleic, omega-3 linolenic and gamma linolenic acids. Evidence suggests that increasing the proportion of these fatty acids in the diet may increase immunity and reduce the risks of heart disease, high blood pressure and arthritis. The best vegetable source of omega-3 EFA in the diet is flax seed. Other sources of EFAs are hemp seeds, nuts, seeds, olives, avocados and cold-water fish.

Expectorant. Herbs that help to relieve mucus congestion from colds. *Examples: coltsfoot, elder, garlic, ginger, hyssop, mullein and thyme.*

Febriguge. Herbs that help reduce fever. *Examples: German chamomile, sage and yarrow.*

Fibre. indigestible carbohydrate. Fiber helps protect against intestinal problems and bowel disorders. *Best sources: raw fruit and vegetables, seeds and whole grains.*

Types of fiber include *pectin,* which reduces the risk of heart disease (by lowering cholesterol) and helps eliminate toxins. It is found mainly in fruits such as apples, berries, citrus fruit, vegetables and dried peas. *Cellulose* prevents varicose veins, constipation, colitis and plays a role in deflecting colon cancer. Because cellulose is found in the outer layer of fruit and vegetables, it is important to buy only organic produce and leave the peel on. The *hemicellulose* in fruits, vegetables and grains aids in weight loss, prevents constipation, lowers risk of colon cancer and helps in removing cancer-forming toxins from the intestinal tract. *Lignin* is a fiber known to lower cholesterol, prevent gallstone formation, and help diabetics. It is found only in fruits, vegetables and Brazil nuts.

When juicing, the pulp or fiber is separated from the pure raw juice and is usually discarded. That is why it is important to include fresh raw fruits and vegetables or pulped drinks for a healthy diet.

Free Radicals. Highly unstable compounds that attack cell membranes and cause cell breakdown, aging and a predisposition to some diseases. Free radicals come from environment causes such as exposure to radiation, UV light, smoking, ozone and certain medications. Free radicals are also formed in the body by enzymes and during energy metabolism. *See also,* **Antioxidants,** page 260.

Flatulence. The gas caused by poor digestion. *See* **Carminative,** page 260.

Food combining. *See* Appendix B, page 256.

Hepatic. Herbs that strengthen, tone and stimulate secretive functions of the liver. *Examples: dandelion, lemon balm, milk thistle, rosemary and turmeric.*

Hypotensive. Herbs used to lower blood pressure. *Examples: garlic, hawthorn, linden flower and yarrow.*

Isoflavones. Isoflavones are phytoestrogens, the plant versions of the human hormone estrogen. Found in nuts, soybeans and legumes, isoflavones help to prevent several cancers, including pancreatic cancer and cancer of the colon, breast and prostate, by preserving vitamin C in the body and acting as antioxidants.

Lactose intolerance. Deficiency of the enzyme lactase which breaks down lactose, a sugar contained in milk from humans and animals. Without sufficient lactase, the sugar ferments in the large intestine causing bloating, diarrhea, abdominal pain and gas.

Laxative. Herbs that stimulate bowel movement should to be used for short term only. *Examples: dandelion root, licorice root, rhubarb and yellow dock.*

Macrobiotic diet. Eating whole food that is seasonal, and produced locally. Whole grains, vegetables, fruit (except tropical fruit), legumes and beans, small amounts of fish or organic meat, sea herbs and nuts and seeds are foods that are appropriate for North Americans.

Milk allergy. Many individuals, especially babies and young children, have allergic reactions to the protein in milk. Reactions include wheezing, eczema, rash, mucous build-up and asthma-like symptoms.

Mucilage. A thick, sticky glue-like substance, found in high concentrations in some herbs, that contains and helps spread the active ingredients of herbs, while soothing inflamed surfaces. *Examples: comfrey root, marshmallow root and slippery elm root.*

Nervine. Herbs used to ease anxiety and stress, and nourish the nerves, by strengthening nerve fibers. *Examples: German chamomile, lemon balm, oats, skullcap, St. John's wort, thyme, valerian and vervain.*

Nonreactive cooking utensils. The acids in foods can react with certain materials and promote the oxidation of some nutrients, as well as discolor the material itself. Nonreactive materials suitable for brewing teas include glass, enamel-coated cast iron or enamel-coated stainless steel. While cast iron pans are recommended for cooking (a meal cooked in unglazed cast iron can provide 20% of the recommended daily iron intake), and stainless steel is a nonreactive cooking material, neither is recommended for brewing or steeping teas.

Organosulfides. Compounds that have been shown to reduce blood pressure, lower cholesterol levels, and reduce blood clotting. *Examples: garlic and onions.*

Phytochemicals. Chemicals from a plant. Phyto, from the Greek, means "to bring forth", and is used as a prefix to designate "from a plant."

Protein. The dietary building block of body tissues. Protein is necessary for healthy growth and repair of cells, for reproduction and for protection against infection. Protein consists of 22 different amino acids, (called "essential amino acids") 8 of which are especially important because they can not be manufactured by the body.

A food that contains all 8 essential amino acids is said to be a complete protein. Protein from animal products — meat, fish, poultry, dairy products — is complete. The only accepted plant source of complete protein is soybeans and soy products, but research is establishing new theories that the protein content of legumes may be complete enough to replace animal protein.

A food that contains some, but not all 8, essential amino acids is called an incomplete protein source. Nuts and seeds, legumes and cereals and grains are plant products that provide us with incomplete protein. If your meals include foods from two complementary incomplete protein sources, your body will combine the incomplete proteins in the right proportions to make a complete protein. For example, many cultures have a tradition of using legumes and whole grains in dishes. Scientifically, this combination provides a good amino-acid (complete protein) balance in the diet because legumes are low in methionine and high in lysine, while whole grains are high in methionine and low in lysine. When eaten together, the body combines them to make complete protein. Nuts and seeds must be paired with dairy or soy protein in order to provide complete protein.

Purgative. Substances that promote bowel movement and increased intestinal peristalsis. *Example: yellow dock.*

Rhizome. Underground stem, usually thick and fleshy. *Examples: ginger and turmeric.*

Ripen. When applied to frozen desserts, means to allow to soften in the refrigerator.

Rubefacient. Herbs that, when applied to the skin, stimulate circulation in that area, bringing a good supply of blood to the skin, and increasing heat in the tissues. *Examples: cayenne, garlic, ginger, horseradish, mustard seed, oils of rosemary, peppermint, thyme and wintergreen.*

Sedative. Herbs that have a powerful quieting effect on the nervous system to relieve tension and induce sleep. *Examples: German chamomile, lettuce, linden, lavender and valerian.*

Stimulant. Herbs that have the effect of focusing the mind and increasing activity. *Examples: basil, cayenne, cinnamon, peppermint and rosemary.*

Styptic. Herbs causing capillaries to contract and thereby stop superficial bleeding. *Examples: calendula and cayenne.*

Tannin. A chemical component in herbs that causes astringency (see **Astringency**, page 260) and helps staunch internal bleeding. *Examples: coffee, tea, vervain and witch hazel.*

Therapeutic dose. Amount recommended by herbalist for healing certain ailments, usually higher and for longer periods of time than herbs used in cooking (which maintain health). Standardized amounts of specific herbs are used.

Tea. Strictly speaking, tea is defined as a solution made by pouring boiling water on the dried, fermented leaves and stems of a tea plant (green or black tea). In a broader sense, tea can be any solution made by pouring boiling water on a plant's leaves, petals or stems.

Tincture. A liquid herbal extract made by soaking a herb(s) in a solvent (usually alcohol) to extract the plant's medicinal components. Some herbalists maintain tinctures are the most effective way to take herbs because they contain a wide range of the plants chemical constituents and are easily absorbed.

Tisane. The "official" term used for steeping fresh or dried herbs in boiling water. The term is interchangeable with "tea" when herbs are used.

Tonic. See page 249.

Vasodilator. A herb that relaxes blood vessels, providing the benefits of increased circulation to the arms, hands, legs, feet and brain. *Examples: peppermint and sage.*

Volatile oil. Essential components found in the aerial parts of herbs. Often extracted to make "essential oils", volatile oils are antiseptic, easily assimilated and very effective in stimulating the body parts to which they are applied.

Vulnerary. A herbal remedy that helps to heal external wounds and reduce inflammation. *Examples: aloe vera, calendula, comfrey, marshmallow root and slippery elm bark powder.*

Wildcrafting. The practice of gathering herbs from the wild. Many plants today are endangered because of excessive wildcrafting. To avoid contributing to this problem, buy herbs that are organically cultivated.

BIBLIOGRAPHY

A Field Guide to Medicinal Plants, Stephen Foster and James A. Duke, New York: Houghton-Mifflin Company, 1990 ISBN 0-395-46722-5

Bartram's Encyclopedia of Herbal Medicine, Thomas Bartram, Dorset: Grace Publishers, 1995 ISBN 0-9515984-1-4

Encyclopedia of Natural Medicine, Michael Murray, N.D. and Joseph Pizzorno, N.D., Rocklin, CA: Prima Publishing, 1991 ISBN 1-55958-091-7

Food Your Miracle Medicine, Jean Carper, New York: Harper Collins Publishers, Inc, 1993 ISBN 0-06-018321-7

Healing Plants, A Medicinal Guide to Native North American Plants and Herbs, Ana Nez Heatherley, Toronto: Harper Collins Publishers Ltd., 1998 ISBN 0-00-638617-2

Healing Wise, Susun Weed, Woodstock, NY: Ash Tree Publishing, 1989 ISBN 0-9614620-2-7

Healing with Herbal Juices, Siegfried Gursche, Vancouver: Alive Books, 1993 ISBN 0-486-22798-7

Healing with Whole Foods: Oriental Traditions and Modern Nutrition, Paul Pitchford, Berkeley: North Atlantic Books, 1993 ISBN 0-938190-64-4

Herbal Remedies for Women, Amanda McQuade Crawford, Rocklin, CA: Prima Publishing, 1997 ISBN 0-7615-0980-1

Herbal Tonics, Daniel B. Mowrey, Ph.D., New Canaan, CT: Keats Publishing Inc., 1993 ISBN 0-87983-565-6

Identifying and Harvesting Edible and Medicinal Plants, Steve Brill with Evelyn Dean, New York: Hearst Books, 1994 ISBN 0-688-11425-3

Meals that Heal, Lisa Turner, Rochester, VT: Healing Arts Press, 1996 ISBN 0-89281-625-2

Nutritional Healing, Denise Mortimer, Boston: Element Books Inc., 1998 ISBN 1-86204-176-8

Nutritional Influences on Illness, Melvyn Werbach M.D., Tarzana, CA: Third Line Press, 1996 ISBN 0-9618550-5-3

Rodale's Basic Natural Foods Cookbook, Charles Gerras, Editor, Emmaus, PA: Rodale Press, 1984 ISBN 0-87857-469-7 (see pages 266 – 267, "how to make soymilk and tofu")

The Complete Book of Ayurvedic Home Remedies, Vasant Lad, New York: Three Rivers Press, 1998 ISBN 0-609-80286-0

The Complete Woman's Herbal, Anne McIntyre, New York: Henry Holt and Company, 1995 ISBN 0-8050-3537-0

The Green Pharmacy, James Duke, Ph.D., Emmaus, PA: Rodale Press, 1997 ISBN 0-312-96648-2

The Healing Herbs Cookbook, Pat Crocker, Toronto: Robert Rose, 1996 ISBN 0-7788-0004-0

The Lactose-Free Family Cookbook, Jan Main, Toronto: Macmillan Canada, 1996 ISBN 0-7715-7374-x

The Multiple Sclerosis Diet Book, Dr. Roy Swank, New York: Bantam Doubleday Dell Publishing Group Inc., 1977 ISBN 0-385-23279-9

The Natural Pregnancy Book, Aviva Jill Romm, Freedom, CA: The Crossing Press Inc., 1997 ISBN 0-89494-819-2

The New Holistic Herbal, David Hoffman, Rockport, MA: Element Inc., 1992 ISBN 1-85230-193-7

SOURCES

HERB AND ORGANIC ASSOCIATIONS/ ORGANIZATIONS/INFORMATION

American Botanical Council
P.O. Box 144345
Austin Texas,
78714-4345
Tel (512) 926 4900
www.herbalgram.org

Canadian Herb Society
5251 Oak Street
Vancouver BC
Canada V6M 4H1
A network of herb enthusiasts

Canadian Organic Growers (COG)
Box 6408, Station J
Ottawa, ON
Canada K2A 3Y6
Tel (613) 231 9047
www.cog.ca
Canada's national information network for organic farmers, gardeners and consumers.

Herb Society of America
9019 Chardon Road
Kirtland, OH 44094
Tel (440) 256-0514
Fax (440) 256-0541
www.herbsociety.org
A well organized group of herb enthusiasts with 6 Districts and many active local units.

Inforganics
Contact: Jeff Johnston
P.O. Box 95
Riverport, NS
Canada B0J 2W0
info@infoganics.com
www.infoganics.com/Food/food/htm
A marketing and services business dedicated to the success of organic farmers and businesses that deal with organics in Canada and around the world. Listings for the following are included at this site:
- *organic farmers*
- *organic bakers & caterers*
- *organic processors*
- *organic exporters*
- *organic food retailers*
- *organic food distributors*
- *CSA and green/brown box programs*
- *farmers' markets*

International Herb Association
910 Charles Street
Fredericksburg, VA 22401
Tel (540) 368-0590
Fax (540) 370-0015
www.iherb.org
A professional organization of herb growers and business owners.

Ontarbio
RR#1
Durham, Ontario
N0G 1R0
Tel (519) 369 5316

Organic Consumers' Association
6101 Cliff Estate Road
Little Marais
MN 55614
Tel (218) 226 4164
Fax (218) 226 4157
www.purefood.org
Excellent tips, information on a wide range of food issues

Organic Trade Association (OTA)
Contact: Linda Lutz, Resource Co-ordinator,
P.O. Box 547
Greenfield, MA 01302-0547
Tel (413) 774 7511
Fax (413) 774 6432
www.ota.com
Promotes awareness and understanding of organic production, as well as providing a unified voice for the industry.

ORGANIC HERBS: PLANTS, DRIED HERBS, TINCTURES

Christina's Hemp Products
R.R.#4, Killaloe, ON
Canada K0J 2A0
Tel (613) 757 3044
Hemp seed (whole), hemp nut (dehulled seed), hemp oil, non-dairy frozen treats

Frontier Natural Products Co-operative
2990 Wilderness Place, Suite 200
Boulder, CO 80301
Tel (303) 449-8137
Fax (303) 449-8139
www.frontiercoop.com
Supplier of bulk herbs.

Kettleby Herb Farms
15495 Weston Road
R.R.#2, Kettleby, ON
Canada L0G 1J0
Tel (905) 727 8344
Fax (905) 727 1415
ww.webx.ca/kettleby
Organic Herb Farm. Mail order: plants (Canada only), seeds, dried herbs, herbal products and supplies. Display gardens, educational and events programs. Send for free catalogue.

Monteagle Herb Farm
Contact: Tina Sentoukas, herbalist/owner
R.R.#1, Maple Leaf, ON
Canada K0L 2R0
Tel (613) 338 3359
www.go.to/MonteagleHerbfarm
Certified organic (OCPP) medicinal herbs in bulk, tinctures, formulas, ointments and goat's milk soap. Consultations available with Tina Sentoukas, herbalist.

Richters Herbs
357 Highway 47
Goodwood, ON
Canada L0C 1A0
Tel (905) 640 6677
Fax (905) 640 6641
orderdesk@richters.com
www.richters.com
Herb specialists with over 800 varieties, selling herbs since 1969. Mail order seeds, plants, books. Free, full-color catalogue. Free seminars and herbal events.

General Index

For specific herb references, see Herb Index, page 281.
Page numbers in **bold** refer to main entries.

S

T

Herb Index

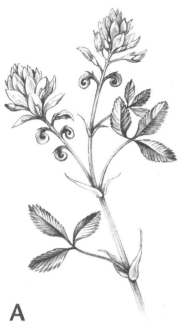

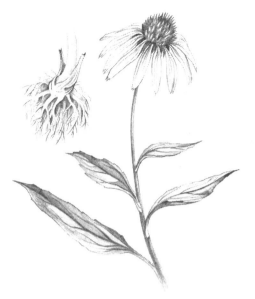

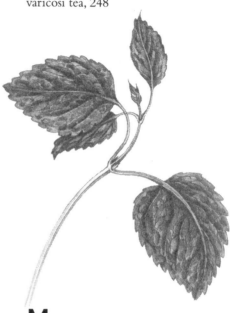

M

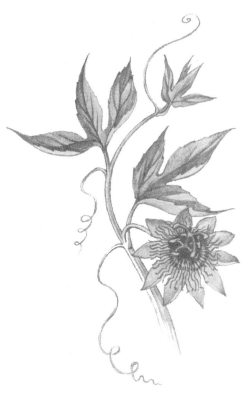

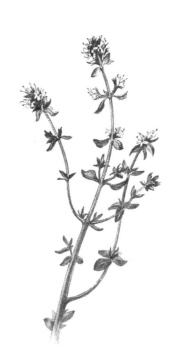